Principles and Practice of Otolaryngology

Principles and Practice of Otolaryngology

Edited by Chad Downs

hayle
medical

New York

Hayle Medical,
750 Third Avenue, 9th Floor,
New York, NY 10017, USA

Visit us on the World Wide Web at:
www.haylemedical.com

ISBN: 978-1-63241-465-6

The publisher's policy is to use permanent paper from mills that operate a sustainable forestry policy. Furthermore, the publisher ensures that the text paper and cover boards used have met acceptable environmental accreditation standards.

Trademark Notice: Registered trademark of products or corporate names are used only for explanation and identification without intent to infringe.

Printed in the United States of America.

Cataloging-in-Publication Data

Principles and practice of otolaryngology / edited by Chad Downs.
    p. cm.
Includes bibliographical references and index.
ISBN 978-1-63241-465-6
1. Otolaryngology. 2. Otolaryngology--Diagnosis. 3. Head--Surgery. 4. Neck--Surgery.
5. Head--Diseases. 6. Neck--Diseases. I. Downs, Chad.
RF46.5 .P74 2017
617.51--dc23

Table of Contents

Preface

In my initial years as a student, I used to run to the library at every possible instance to grab a book and learn something new. Books were my primary source of knowledge and I would not have come such a long way without all that I learnt from them. Thus, when I was approached to edit this book; I became understandably nostalgic. It was an absolute honor to be considered worthy of guiding the current generation as well as those to come. I put all my knowledge and hard work into making this book most beneficial for its readers.

The area of medicine that deals with disease and disorders of the ear, nose and throat region is called otolaryngology. The discipline also encompasses diseases of the adjoining head and neck areas. Otolaryngology is often referred to as a sub-discipline of surgery. This book presents researches and studies performed by experts from varied parts of the world. It aims to provide to its readers a broad spectrum of topics that fall under this field. This book is a compilation of interesting case studies from across the globe that would help in understanding the subject matter in a comprehensive way. It will help the readers in keeping pace with the rapid changes in this field.

I wish to thank my publisher for supporting me at every step. I would also like to thank all the authors who have contributed their researches in this book. I hope this book will be a valuable contribution to the progress of the field.

Editor

Surgical exploration and discovery program: inaugural involvement of otolaryngology – head and neck surgery

Brittany Greene[1], Linden Head[1], Nada Gawad[1,2,3], Stanley J Hamstra[3,4] and Laurie McLean[5*]

Abstract

Background: There is significant variability in undergraduate Otolaryngology – Head and Neck Surgery (OTOHNS) curricula across Canadian medical schools. As part of an extracurricular program delivered jointly with other surgical specialties, the Surgical Exploration and Discovery (SEAD) program presents an opportunity for medical students to experience OTOHNS. The purpose of this study is to review the participation and outcome of OTOHNS in the SEAD program.

Methods: The SEAD program is a two-week, 80-hour, structured curriculum that exposes first-year medical students to nine surgical specialties across three domains: (1) operating room observerships, (2) career discussions with surgeons, and (3) simulation workshops. During observerships students watched or assisted in surgical cases over a 4-hour period. The one-hour career discussion provided a specialty overview and time for students' questions. The simulation included four stations, each run by a surgeon or resident; students rotated in small groups to each station: epistaxis, peritonsillar abscess, tracheostomy, and ear examination. Participants completed questionnaires before and after the program to evaluate changes in career interests; self-assessment of knowledge and skills was also completed following each simulation. Baseline and final evaluations were compared using the Wilcoxon Signed-Rank test.

Results: SEAD participants showed significant improvement in knowledge and confidence in surgical skills specific to OTOHNS. The greatest knowledge gain was in ear examination, and greatest gain in confidence was in draining peritonsillar abscesses. The OTOHNS session received a mean rating of 4.8 on a 5-point scale and was the most popular surgical specialty participating in the program. Eight of the 18 participants were interested in OTOHNS as a career at baseline; over the course of the program, two students gained interest and two lost interest in OTOHNS as a potential career path, demonstrating the potential for helping students refine their career choice.

Conclusions: Participants were able to develop OTOHNS knowledge and surgical skills as well as refine their perspective on OTOHNS as a potential career option. These findings demonstrate the potential benefits of OTOHNS departments/divisions implementing observerships, simulations, and career information sessions in pre-clerkship medical education, either in the context of SEAD or as an independent initiative.

Keywords: Undergraduate medical education, Surgical exploration and discovery, Simulation

* Correspondence: lmclean@toh.on.ca
[5]Department of Otolaryngology Head and Neck Surgery, The Ottawa Hospital, General Campus, 501 Smyth Road, Ottawa, Canada
Full list of author information is available at the end of the article

Background

The pre-clerkship Otolaryngology – Head and Neck Surgery (OTOHNS) curriculum in Canadian undergraduate medical education has been examined recently by the Canadian Society of OTOHNS (CSO) Undergraduate Medical Education (UME) Working Group [1]. The authors found significant variation exists between schools across the country [1]. At the pre-clerkship level, hours dedicated to OTOHNS teaching ranges from 0 to 50, and there is substantial variability in format of teaching delivered [1]. As many as 7 Canadian medical schools provide 10 or fewer hours of formal OTOHNS teaching [1]. Studies have shown that poor early exposure and minimal involvement of surgeons in pre-clerkship education are barriers to creating interest in the field [2-4]. Also, importantly, the majority of medical students predict their specialty choice prior to clerkship [5].

The Surgical Exploration and Discovery (SEAD) program provides more experiential learning opportunities for pre-clerkship medical students interested in surgical careers, through operating room (OR) observerships, career discussions, and simulation-based workshops [6]. The program was founded at the University of Toronto in 2012 and has run successfully there for three years [6]. In June of 2014, the University of Ottawa Skills and Simulation Centre (uOSSC) collaboratively with the University of Ottawa Faculty of Medicine, Department of Otolaryngology – Head and Neck Surgery and Department of Surgery, initiated the first Canadian expansion of the SEAD program. At the University of Ottawa, the program maintained the overall structure of the program as implemented in Toronto, with some variation in specialties included and the workshop content.

OTOHNS is a unique surgical specialty in Canada in that at some institutions it is its own department, while at others it is a division within the Department of Surgery. As such, its inclusion into surgical education programs can be variable. In past SEAD programs at other institutions, OTOHNS was not included in the curriculum. However, as a direct-entry surgical specialty, the inclusion of OTOHNS in the SEAD program is vital to the underlying objective of SEAD: to facilitate informed career decision-making for students interested in surgery. Thus, through the collaborative efforts of both the Department of OTOHNS and the Department of Surgery, OTOHNS was included for the first time in any SEAD program in 2014 at the University of Ottawa.

The purpose of this study is to review the participation and outcome of OTOHNS in the University of Ottawa SEAD program. The findings of this study may help to inform OTOHNS departments and divisions considering implementing simulation-based learning and career information sessions in UME, either in the context of SEAD or as an independent initiative.

Methods

SEAD program curriculum at the University of Ottawa

The SEAD Program is a two-week summer program for students who have completed their first year of medical school. All divisions within the Department of Surgery (General Surgery, Plastic Surgery, Orthopedic Surgery, Urology, Neurosurgery, Cardiac Surgery, Vascular Surgery, Thoracic Surgery) as well as Otolaryngology – Head and Neck Surgery were included. Over the course of the two weeks, students were exposed to nine surgical specialties across three domains:

(1) *Operating room observerships:* students spent one morning (8 am – 12 pm) observing each of the specialties in the OR.
(2) *Career discussions:* over lunch (12 pm – 1 pm) a surgeon provided a career discussion and answered questions on their respective specialty. The discussion covered training, fellowships, scope of practice, daily responsibilities, and work-life balance. Each specialty provided one session.
(3) *Simulation workshop:* each afternoon (1 pm – 4 pm) the specialty providing the career discussion would proceed to run a hands-on, simulation workshop. The goals of the sessions were to provide exposure to common procedures, develop the students' skills, and stimulate interest in the specialty.

At the end of the two week program all students had completed an observership, and participated in a career discussion and simulation for each of the nine participating surgical specialties; the detailed schedule for the program can be found in Additional file 1.

All program participants were given an informational manual (68 pages) at the outset of the program, which provided an overview of the information covered in each of the nine specialties' career discussion and simulation workshop. The OTOHNS segment was 5 pages. It included a description of the specialty, residency and fellowship training programs, brief descriptions of common procedures and an outline of the stations at the simulation workshop. Students were also provided with workshop objectives to guide preparation, and a list of reference books available online to review surgical anatomy prior to their OR observership.

OTOHNS SEAD curriculum
Career discussion

Two otolaryngologists, one with an academic practice and the other primarily community-based, facilitated the lunchtime career discussion. The setting was informal. Participants were encouraged to ask questions.

Simulation workshop

The 3-hour simulation workshop involved four stations. Participants rotated through stations in groups of 4–5, every 45 minutes. Facilitators remained at one station for the duration of the workshop.

Epistaxis Station (two resident facilitators) At this station, there were two plastic head models. Bleeding was simulated through an IV attached inside the nose. Students were provided with a nasal packing tray. Residents provided teaching as per the objectives in Table 1.

Peritonsillar Abscess Station (one resident facilitator) A low fidelity model that was built in-house was used to demonstrate a peritonsillar abscess [7]. A balloon filled with lotion was set behind a latex mold resembling the oropharynx which was then inset within a box to mimic the approach through the oral cavity. Students were provided with a procedure tray. The resident provided teaching as per the objectives in Table 2.

Tracheostomy Station (one staff surgeon facilitator) Cadaveric porcine tracheas were used as models and students were provided with a tracheostomy tray and cuffed tracheostomy tube. Students were paired such that one acted as the primary surgeon and the other as assistant. Students completed the procedure then switched roles. The surgeon provided teaching as per the objectives in Table 3.

Ear Exam Station (one staff surgeon facilitator) The OtoSim™ and a diagram of the temporal bone in cross section were used at this station. Participants had no prior knowledge of ear and its exam. The surgeon provided teaching as per the objectives in Table 4.

Participants

SEAD Program participants consisted of 18 students who had just completed their first year of medical school at the University of Ottawa. Participants were selected based on a written application outlining their desire to participate in a surgical education program; there were 29 students who applied for 18 spots. The number of positions available was determined based on the capacity of each specialty to accommodate students in the ORs.

Participation in the program was voluntary. Institutional ethics approval was received, and written informed consent was obtained from all participants.

Evaluations

Evaluation OTOHNS's involvement in the SEAD program consisted of three components:

(1) Entry questionnaire regarding baseline demographics, surgical experience (e.g. observerships, undergraduate education), and specialties of interest;
(2) Two OTOHNS specific evaluation forms
(3) Exit questionnaire to determine the influence of the program on career interests

OTOHNS evaluation design

Two forms, evaluating participants' reaction to the programming and their learning [8], were provided to students to complete the day after participating in the OTOHNS lunchtime career discussion and afternoon simulation workshop. The same two forms were used to evaluate each of the specialties included in SEAD the day after the specialty-specific career discussion and workshop.

(1) A standardized evaluation form developed and used broadly by the uOSSC to measure participants' reaction to any simulation session held there. The form is based on a 5-point Likert Scale. Students were asked to quantify reactions to overall quality (1 – poor; 5 – excellent), and specific elements of the day such as time, equipment, objectives (1 – strongly disagree; 5 – strongly agree). There was also a space

Table 1 Goals of Epistaxis station

Knowledge	Skills	Attitudes
List the blood supply to the nose.	List/identify the instruments/medications required to perform nasal packing and set up a tray accordingly.	Epistaxis is common and will be encountered by most physicians regardless of specialty.
Identify Kiesselbach's plexus/Little's area.		
Recognize the difference between anterior and posterior epistaxis.	Learn how to hold a nasal speculum, bayonet forceps, nasal suction.	Can be life threatening, Recognize importance of identifying bleeding source and doing a good pack.
List the risk factors for epistaxis.	Learn how to examine the nose (anterior rhinoscopy).	Recognize what constitutes a poor pack.
List and explain the treatment options for acute management of anterior epistaxis.	Learn how to place local anesthetic/vasoconstrictor in the nose.	
List and explain the treatment options for acute management of posterior epistaxis.	Compare and contrast various nasal packs.	
	Learn how to place an anterior pack.	
Describe how to potentially prevent epistaxis.	Review complications of nasal packing.	

Table 2 Goals of Peritonsillar Abscess (PTA) station

Knowledge	Skills	Attitudes
Recognize how infectious tonsillitis may affect other organ systems. Explain how to grade the size of tonsils. Compare and contrast the clinical presentation, diagnosis, and treatment of tonsilloliths, peritonsillar cellulitis, PTA, and mononucleosis.	List/identify the instruments/medications required to drain a PTA and set up a tray accordingly. Identify a PTA. Identify the most likely location of a PTA and the landmarks for your aspiration/incision and drainage. Topically anesthetise the oropharynx. Inject local anesthetic into the soft palate. Incise and drain a PTA. Review complications of PTA drainage.	Peritonsillar abscess drainage is a straightforward procedure that Family Medicine, Emergency, and OTOHNS should be able to perform. Many communities do not have OTOHNS MDs, so the more MDs that can successfully do this procedure, the better the patient care. Understand peritonsillar anatomy so that fear of performing the procedure is decreased

for written comments. The detailed form can be found in Additional file 2.

(2) A second evaluation form was created to evaluate self-reported learning of knowledge and skills as well as reaction. Students were asked to rate their knowledge and confidence (before and after the activity) of different topics in OTOHNS related to each simulation on a 10-point scale (none to very high). Students were asked to describe their reaction to elements of the day on a 5-point Likert Scale (Strongly Disagree to Strongly Agree). The detailed form can be found in Additional file 3.

Career interest questionnaire design

As part of the entry questionnaire, students were asked to indicate which surgical specialties they were interested in pursuing as a career. The 9 surgical specialties of the program were listed as options. Students could select as many as they wanted. The identical question was repeated on the exit questionnaire.

Statistical analysis

The Wilcoxon Signed-Rank test was used to compare non-parametric paired data for differences in baseline and final test results. A p value of < 0.05 was indicative of statistical significance. All statistical evaluation was performed with SPSS software.

Results

Eighteen first-year medical students completed the SEAD Program. Baseline demographics and surgical experience of the participants are outlined in Table 5.

Students' self-reported change in knowledge over the course of the program is reported in Table 6. There was a significant difference between the pre- and post-activity measures on all knowledge dimensions. The overall mean difference in knowledge pre and post was 3.0, with knowledge in ear examination experiencing the largest change at 5.2; the smallest change was observed in knowledge of development needs.

Students' self-reported change in confidence in clinical skills over the course of the program is reported in Table 7. There was a significant difference between the pre- and post-activity measures on all confidence dimensions. The overall mean difference in confidence pre and post was 3.9, with confidence in draining peritonsillar abscess experiencing the largest change at 4.9; the smallest change was observed in overall confidence in surgical skills.

Student feedback about the simulation session and career talk is reported in Table 8 and Figure 1. Students rated the session very positively, with an overall mean of 4.8 (5-point scale). The OTOHNS session was the highest rated session over the course of the two-week program; session ratings ranged from 4.0 to 4.8.

The median net change in interest was −1 overall, for all specialties (Table 9). At baseline and following the program, OTOHNS had the largest number of interested

Table 3 Goals of Peritonsillar Abscess (PTA) station

Knowledge	Skills	Attitudes
Identify the parts of a tracheostomy tube including: inner cannula, introducer, tracheostomy tube, phalanges, tracheostomy tie, cuff, and cork. Compare and contrast tracheostomy and cricothyroidotomy. List three indications for placement of a tracheostomy tube.	List/identify the instruments/medications required to perform a tracheostomy/cricothyroidotomy and set up a tray accordingly. Identify the landmarks for a tracheostomy/cricothyroidotomy. Carry out a stepwise approach to a tracheostomy/cricothyroidotomy. Learn how to safely change a tracheostomy tube. Review complications of tracheostomy/cricothyroidotomy (acute and chronic).	Airway obstruction is life threatening. Be safe and calm under pressure. Important to work as a team. Consider multidisciplinary care (respiratory therapy, nursing, anaesthesia).

Table 4 Goals of Peritonsillar Abscess (PTA) station

Knowledge	Skills	Attitudes
Identify structures of the external and middle ear.	Properly use an otoscope.	Gain proficiency in basic otoscopy.
	Perform an otologic exam.	
	Identify landmarks of the external and middle ear (normal and diseased).	

students (10). Over the course of the program two students lost interest in OTOHNS as a potential career path and two new students gained interest, for an overall net change of 0.

Discussion

Inclusion of OTOHNS in the SEAD program is novel to the University of Ottawa. While the SEAD program is relatively new itself, it presents a unique opportunity to provide meaningful exposure to the surgical specialties for medical students early in their training. Given that there is substantial variability in OTOHNS undergraduate

Table 5 Baseline demographics and surgical experience of SEAD participants (n = 18)

Gender	Male	7
	Female	11
Age	20 to 22	12
	23 to 25	2
	>25	4
Education	Bachelor's degree	14
	Master's degree	3
	PhD	1
Cases observed prior to participating in SEAD program	0	0
	1 to 5	5
	6 to 10	6
	11 o 15	1
	16 to 20	5
	>20	1
Number of surgical specialties observed prior to participating in SEAD program	Mean	2.22
	Median	2
	Range	4
Interest in a surgical career prior to participating in SEAD program	Very interested	13
	Somewhat interested	5
	Not interested	0
Learned suturing skills prior to participating in SEAD program	No	4
	Yes, before medical school	2
	Yes, suturing workshops in medical school	12
Participated in Simulation Session(s) prior to participation in SEAD program	No	16
	Yes	2

Table 6 Self-reported knowledge of key concepts

	Before activity, mean (SE)	After activity, mean (SE)	Difference mean (SE)	p-value
1. Knowledge of Otolaryngology - Head and Neck Surgery as a Career	4.7 (0.4)	7.8 (0.2)	3.1 (0.4)	<0.001
2. Knowledge of Epistaxis	5.9 (0.4)	8.3 (0.2)	2.4 (0.4)	<0.001
3. Knowledge of Airway Obstruction and Tracheostomy	5.1 (0.4)	8.0 (0.3)	2.9 (0.3)	<0.001
4. Knowledge of Examining the Ear	2.1 (0.3)	7.3 (0.4)	5.2 (0.4)	<0.001
5. Knowledge of Tonsillitis, Peritonsillar Cellulitis and Peritonsillar Abscess	5.2 (0.4)	8.3 (0.3)	3.1 (0.4)	<0.001
6. Knowledge of your own strengths and development needs	5.6 (0.5)	7.3 (0.3)	1.7 (0.5)	0.003
Mean	**4.8 (0.2)**	**7.8 (0.1)**	**3.0 (0.2)**	<0.001

Table 7 Self-reported confidence in clinical skills

	Before activity, mean (SE)	After activity, mean (SE)	Difference mean (SE)	p-value
1. Confidence in your ability to manage epistaxis	3.2 (0.4)	7.2 (0.3)	3.9 (0.4)	<0.001
2. Confidence in your ability to perform a	tracheostomy	2.0 (0.3)	5.8 (0.4)	3.8 (0.3)
<0.001				
3. Confidence in your ability to examine the ear	2.4 (0.5)	7.1 (0.5)	4.7 (0.5)	<0.001
4. Confidence in your ability to drain a peritonsillar abscess	2.0 (0.3)	6.9 (0.4)	4.9 (0.4)	<0.001
5. Confidence in overall surgical skills	4.3 (0.5)	6.5 (0.3)	2.2 (0.5)	0.001
Mean	**2.8 (0.2)**	**6.7 (0.2)**	**3.9 (0.2)**	<0.001

Table 8 Student feedback of simulation session

Domain	Mean (SE)
Overall quality	4.7 (0.1)
Clear & informative lecture/demo	4.7 (0.1)
Clear objectives	4.9 (0.1)
Objectives met	4.8 (0.1)
Instructor knowledgeable & informed	5.0 (0.0)
Time	4.6 (0.2)
Feedback	4.8 (0.1)
Teaching ratio	4.9 (0.1)
Equipment	4.7 (0.2)
Mean	**4.8 (0.04)**

medical education at the pre-clerkship level, including OTOHNS in the SEAD program creates an interesting platform to enhance students' learning and promote it as a career choice.

Building OTOHNS knowledge and confidence

OTOHNS learning in the SEAD program is significant and valuable to participants. According to self-reported rating of knowledge in the four simulation stations, participants report a significant improvement. Students also report a significant improvement in their confidence to perform the skills learned in each of the stations. As expected, at baseline, students rated their knowledge higher than their confidence to perform the corresponding skill. A greater magnitude of growth in confidence was noted than in knowledge. Significant gains in skill-related confidence were observed after just 45 minutes of simulation for each skill.

The largest gain in knowledge was documented for the ear exam station. Ear anatomy and pathology is taught primarily in the second year of the pre-clerkship curriculum. The other 3 stations had corresponding 60–90 minute lectures on the content in the first year of the pre-clerkship

curriculum. Consequently, the OtoSim™ was many students' first exposure to the anatomy of the ear. Access to simulation-based learning for pre-clerkship medical students is highly limited. In the future, it may be worthwhile integrate simulation-based learning into the core curriculum.

The largest gain in confidence was in draining a PTA. While learning of attitudes was not directly measured, the large gain in confidence may act as a surrogate measure. Students seem to have learned the attitude that PTA drainage is a straightforward procedure that does not always require a specialist. After the workshop, participants rated their confidence in ability to perform a tracheostomy lowest, compared to the other stations. This suggests students have some insight into their skills as well as risks and complications of procedures.

OTOHNS career interest

Among SEAD students there was a very strong interest in OTOHNS as a potential career path; at the outset and close of the program, OTOHNS had the highest number of interested students of all surgical specialties. It is important to note that the level of interest among SEAD participants is likely not representative of level of interest among the entire first-year class. The competitive application process for a limited number of spots in this extracurricular program creates a selection bias for students who have already identified an interest in surgical specialties. The source of this interest among surgically inclined students could be a result of the relatively strong presence of OTOHNS in the University of Ottawa UME pre-clerkship curriculum. In the pre-clerkship curriculum there are 50 hours of OTOHNS instruction, which is the highest amount of OTOHNS pre-clerkship instruction offered at any Canadian medical school [9].

Despite high interest levels in pre-clerkship, historically, there has been an average of two students from the

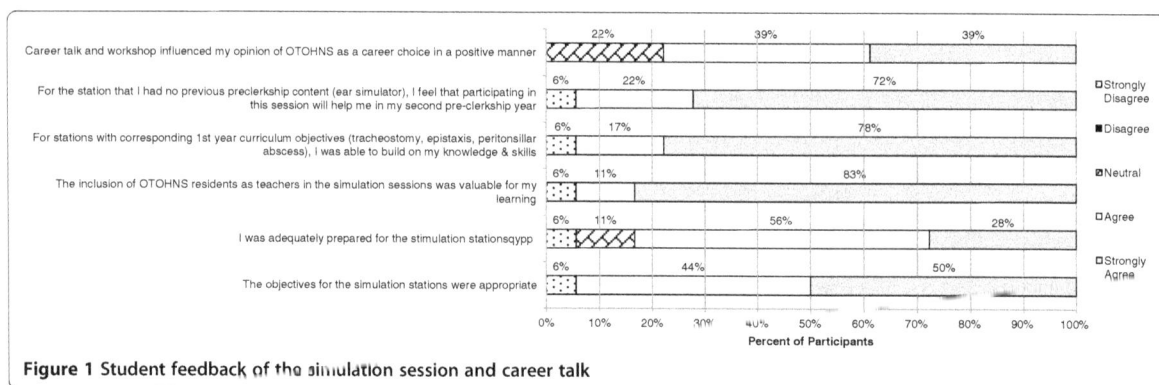

Figure 1 Student feedback of the simulation session and career talk

Table 9 Interest by surgical specialty before and after SEAD

Surgical specialty	No. interested at baseline	Final no. Interested	No. that developed a new interest	No. that ruled out a prior interest	Net change in no. interested
OTOHNS	10	10	2	2	0
Plastic surgery	7	8	1	0	+1
Orthopaedic surgery	9	7	1	3	−2
Cardiac surgery	6	2	0	4	−4
Vascular surgery	7	9	5	3	+2
Neurosurgery	2	4	3	1	+2
Thoracic surgery	7	2	2	7	−5
General surgery	10	9	2	3	−1
Urology	5	3	1	3	−2
Median	**7**	**7**	**2**	**3**	**−1**

University of Ottawa to apply to OTOHNS as a first choice residency program [10]. This is the first time that there is an indication of the number of first year students interested in OTOHNS. Although there are limitations in comparing these two groups of students, as SEAD participants could select several specialties on the questionnaire, the observation suggests that there is attrition of candidates from the University of Ottawa considering OTOHNS as a career choice as they progress through their undergraduate education. There could be several factors contributing to this phenomenon. First, OTOHNS is highly represented in pre-clerkship at the University of Ottawa, with significant lecture and workshop time. Conversely, students' main exposure to many of the other surgical specialties, such as plastic surgery and vascular surgery, occurs in clerkship. Thus, the high initial rate of interest may simply be because of early exposure to OTOHNS. Secondly, OTOHNS is a highly competitive specialty with only 30 residency positions available across Canada [10]. It is possible that some students self-select out of vying for an OTOHNS residency position. Third, it can be expected that as students explore other surgical and medical specialties, they modify their career interests as they make a more informed decision. While it has been documented that most students change their career choice between matriculation and graduation [11], it is unknown if other specialties see similar reductions in interest level throughout the undergraduate medical curriculum.

It is also important, however, to examine the role of clerkship in career decision-making as it has been demonstrated that positive clerkship experiences have a positive impact on preferences and attitudes towards a specialty as a career [12]. Compared to other surgical clerkship rotations (excluding Ophthalmology), where students are assigned to a discrete team (surgical clerk, junior resident, senior resident), the OTOHNS clerkship at the University of Ottawa is one week in duration. Students rotate through the different subspecialties of OTOHNS

to obtain broad exposure. The amount of exposure to surgical aspects of OTOHNS is highly variable between individual students. These data provide an interesting opportunity for further investigation into the delicate balance of broad specialty exposure and the team participation. It also gives pause about opportunities for student exposure to OTOHNS in other Canadian programs that have no mandatory OTOHNS clerkship rotation.

Interesting to note, there was a median net loss in interest in surgery as a career choice by −1. Although some could criticize that the SEAD program resulted in one less student being interested in surgery, it should be viewed as a positive outcome in that one student has been provided the early opportunity to make a more informed career choice—a choice that has a better chance of resulting in a well-matched, well-suited physician who truly enjoys his/her career.

Curriculum feedback and future opportunities
The participants' reaction to OTOHNS as part of the SEAD program was very positive. Overall, the session was rated a mean of 4.8 on a 5-point scale and was the highest rated session over the course of the program. The OTOHNS workshop was most closely tied to the UME curriculum objectives; 94% of participants found the objectives appropriate. Appropriately tailored objectives may have set the students up for success, which led to high satisfaction with the session. It is also possible the rating could be inflated by its timing in the context of the whole SEAD program, as it was the first specialty-specific workshop (immediately following the two days of introductory skills).

When evaluating different elements of the program on a Likert scale, the most participants stated they 'strongly agree' that having residents as teachers in the simulation session was valuable for their learning. Residents can provide instruction that is appropriate for the learner's level as they are of similar tenure. It also provides the added benefit of creating an opportunity for participants to ask more candid questions about the demands of the training program and lifestyle. For residents, leading stations at the workshop for SEAD participants creates a low-risk environment for them to develop their teaching skills.

Although the OTOHNS simulation was well received by students, evaluation of written and verbal feedback from various stakeholders (workshop facilitators, participants, simulation technicians) provides direction for opportunities to improve future sessions.

The PTA model was composed of a low-fidelity latex mold (designed to resemble the oropharynx) [7]. Creating a latex mold with representative anatomy proved challenging, hence it may be worthwhile to create a second-generation simulator based on lessons learned from this session (ie. use a simple printed image of the oropharynx in lieu of the mold). Given that the model is low tech and low cost, ideally the student:simulator ratio would approximate 1:1, ensuring that all students have ample opportunity to develop their skills. Overall, the model was an excellent tool for simulating a PTA and could potentially be used as a simulation for Emergency Medicine physicians as PTA is a common presentation to the Emergency Department.

Several students identified the tracheostomy station as the most exciting part of the simulation. In future sessions, it will be important to ensure that there are sufficient models to allow students to both perform and assist in the simulation. Also, it would be helpful to have examples of the numerous tracheostomy models that exist as well as the cricothyroidotomy kit that is found in the ED; this would serve to familiarize students with elements that they may encounter in their clerkship training. Similarly, for the epistaxis simulation it would be beneficial to orient students to headlights, Rapid Rhino, Nasal Epistaxis Double Balloon Catheter, and Floseal.

The OtoSim™ was well received by students, however given that they had no prior knowledge of ear anatomy and pathology, a brief online learning module completed the evening before might allow students to develop an understanding of basic anatomy in advance, allowing Oto-Sim™ to be an opportunity to apply their knowledge clinically.

Two stations that were not included in the simulation curriculum that would be interesting to explore the feasibility of for future sessions are a flexible fiberoptic laryngoscopy and a foreign body airway.

In the future, it would be valuable to formally evaluate the program feasibility from the preceptors' perspective. However, from informal discussions with staff and residents, the additional burden of work was well distributed. The program is a student-led initiative. Each specialty was assigned a second-year medical student liaison that worked with the lead staff surgeon to organize their respective specialty's participation. Two

weeks of OR observerships had minimal impact on the surgeons' daily schedule. Student leaders arranged the logistics of observership scheduling. Simulations were designed in collaboration with the simulation centre staff, surgeons, and student liaisons. Student liaisons developed the instructional manual. While the entire program was two weeks long, each speciality was only required to lead one afternoon, a 4-hour time commitment from 1–2 staff surgeons per specialty, to provide a career discussion and a workshop for all program participants. The cost of administering the program was divided between student participation fees, an external grant, and department funding, such that it was affordable for all parties involved. The majority of the cost was attributable to simulation centre rental fees, which would vary between institutions. The SEAD program has run successfully for 3 years at the University of Toronto, and now at the University of Ottawa. As evidence builds to support program's value, future iterations may explore modifications to the core structure such that more students can be included, without compromising the quality of the experience.

Conclusions
The inclusion of OTOHNS in the SEAD program at the University of Ottawa seemed to have been a success for all stakeholders. Students had the opportunity to develop their OTOHNS specific knowledge and surgical skills as well as refine their perspective on potential career options. The Department of OTOHNS had the opportunity build upon its formal UME curriculum as well as introduce concepts and skills to engaged students. OTOHNS residents also were provided a unique opportunity for teaching while providing a "real-life" perspective for students about OTOHNS residency. With continued expansion of the SEAD program to other medical schools, inclusion of OTOHNS should be considered to provide interested students with well-rounded exposure to OTOHNS and other surgical disciplines. Even in the absence of the SEAD program, an isolated OTOHNS simulation session and career discussion could provide many similar benefits for students and the Department alike.

Additional files

Additional file 1: SEAD program schedule.
Additional file 2: Student evaluation form.
Additional file 3: OTOHNS specific student evaluation form.

Abbreviations
OTOHNS: Otolaryngology – Head and Neck Surgery; CSO: Canadian Society of OTOHNS; UME: Undergraduate Medical Education; SEAD: Surgical Exploration and Discovery; OR: Operating room; uOSSC: University of Ottawa Skills and Simulation Centre.

Competing interests
The author(s) declare that they have no competing interests.

Authors' contributions
BG and LH were jointly responsible for study conception, design and
execution of the SEAD program, data collection and manuscript preparation.
NG was responsible for originally developing the SEAD program at the
University of Toronto, providing guidance on its execution at the University
of Ottawa, and critically reviewing the manuscript. SJH was responsible for
guiding the execution of the SEAD program and critically reviewing the
manuscript. LM was responsible for designing and executing the OTOHNS
specific element of the SEAD program, conceiving and guiding the study
design, and was integrally involved in manuscript preparation. All authors
read and approved the final manuscript.

Acknowledgements
The authors would like to thank the University of Ottawa Skills and
Simulation Centre (uOSSC), the University of Ottawa Faculty of Medicine, and
the University of Ottawa Department of Surgery for their combined efforts
and contributions in the execution of the Surgical Exploration and Discovery
(SEAD) program. The authors also acknowledge the University of Toronto
Medical School Faculty (Dr. James Rutka, Chair of Department of Surgery; Dr.
George Christakis, Director of Undergraduate Surgical Education; Dr. David
Latter, Vice-Chair of Education) who, along with Dr. Nada Gawad, originally
developed the SEAD Program.

Author details
[1]University of Ottawa Faculty of Medicine, 451 Smyth Road, Ottawa, Canada.
[2]University of Toronto Department of Surgery, Faculty of Medicine, 1 King's
College Circle, Medical Sciences Building, Room 2109, Toronto, Canada.
[3]Department of Surgery, The Ottawa Hospital, General Campus, 501 Smyth
Road, Ottawa, Canada. [4]University of Ottawa Skills and Simulation Centre,
The Ottawa Hospital, Civic Campus, Loeb Research Building, 1st floor, 725
Parkdale Avenue, Ottawa, Canada. [5]Department of Otolaryngology Head and
Neck Surgery, The Ottawa Hospital, General Campus, 501 Smyth Road,
Ottawa, Canada.

References
1. Fung K, McLean L. Variation in Otolaryngology - Head and Neck Surgery
    Undergraduate Medical Education in Canada. In: Canadian Society of
    Otolaryngology - Head and Neck Surgery Undergraduate Medical Education
    Working Group. 2009. p. 1.
2. Polk HC. The declining interest in surgical careers, the primary care mirage,
    and concerns about contemporary surgical education. Am J Surg.
    1999;178:177–9.
3. O'Herrin JK, Lewis BJ, Rikkers LF, Chen H. Why do students choose careers in
    surgery? J Surg Res. 2004;119:124–9.
4. Scott IM, Matejcek AN, Gowans MC, Wright BJ, Brenneis FR. Choosing a
    career in surgery: factors that influence Canadian medical students' interest
    in pursuing a surgical career. Can J Surg. 2008;51:371–7.
5. Zeldow P, Preston R, Daughterty S. The decision to enter a medical
    specialty: timing and stability. J Med Educ. 1992;26:327–32.
6. Gawad N, Moussa F, Christakis GT, Rutka JT. Planting the "SEAD": early
    comprehensive exposure to surgery for medical students. J Surg Educ.
    2013;70:487–94.
7. Taylor SR, Chang CWD. Novel peritonsillar abscess task simulator.
    Otolaryngol Neck Surg. 2014;151:10–3.
8. Kirkpatrick DL, Kirkpartick JD. Evaluating Training Programs. Thirdth ed.
    San Francisco: Berrett-Koehler Publishers; 2009.
9. Kelly K, Fung K, Mclean L. Canadian Otolaryngology - Head and Neck
    Surgery clerkship curricula/: evolving toward tomorrow ' s learners.
    J OTOHNS. 2013;42:33–40.
10. Canadian RMS. Statistics from the Match 2002 – 2014. Ottawa; 2014
11. Compton MT, Frank E, Elon L, Carrera J. Changes in U.S. medical students'
    specialty interests over the course of medical school. J Gen Intern Med.
    2008;23:1095–100.
12. Al-Heeti KNM, Nassar AK, Decorby K, Winch J, Reid S. The effect of general
    surgery clerkship rotation on the attitude of medical students towards
    general surgery as a future career. J Surg Educ. 2012;69:544–9.

2

Frontal recess anatomy in Japanese subjects and its effect on the development of frontal sinusitis: computed tomography analysis

Kazunori Kubota[1,2*], Sachio Takeno[1] and Katsuhiro Hirakawa[1]

Abstract

Background: Comprehensive understanding of frontal recess anatomy is essential for the successful treatment of patients with frontal sinus disease. This study was designed to determine the prevalence of specific frontal recess cells in Japanese subjects and the association of these cells with the development of frontal sinusitis.

Methods: Frontal recess anatomy was analyzed using high-resolution spiral computed tomography images of paranasal sinuses from December 2008 through September 2011. The distribution of various frontal recess cells in patients with and without frontal sinusitis was compared by logistic regression analysis.

Results: A total of 150 patients met the criteria, and 300 sides were analyzed. Agger nasi cells were present in 88.0 % of sides; frontal cell types 1 (FC1), 2 (FC2), 3 (FC3), and 4 (FC4) were present in 37.0 %, 6.3 %, 4.3 %, and 1.3 %, respectively; supraorbital ethmoid cells in 6.0 %, suprabullar cells in 37.0 %, frontal bullar cells (FBC) in 7.0 %, and interfrontal sinus septal cells in 8.6 %. Multiple logistic regression analysis showed that the presence of FBCs was significantly associated with the development of frontal sinusitis ($p = 0.043$).

Conclusions: The frequencies of frontal recess cells in Japanese adult patients were similar to those reported for other East Asian adult populations, including Chinese, Korean, and Taiwanese. Anatomically, FBCs may show a greater association with the development of frontal sinusitis than other frontal recess cells.

Keywords: Frontal recess cells, Frontal recess anatomy, Frontal sinusitis

Background

Advances in endoscopic visualization and high-resolution computed tomography (CT) have enhanced the understanding of frontal recess anatomy. Before frontal sinus surgery, the variable frontal recess cells in each patient must be analyzed to plan a strategy for dissecting all cells disturbing the nasofrontal recess, including drainage of the frontal sinus. Frontal recess cells consist of a combination of cells, including agger nasi cells (ANCs), frontal cell types (FCs) 1 to 4, suprabullar cells (SBCs), supraorbital ethmoid cells (SOECs), frontal bullar cells (FBCs), and intersinus septal cells (IFSSCs) [1]. In healthy persons, the FC3 and FBC extend into the frontal sinus and narrow

the nasofrontal recess, defined as the pathway draining the frontal sinus (Fig. 1). In patients with frontal sinusitis, the FC3 is positioned next to the orbit, and the FBC lies along the skull base (Fig. 2). Because of the complexity of the frontal recess and the risk during surgery of injuring the orbit and skull base, a comprehensive understanding of frontal recess anatomy is essential for treating frontal sinus disease successfully.

Although CT has been used to assess frontal recess pneumatization patterns [1–7], few studies in English have focused on Japanese adult populations. This study used high-resolution CT images to analyze Japanese patients with frontal sinusitis. We hypothesized that Stammberger's theory may apply to the development of frontal sinusitis, and paid particular attention to FC3s, FC4s, SBCs, SOECs, and FBCs, which can narrow the ventilation pathway of the frontal sinus. The purpose of this study was to clarify the association of various frontal

* Correspondence: kazunokubota@gmail.com
[1]Department of Otolaryngology, Head and Neck Surgery, Division of Clinical Medical Science, Programs for Applied Biomedicine, Graduate School of Biomedical Sciences, Hiroshima University, Hiroshima, Japan
[2]Department of Otorhinolaryngology, Hiroshima University School of Medicine, 1-2-3 Kasumi, Minami-ku, Hiroshima 734-8551, Japan

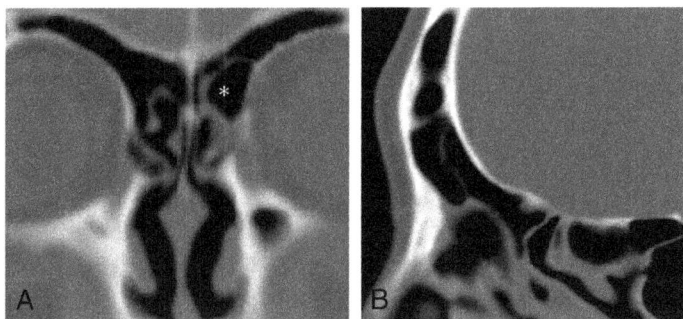

Fig. 1 Computed tomography (CT) images of a healthy frontal sinus. **a** Coronal CT showing a left frontal cell type 3 (FC3) (*). **b** Sagittal CT showing a frontal bullar cell (FBC) (+)

recess cells with the development of frontal sinusitis in Japanese patients by determining cell frequency in those with and without frontal sinusitis.

Methods

The study was performed at the Department of Otorhinolaryngology–Head and Neck Surgery, Hiroshima University Hospital, Hiroshima, Japan. Between December 2008 and September 2011, 150 consecutive patients underwent CT of the nasal cavities and paranasal sinuses. Spiral CT scans of the nasal cavities and paranasal sinuses were performed on a Toshiba Aquilion CT scanner (Toshiba Medical Systems, Tokyo, Japan) with 1-mm-thick axial cuts. The following scanning parameters were used: kV 120, mA 200, window level 2000, central level 500. The CT data were reconstructed into coronal and sagittal images at a computer workstation. Imaging angles, contrast, and brightness were adjusted on the computer workstation to improve bony detail, which was especially useful for identifying severely diseased frontal recess cells in patients with rhinosinusitis.

The 150 patients consisted of 50 patients with chronic rhinosinusitis and 100 controls, including 50 patients with allergic rhinitis without chronic rhinosinusitis and

50 normal individuals with no nasal symptoms. Exclusion criteria included previous sinus surgery, age <18 years, maxillofacial fracture, and/or sinonasal malignancy. CT images on which it was difficult to identify the delicate structures of the frontal sinus because of excessive motion or beam hardening artifacts were also excluded. Frontal sinusitis was defined as mucosal thickening >3 mm involving the entire frontal sinus or its dependent portions and the presence of symptoms. Fullness or heaviness of the frontal head, frontal pain, and 15 other sinonasal symptoms were also evaluated using the modified Sino-Nasal Outcome Test-22 scoring system, with scores ranging from 0 to 5; the average scores of fullness or heaviness of the frontal head and of frontal pain symptoms are shown in Fig. 3 as representative of frontal sinusitis patients.

The 300 sides of the 150 patients were categorized into three groups, based on the findings of frontal sinusitis on CT images and the presence of chronic rhinosinusitis (Table 1). Images were evaluated for the presence of ANCs, FCs, SBCs, SOECs, FBCs, and IFSSCs. FC types were determined according to modifications of previous criteria [1], which clarified the definitions of several types of frontal recess cells. The Lund–Mackay score of each paranasal sinus shadow was evaluated in

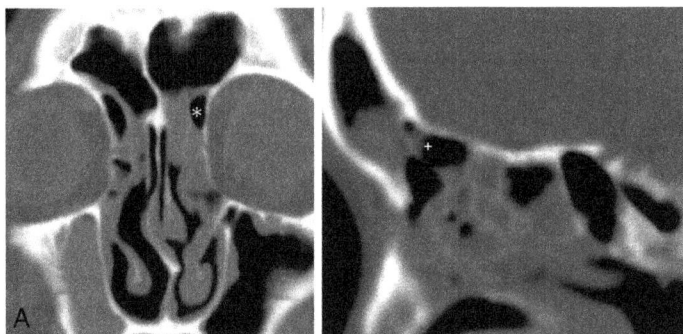

Fig. 2 CT images of a patient with frontal sinusitis. **a** Coronal CT showing a left FC3 (*). **b** Sagittal CT showing an FBC (+)

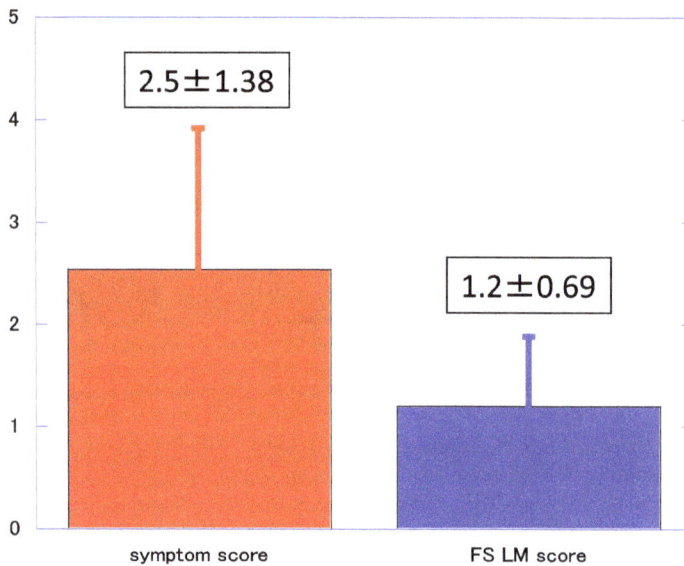

Fig. 3 Symptom and Lund–Mackay scores of patients with frontal sinusitis. Symptom score was based on the SNOT-22. FS LM score: frontal sinus Lund–Mackay score

all patients and compared in patients with and without frontal sinusitis [8]. To minimize variations in interpretation, each CT scan was evaluated jointly by two trained ear–nose–throat (ENT) surgeons, with any disagreements resolved by consensus.

Statistical analyses were performed using Excel Statistics 2010 (Shakai Jouhou Corp. Tokyo, Japan). Multivariate logistic regression analyses were performed to identify factors associated with frontal sinusitis. The odds ratio (OR) and 95 % confidence interval (CI) were calculated for each factor. ANCs, FC1–FC4s, SBCs, SOECs, FBCs, and IFSSCs were chosen as predictive variables. A p value <0.05 was considered statistically significant for all measurements. The protocol was approved by ethical committee of epidemiological research at Hiroshima University (No. 1063).

Results

A total of 300 sides from 150 patients were assessed (Table 1). Seventy sides, 50 from men and 20 from women, showed evidence of frontal sinusitis, whereas 230 sides did not. The mean symptom score of patients with frontal sinusitis was 2.5 ± 1.38 and the Lund–Mackay score of their frontal sinuses was 1.2 ± 0.69 (Fig. 3). Fourteen patients (14 sides) had unilateral frontal sinusitis and 28 (56 sides) had bilateral frontal sinusitis. Patients with frontal sinusitis were older (57.8 ± 13.8 years) than those without frontal sinusitis (41.3 ± 17.5 years), but the difference was not significant ($p = 0.469$). Mean Lund–Mackay score (7.9 ± 2.4 vs. 5.5 ± 1.8, $p = 0.000$) and mean anterior ethmoid score (1.8 ± 0.45 vs. 1.4 ± 0.55, $P = 0.001$) were significantly higher in patients with than without frontal sinusitis.

In categorizing frontal recess cells, we found ANCs in 265 sides (88.0 %) and FCs in 147 (49.0 %), with FC1s in 111 sides (37.0 %), FC2s in 19 sides (6.3 %), FC3s in 13 sides (4.3 %), and FC4s in four sides (1.3 %). SBCs, SOECs, FBCs, and IFSSCs were observed in 111 (37.0 %), 18 (6.0 %), 21 (7.0 %), and 26 (8.6 %) sides, respectively (Table 2). In comparing the percentage of frontal recess

Table 1 Data for 150 patients undergoing computed tomography

	CRS(+)		CRS(−)	Total
	Frontal sinusitis (+)	Frontal sinusitis (−)		
Age (years ± SEM)	57.8 ± 13.8	41.3 ± 17.5	47.0 ± 19.4	51.1 ± 18.4
Distinguishable sides	70	30	200	300
Male: Female	50:20	14:16	100:100	164:136
Lund-Mackay score (±SEM)	7.9 ± 2.4	5.5 ± 1.8	0.19 ± 0.64	2.6 ± 3.6
Anterior ethmoid score (±SEM)	1.8 ± 0.45	1.4 ± 0.55	0.025 ± 0.16	0.58 ± 0.84

CRS = chronic rhinosinusitis; SEM = standard error of the mean

Table 2 Incidence of frontal recess cells in various populations

Cell types	Our cases Japanese; 300 sides, no. (%)	Taiwanese; 363 sides, no. (%)	Chinese, 404 sides, no. (%)	Korean, 114 sides, no. (%)	Caucasian, 82 sides, no. (%)
ANC	265 (88.0)	323 (89.0)	380 (94.1)	107 (94.0)	71 (86.6)
FC1	111 (37.0)	78 (21.5)	98 (24.4)	26 (22.8)	29 (35.4)
FC2	19 (6.3)	38 (10.5)	28 (7.0)	16 (14.0)	17 (20.7)
FC3	13 (4.3)	28 (7.7)	33 (8.2)	9 (7.9)	7 (8.5)
FC4	4 (1.3)	0 (0)	0 (0)	0 (0)	0 (0)
SBC	111 (37.0)	142 (39.1)	148 (36.6)	45 (39.5)	9 (11.0)
SOEC	18 (6.0)	28 (7.7)	22 (5.4)	3 (2.6)	53 (64.6)
FBC	21 (7.0)	23 (6.3)	36 (9.0)	16 (14.0)	5 (6.1)
IFSSC	26 (8.6)	35 (9.6)	25 (12.4)	10 (8.8)	6 (7.3)

cells in patients with [CRS(+)] and without [CRS(−)] chronic sinusitis (Fig. 4), we found a significant difference in the presence of FC1s. In addition, the presence of FBCs was significantly higher in the CRS(+) than in the CRS(−) group. There was no difference in the distribution of frontal recess cells between normal controls and patients with allergic rhinitis. Multivariate analysis showed that the presence of FBCs was strongly associated with an increased frequency of frontal sinusitis ($p = 0.043$) (Table 3).

Discussion

The frontal recess is a complex space that resembles an inverted funnel or cone, with the apex at the frontal ostium. This space is filled by various anterior ethmoid or frontal recess cells [9]. Because of the intrinsic anatomic complexity of this narrow space, comprehensive knowledge of frontal recess anatomy is required prior to surgery.

In investigating the prelavence of frontal recess cells on CT images, we found that the prevalence of ANCs was 88.0 %, similar to previous findings [1–4]. Although we found that the prevalence of FC1s in Japanese patients was almost as high as in Caucasians, the prevalence of other frontal cells (FC2–FC4s), especially FC2s, was in line with findings in other Asian populations. FC4s are independent of the appearance of ANCs [1]. Previous studies have reported FC4s in 16 (2.1 %) of 768 subjects [5] and in 3 (3.1 %) of 98 frontal recesses [6], making FC4s quite rare among frontal recess cells. In our study, nearly half (48.9 %) of the Japanese subjects had frontal cells.

Similar to findings in other East Asian populations, SBCs were more frequent while SOECs were less frequent, in Japanese than in Caucasian patients [1–4]. Although the prevalence of these frontal recess cells in our study population was more consistent with those in Chinese, Korean, and Taiwanese populations than with those in Caucasians, the prevalence of FC1s (37.0 %) in Japanese patients was closer to that in Caucasians

(35.4 %) than in Taiwanese (21.5 %), Chinese (24.4 %), and Korean (22.8 %) groups. The latter discrepancy may be due to racial differences between Japanese and other East Asian populations [3].

The pathophysiology of frontal sinusitis is associated with ventilation of the sinus via the sinus ostium. The size of the frontal sinus ostium is key to frontal sinus drainage. Generally, frontal recess cells and their inflammation can influence frontal sinus ventilation by narrowing the frontal sinus drainage pathway. Because frontal cells may be associated with frontal sinus inflammation, we assessed whether frontal recess cells were associated with frontal sinusitis in Japanese subjects.

The association between the presence of anterior frontal recess cells (ANCs and FC1–FC4s) and the development of frontal sinusitis is unclear. Enlargement of ANCs has been found to correlate with a decrease on CT in the anteriroposterior size of the nasofrontal recess, involved in the frontal sinus drainage pathway. The association between a requirement for revision sinus surgery in patients with frontal sinusitis and agger nasi disease was highly statistically significant. Failure to address agger nasi disease can contribute to failure of the primary surgery [10]. An analysis of 768 coronal CT scans showed that the prevalence of frontal mucosal thickening was higher in individuals with frontal cells of any type than in individuals without frontal cells, with the prevalence of FC3 and FC4 differing significantly [5].

Another study, however, found no difference in the frequency of frontal sinusitis on sides with and without frontal cells [6]. Moreover, the incidence of frontal sinusitis was not increased in patients with persistent ANCs undergoing revision surgery, and the diameters and areas of the frontal isthmus were similar in sinuses with various types of frontal cells.

In assessing the frontal recess cells posterior and posterolateral to the frontal recess (FBCs, SBCs, SOECs), our multivariate analysis suggested that the prevalenc of FBCs was associated with the development of frontal

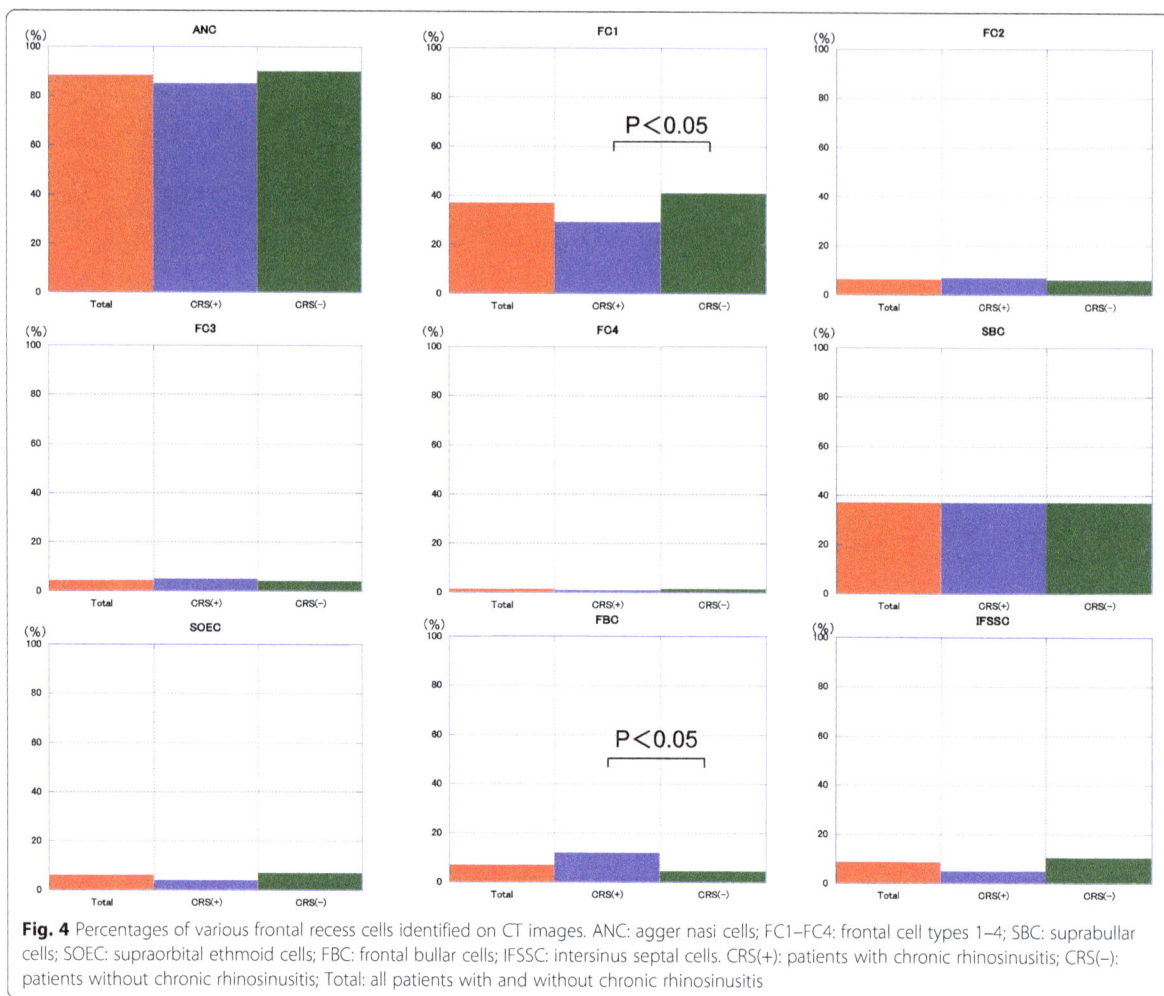

Fig. 4 Percentages of various frontal recess cells identified on CT images. ANC: agger nasi cells; FC1–FC4: frontal cell types 1–4; SBC: suprabullar cells; SOEC: supraorbital ethmoid cells; FBC: frontal bullar cells; IFSSC: intersinus septal cells. CRS(+): patients with chronic rhinosinusitis; CRS(−): patients without chronic rhinosinusitis; Total: all patients with and without chronic rhinosinusitis

Table 3 Statistical analysis of the effect of various frontal recess cells on the development of frontal sinusitis

Variable	CRS (+) 100 sides, no. (%)		CRS (−) 200 sides, no. (%)	Univariate analysis			Multivariate analysis		
	FS (+)	FS (−)		OR	95 % CI	P value	OR	95 % CI	P value
FBC	9 (13)	3 (10)	9 (4.5)	2.63	1.06–6.52	0.038*	2.56	1.03–6.38	0.043*
ANC	60 (86)	26 (87)	179 (89.5)	0.75	0.34–1.64	0.469			
FC1	21 (30)	8 (27)	82 (41)	0.65	0.37–1.15	0.14			
FC2	5 (7.1)	2 (6.7)	12 (6)	1.16	0.40–3.35	0.779			
FC3	4 (5.7)	1 (3.3)	8 (4)	1.46	0.44–4.89	0.54			
FC4	2 (2.9)	0 (0)	2 (1)	3.29	0.46–23.8	0.238			
SBC	22 (31)	15 (50)	74 (37)	0.77	0.44–1.35	0.358			
SOEC	4 (5.7)	0 (0)	14 (7)	1.26	0.43–3.66	0.673			
IFSSC	3 (4.3)	2 (6.7)	21 (11)	0.40	0.12–1.36	0.14			

FS frontal sinusitis, *OR* odds ratio, *CI* confidence interval. Asterisk indicates significance at p < 0.05

sinusitis. FBCs are characterized by pneumatization along the skull base in the posterior frontal recess and extend through the frontal ostium into the true frontal sinus. FBCs are significantly associated with the narrow antero-posterior diameter of the frontal ostium and frontal recess [2]. In frontal recesses that have FBCs, this anatomic tendency may play a role in narrowing the frontal sinus drainage pathway, resulting in significant obstruction.

Although anatomic variations in the frontal recess are likely to play a role in frontal sinusitis, mucosal inflammatory processes are also likely to be an important etiologic factor [6, 11, 12]. Allergies, asthma, and tobacco smoking can affect the nasal mucosa and lead to poorer outcomes of functional endoscopic sinus surgery, despite meticulous handling of the frontal ostium mucosa and preservation of the natural outflow tract [13]. An evaluation of 289 frontal recesses at the time of revision surgery found that 193 (66.8 %) had mucosal edema or polyposis obstructing the frontal recess [11]. In the absence of anatomic reasons for obstruction, mucosal inflammatory disease in the frontal recess should be considered a medical rather than a surgical problem. Seven major factors were associated with frontal sinusitis: mucosal disease (67 %); retained ethmoid cells (53 %); lateralized middle turbinates (30 %); retained ANCs (13 %); scar tissue (12 %); retained frontal cells (8 %); and neo-osteogenesis (7 %), with most frontal recesses having more than one factor (average 1.6) [11]. Frontal sinusitis is therefore caused by multiple factors, including anatomic variations, mucosal inflammation, and sinonasal polyposis. Further investigations are needed to understand the effects of anatomic variants of frontal recess cells on frontal sinusitis.

Conclusions
The frequencies of frontal recess cells in Japanese adult patients were similar to those reported for other East Asian adult populations, including Chinese, Korean, and Taiwanese patients. Frontal bullar cells may have more influence on the development of frontal sinusitis than other frontal recess cells.

Consent
Written informed consent was obtained from the patient for the publication of this report and any accompanying images.

Competing interests
This research was supported by a grant from Hiroshima University Ryokufukai.

Authors' contributions
KK, ST, and KH evaluated CT images, counted the number of frontal cells, and determined the Lund–Mackay scores. KK performed the statistical analysis. ST and KH conceived the study, participated in its design and coordination, and helped draft the manuscript. All authors read and approved the final manuscript.

Authors' information
KK: Graduate Student in Otorhinolaryngology–Head and Neck Surgery, Hiroshima University
ST: Assistant Professor of Otorhinolaryngology–Head and Neck Surgery, Hiroshima University
KH: Professor of Otorhinolaryngology–Head and Neck Surgery, Hiroshima University

Acknowledgement
We thank Ms. Ai Kashima for her technical assistance.

References
1. Lee WT, Kuhn FA, Citardi MJ. 3D computed tomographic analysis of frontal recess anatomy in patients without frontal sinusitis. Otolaryngol Head Neck Surg. 2004;131:164–73.
2. Lien CF, Weng HH, Chang YC, Lin YC, Wang WH. Computed tomographic analysis of frontal recess anatomy and its effect on the development of frontal sinusitis. Laryngoscope. 2010;120:2521–7.
3. Cho JH, Citardi MJ, Lee WT, Sautter NB, Lee HM, Yoon JH, et al. Comparison of frontal pneumatization patterns between Koreans and Caucasians. Otolaryngol Head Neck Surg. 2006;135:780–6.
4. Han D, Zhang L, Ge W, Tao J, Xian J, Zhou B. Multiplanar computed tomographic analysis of the frontal recess region in Chinese subjects without frontal sinus disease symptoms. ORL J Otorhinolryngol Relat Spec. 2008;70:104–12.
5. Meyer TK, Mehmet K, Smith MM, Smith TL. Coronal computed tomography analysis of frontal cells. Am J Rinol. 2003;17:163–8.
6. DelGaudio JM, Hudgins PA, Venkatraman G, Beningfield A. Multiplanar computed tomographic analysis of frontal recess cells. Arch Otolaryngol Head Neck Surg. 2005;131:230–5.
7. Zhang L, Han D, Ge W. Computed tomographic and endoscopic analysis of supraorbital ethmoid cells. Otolaryngol Head Neck Surg. 2007;137:562–8.
8. Lund VJ, Mackay IS. Staging in rhinosinusitis. Rhinology. 1993;31:183–4.
9. Bent JP, Cuilty-Siller C, Kuhn FA. The frontal cell as a cause of frontal sinus obstruction. Am J Rhinol. 1994;8:185–91.
10. Bradley DT, Kountakis SE. The role of agger nasi air cells in patients requiring revision endoscopic frontal sinus surgery. Otolaryngol Head Neck Surg. 2004;131:525–7.
11. Otto KJ, DelGaudio JM. Operative findings in the frontal recess at time of revision surgery. Am J Otolaryngol. 2010;31:175–80.
12. Han JK, Tamer G, Lee B, Gross CW. Various causes for frontal sinus obstruction. Am J Otolaryngol. 2009;30:80–2.
13. Friedman M, Bliznikas D, Vidyasagar R, Joseph NJ, Landsberg R. Long-term results after endoscopic sinus surgery involving frontal recess dissection. Laryngoscope. 2006;116:573–9.

3

A new diagnostic vestibular evoked response

Zeinab A Dastgheib[1*], Brian Lithgow[2], Brian Blakley[3] and Zahra Moussavi[4]

Abstract

Objective: To describe the development of a new clinically applicable method for assessing vestibular function in humans with particular application in Meniere's disease.

Study design: Sophisticated signal-processing techniques were applied to data from human subject undergoing tilts stimulating the otolith organs and semicircular canals. The most sensitive representatives of vestibular function were extracted as "features".

Methods: After careful consideration of expected response features, Electrovestibulography, a modified electrocochleography, recordings were performed on fourteen Meniere's patients and sixteen healthy controls undergoing controlled tilts. The data were subjected to multiple signal processing techniques to determine which "features" were most predictive of vestibular responses.

Results: Linear discriminant analysis and fractal dimension may allow data from a single tilt to be used to adequately characterize the vestibular system.

Conclusion: Objective, physiologic assessment of vestibular function may become realistic with application of modern signal processing techniques.

Keywords: Meniere's disease, EVestG, Vestibular response, Classification, Fractal dimension

Introduction

Vestibular disorders are among the most common reasons that patients seek the advice of a physician, yet the diagnosis of dizziness largely relies on the patient history. The patient history is subjective and its reproducibility has not been validated. Significant physiologic disruptions of neurological function should cause repeatable, measureable changes in neural activity. We believe that sophisticated and objective measurement of these changes should be diagnostic and should reveal underlying pathologic mechanisms. This paper outlines the application of advanced statistical signal processing techniques from the fields of engineering and statistics to understand normal and pathologic vestibular function using Meniere's disease as a prototype.

Evoked potentials have been successfully applied to diagnose auditory disorders but may be difficult for vestibular diagnosis. Auditory evoked potentials typically involve temporal averaging of several hundred auditory stimuli which may be problematic in vestibular stimuli. On the other hand, when observing the averaging process of auditory evoked potentials in real time, the first response or two are often adequate to see the general nature of the response. It would seem then that the first response or two should contain diagnostic information if it could be extracted. With this observation in mind is seems plausible that sophisticated signal processing techniques might be able tease out enough information from a few tilts to permit recognition of repeatable patterns of waveforms that could be diagnostically useful.

Electrocochleography (ECoG) is a diagnostic evoked-potential method that records an excitatory 'gross' evoked response by averaging responses to a series of auditory clicks [1-3]. A useful, analagous vestibular test would directly measure the dynamic response of the vestibular system to both excitatory and inhibitory inputs, and derive a measure of its dynamic range. Electrovestibulography (EVestG) [4,5] is similar to ECoG but the multiple acoustic stimuli are replaced by one or two passive whole body tilts in a hydraulically controlled chair located in an electrically and acoustically shielded chamber. The EVestG signal is recorded during dynamic and static phases via

* Correspondence: umdastgh@myumanitoba.ca
[1]Department of Electrical & Computer Engineering, University of Manitoba, Room E3-512 Eng. Bldg., 75A Chancellor's Circle, Winnipeg, MB R3T 5V6, Canada
Full list of author information is available at the end of the article

ECoG electrodes resting near the tympanic membrane of both ears [6]. Figure 1, shows the recording system with the hydraulic chair. A proprietary software algorithm called the "Neural Event Extraction Routine (NEER)" [5] has been developed to extract the field potential (FP) signals from the EVestG recordings. NEER algorithm derives two signals from the recording raw signals: the averaged response of FPs and the time intervals between the FPs. Pattern recognition techniques applied to EVestG signals have shown very encouraging results in other neurological diagnostic applications such as Parkinson's disease, depression, and schizophrenia disorder by other studies [7-9]. In this paper will apply EvestG techniques to Meniere's disease patients with a view to developing an objective test for the disorder.

Usually several features as biomarkers are extracted from the output of the NEER algorithm on the EVestG signals. Most diagnostic tests measure the signals' most important parameters to classify a system as normal or abnormal. The "feature" extraction technique utilizes many quantitative criteria from the signal to categorize the response. Extracted criteria may be statistical parameters, calculations of some characteristic of the waveform or derivations from multiple other sources. The technique of "feature extraction" is similar to that used in cochlear implants. Herein, we apply it to vestibular function. A major difficulty in measuring biological electrical potentials is the signal-to-noise ratio. We are trying to detect a small signal in the midst of tremendous electrical noise from nerve, muscle and other cells. In this paper we discuss the clinical utility of NEER algorithm and EVestG extracted signals. First we briefly describe of the key concepts. Further details can be found in the Additional file 1.

Features

In signal processing, features are quantities that are associated with a signal or a process. Features may be statistical measures such as the mean, standard deviation, skewness, kurtosis, etc. of a statistical process, or they may be other quantitative measures representing fractal nature, power distribution, etc. of a signal or process. In addition to statistical features, this report includes features representing fractal dimension (FD) as assessed by the Higuchi fractal dimension (HFD), and entropy-based dimensions such as the Information dimension (DI) [10] and the Correlation dimension (DC). These features were extracted from the FP and timing intervals of the EVestG recordings from patients undergoing EVestG testing.

Fractal dimension calculation (FD) can be interpreted as the "degree of meandering" (roughness, brokenness, irregularity or singularity) of an object. Another interpretation of a fractal dimension is that it is the critical exponent in a power-law relation [10,11]. Fractal dimension mathematically refers to a non-integer or fractional dimension

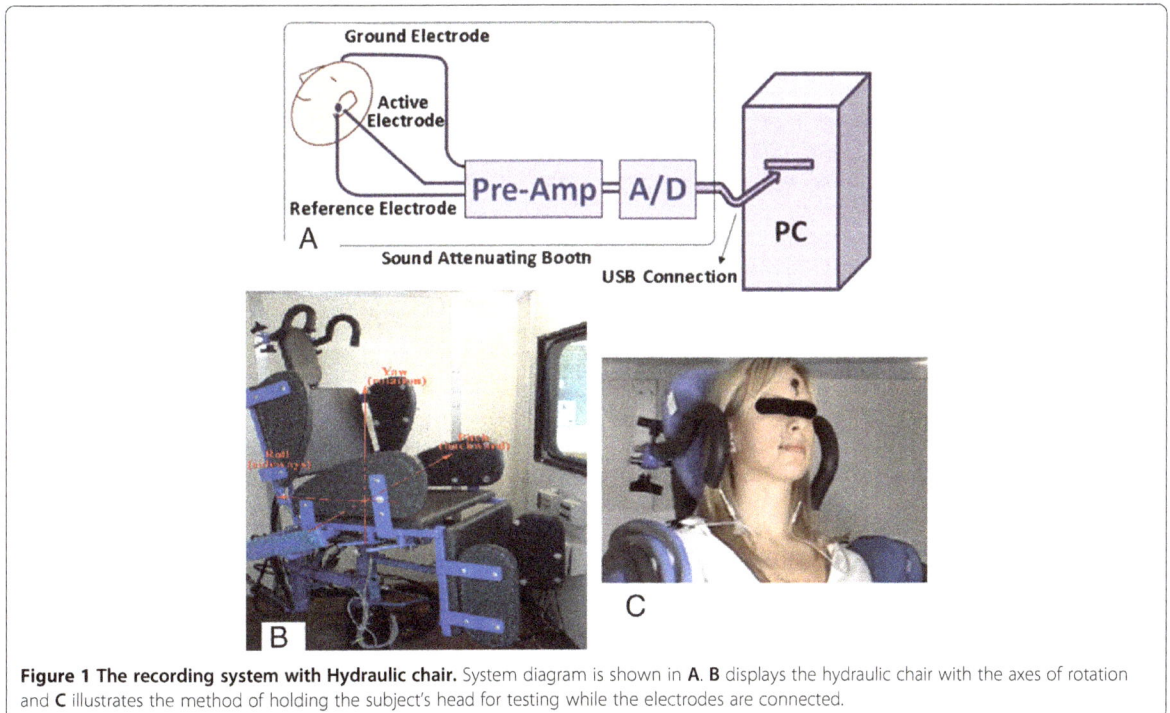

Figure 1 The recording system with Hydraulic chair. System diagram is shown in **A**. **B** displays the hydraulic chair with the axes of rotation and **C** illustrates the method of holding the subject's head for testing while the electrodes are connected.

of a self-similar (or a self-affine) object [10]. The self-similarity (or self-affinity) of the object is confirmed if a portion of the object is exactly (or statistically) a scaled down version of itself.

FD analysis is widely used as an analytical tool in a variety of research areas particularly biological signal processing [11]. It measures the irregularity, the complexity and the self-similarity of a signal. The more complex the signal, the higher the FD value will be. Two effective methods for FD calculation are the Higuchi fractal dimension and Entropy based fractal dimension (see Additional file 1 for details).

Higuchi Fractal Dimension (HFD) is well suited for studying signal fluctuation in one dimension [12]. HFD, proposed in 1988, is an efficient algorithm for measuring the FD of discrete time series [13]. HFD has been established as a method to characterize the morphological complexity of biological signals [14].

Entropy-Based Fractal Dimensions - Entropy can be defined as the amount of information needed to specify the state of a system [10]. Entropy is known as the measure of disorder in physical systems, or an amount of information that may be gained by observations of disordered systems [15]. Entropy-based fractal dimensions can deal with fractals objects which have non-uniform distributions, while the morphological fractal dimensions such as HFD deal with the shape of a projection of the fractal only. This is understandable because the morphological dimensions are purely metric and not probabilistic concepts. The information dimension (DI) and correlation dimension (DC) are special cases related to generalized entropy concept as introduced by Alfred Renyi in 1955 [16]. Both dimensions are improvements of the geometric definition of a fractal object (See Additional file 1).

The DI reveals the expected spread in the non-uniform probability distribution of the fractal objects, but not its correlation. The DC was introduced to address this problem. Both DI and DC represent a weighted average measure of the actual distribution of self-information over the fractal object (See Additional file 1).

Linear Discriminant Analysis (LDA) is a mathematical technique that utilizes features to classify objects or signals into one or more classifications. Each object/signal has certain features that may be relevant in classifying that object/signal; some of these features can be more important predictors than others. In this study, we are trying to classify patients as with either Meniere's disease or no Meniere's disease.

Minimal-redundancy-maximal-relevance (mRMR) feature selection method [17] is a method of ranking features based on the two criteria of minimum redundancy and maximum relevancy; thus allowing to choose the most relevant and least redundant features as the best set of features for classification.

Methods
EVestG research labs have been established for human testing at Alfred Hospital in Melbourne Australia and Riverview Health Center in Winnipeg, Canada. In this study, however, only data recorded at Alfred Hospital in Australia has been used. The EVestG signal acquisition apparatus is illustrated in Figure 1.

Study subjects
EVestG data of 14 Meniere's patients (54.2 ± 9.7 years, 4 males) and 16 healthy individuals (56.1 ± 5.5 years, 7 males) from the EVestG lab at the Alfred Hospital, Melbourne, Australia, were used as the training data to design the diagnostic algorithm. Ethics approval was granted by the Health Research Ethics Board of Alfred Hospital, and all study subjects signed an informed consent form prior to the experiments.

EVestG protocol
A complete EVestG recording [4,5] includes passive lateral whole body tilts, up/down movements, rotations from the sitting position and up/down movements and rotations from the supine position. This paper will report data for right and left lateral tilts only. Tilts were symmetric movements moving over 3 seconds from the upright sitting position to a position 45 degrees from the vertical to the right, then upright and then to the left. The EVestG signal was recorded at a sampling rate of 41666 Hz.

Table 1 shows the timing segments and names for a tilt to the right and back to the upright position. The labels for the segments in Table 1 are those from the original EvestG description in the literature that relate to EvestG in general, rather than specific application to the ear. Following this tilt to the right, a tilt to the left is performed with the same naming system. Rightward tilts are referred to as right ipsilateral (IP) and left contralateral (CT). In different segments of the motion, there are "periods of interest" that are the critical time periods for analysis as indicated in Figure 2.

The NEER [5] algorithm extracts data from the neural response. Each tilt's recorded data results in two main signals, an average field potential (FP) and its firing pattern for each time segment (see Table 1) for each ear. In this study, we only used signals of the contralateral and ipsilateral side tilt stimuli that presumably stimulate otolith and semicircular canals.

Signal analysis
An average field potential is illustrated in Figure 3 top. Each FP fires many times representing its firing pattern. The firing pattern of the FP is presented by 1) the time intervals between each two successive FP occurrences, as in Figure 3 lower left, and 2) the probability distribution

Table 1 Labeling of components of EvestG test

Segment	Period of Interest (POI) of the segment (See Figure 2)	Name of POI
20 s background recording	the final 1.5 s	BGi
3 s lateral tilt to the right (about 40 degrees)	first half, 1.5 s, the acceleration phase	On AA
	second half, 1.5 s the deceleration phase	On BB
17 s rest in the tilted position	final 1.5 s just before returning to center	RTC BGi
3 s returning back to center	the first 1.5 s	RTC OnAA
	the second 1.5 s	RTC OnBB
17 s rest at the center position before a new tilt	Transition to Steady State	RTC OnSS

Labeling of components of EvestG test.

function (pdf) of the time intervals estimated by the histogram of time interval data as shown in Figure 3 lower right.

We investigated the changes in the differences among different time segments for each tilt signal to examine the effects of dynamic changes from resting to acceleration or deceleration phases of the time segment, and also the differences between the two phases (acceleration/deceleration) of chair movement as well as differences between the right and left symmetry (L-R).

The NEER algorithm [5] removes segments of the original signal that are corrupted by large artifact (due to hydraulic chair, muscle artifact, movements, poor electrode contact, etc.); therefore, not all the segments were precisely of 1.5 s duration. We excluded the segments shorter than 1.36 s. Thus, it was possible that not every subject have all the extracted features.

Feature extraction

We calculated the mean, mean of the absolute value, variance (Var), skewness, kurtosis, HFD, entropy-based dimensions such as the Information dimension (DI) and the Correlation dimension (DC), the total energy and the average power of the aforementioned intervals for the range of 100–11000 Hz of the pre- and post-potential regions of every FP signal. Also the depth of the AP point was selected as suggested in [6].

From the time interval of the FP's firing pattern signals (Figure 3 lower left), we calculated the mean, standard deviation (Std), skewness, kurtosis, mode, median, the DI, DC, HFD. We also calculated the average number of the time intervals less than 0.5 msec, and the correlation of the probability distribution function (PDF) of the time interval signals (Figure 3 lower right) with the relevant FP signals (Figure 3 top) as another feature.

Overall, we calculated over 40 features to consider. The features are grouped in three categories based on which signal they were calculated: 1) the features from from the field potential signals, 2) the features from one of the firing pattern representations, and 3) the features from the correlation calculation between the pdf of the time interval signals and FPs. The names of the features are summarized for the sake of space. For example, the names of "Pre Kurtosis", "Pre mean abs", or "Pre Energy"

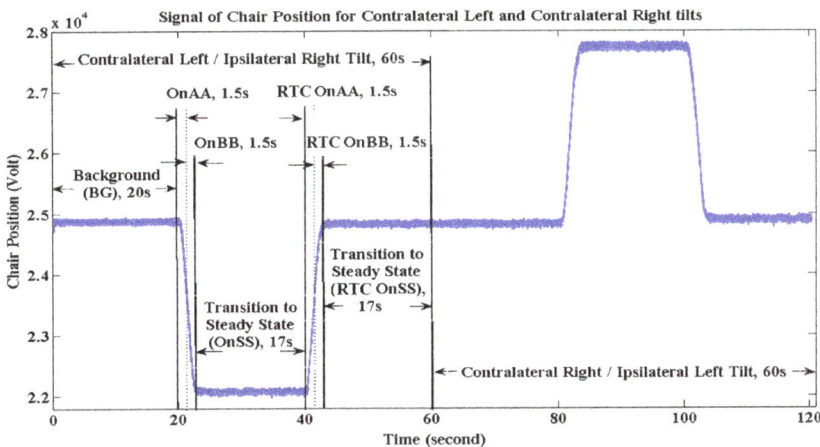

Figure 2 The chair movement pattern during the side tilt.

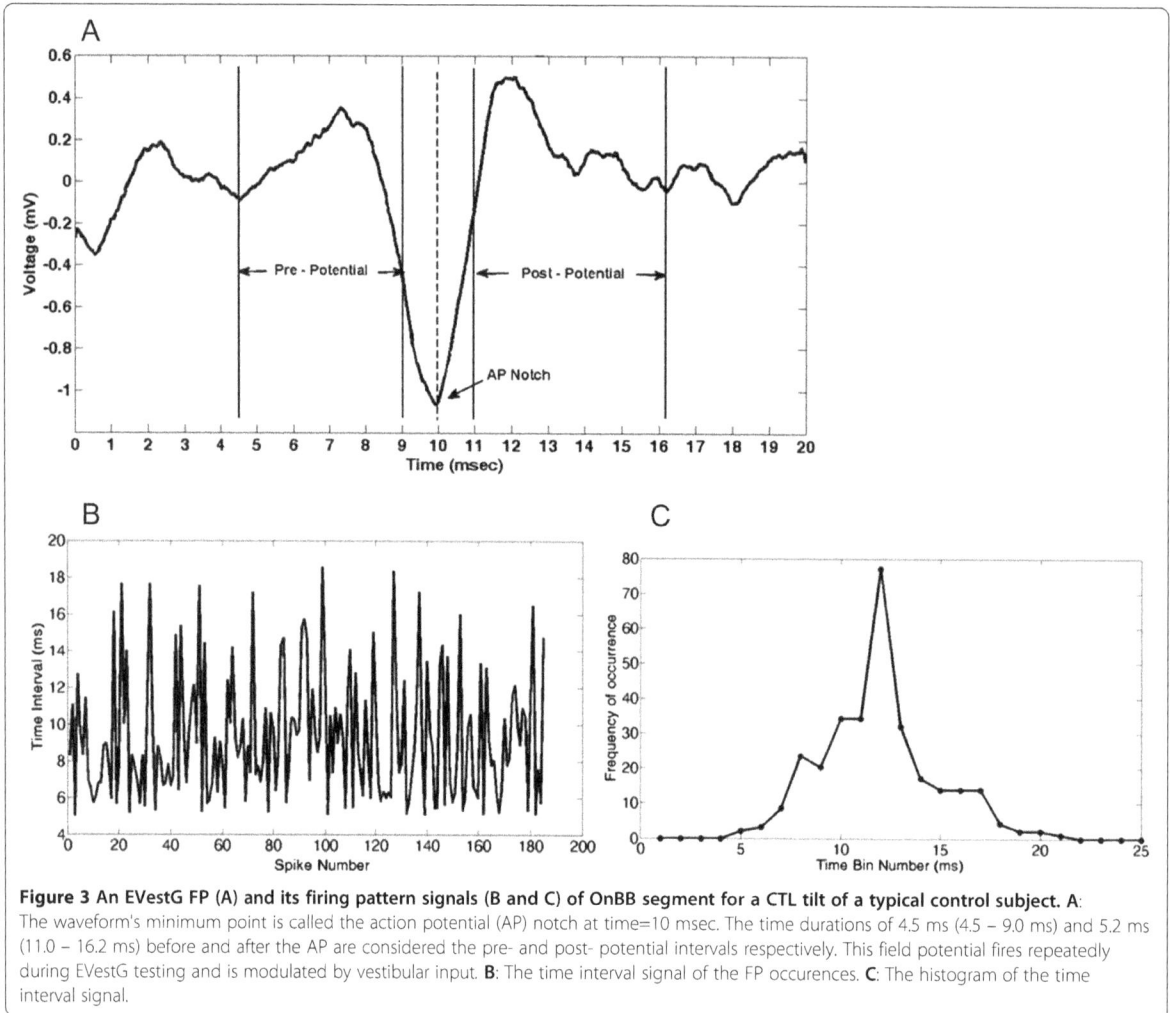

Figure 3 An EVestG FP (A) and its firing pattern signals (B and C) of OnBB segment for a CTL tilt of a typical control subject. **A**: The waveform's minimum point is called the action potential (AP) notch at time=10 msec. The time durations of 4.5 ms (4.5 – 9.0 ms) and 5.2 ms (11.0 – 16.2 ms) before and after the AP are considered the pre- and post- potential intervals respectively. This field potential fires repeatedly during EVestG testing and is modulated by vestibular input. **B**: The time interval signal of the FP occurences. **C**: The histogram of the time interval signal.

show that the features are found by calculation of the kurtosis, mean of absolute value, or total energy (from the entire frequency range) of the pre potential interval of the mentioned original segment.

A t-test was used to assess the statistical significance of differences for CT tilt and IT tilt between Meniere's patients and controls. Then, we ran the mRMR algorithm on these 39 statistically significant features, and selected 5 top features (from every tilt) as the best features for classification.

Classification (Average Voting Classifier)

Each selected feature was used in a single feature classifier using linear discriminant classification algorithm (LDA) [18]. We used leave-one-out routine [18] for training classifiers. Then, we considered each feature as a symptom, and used a heuristic method for a final classification, called Average Voting Classifier, in which

every feature has "a vote" for the test subject as either Meniere's (vote = 1) or non-Meniere's (vote = 0) based on the LDA classifier, and the final classification is based on the average vote of all the selected best features. In this way, the final vote represents the probability that the test subject is a Meniere's or non-Meniere's patient. If that probability is greater than 0.5, the subject is classified as a Meniere's patient; otherwise as non-Meniere's.

Results

Of the features extracted from the side tilt signals, 39 (22 from CT tilt and 17 from IT tilt) were found significantly different among the Meniere's patients and controls (t-test, $p < 0.05$). The proposed Average Vote Classifier resulted in 85.7%, 75% and 80% sensitivity, specificity and accuracy, respectively assuming the clinical diagnosis as the "gold standard" (Figure 4), which are encouraging in this first attempt. The five best features for IT and CT tilts

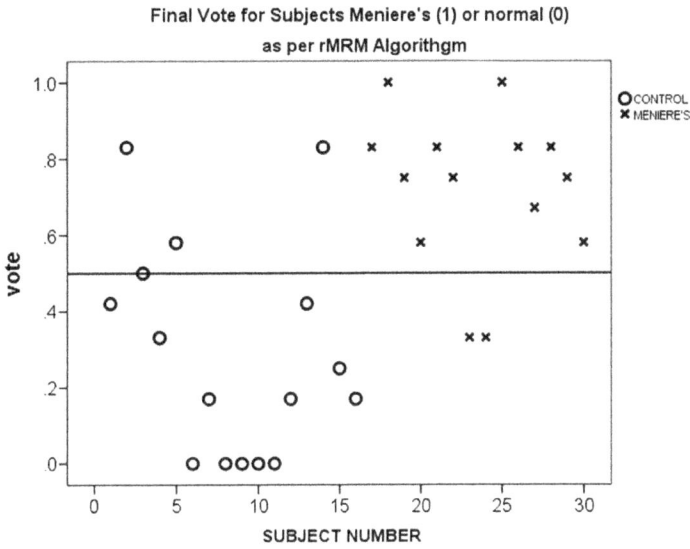

Figure 4 Final Vote classification results of the training subjects for side (CT&IT) tilt for 30 subjects (14 Meniere's patients and 16 normals). If the probability is greater than 0.5 (above the reference line in the figure) the subject would be classified as a Meniere's patient, otherwise the subject would be classified as normal. Sensitvity, specificity and accuracy were 85.7%, 75% and 80% respectively.

identified by the mRMR algorithm and used for classification, are shown in Table 2.

The features that extracted in this study represented some consistent variations. Fractal dimension calculation (DI, and CI) over both firing patterns and FP signals showed higher values for control subjects compared to those of the Meniere's subjects. This may imply the higher complexity in control subjects' data compared to Meniere's patient, which is congruent with the observed pattern of fractal dimension features calculated from other biological signals [19].

Table 2 Five best features for CT (Feature 1–5), and IT (Feature 6–10) tilts

Feature Number	Feature Name	Original Signal	p_value
1	Post skewness	OnBB - R	0.007
2	Ap height	RTC OnAA - RTC OnBB - L-R	0.028
3	ID of Time Interval Signal	OnBB – L + R	0.007
4	Correlation	OnBB - L-R	0.048
5	Correlation	RTC OnBB - R + L	0.0079
6	Pre energy	RTC BGi - L	0.0046
7	Post HFD	RTC OnAA - R	0.0066
8	Post mean	BGi - OnBB - R	0.006
9	CD of Time Interval Signal	BGi - OnBB - R	0.0071
10	Correlation	RTC OnBB - L	0.017

Moreover, the correlation between the FP and the pdf of FP's firing signal demonstrated positive values in Meniere's patients, while negative ones were observed in controls. Also, the AP was lower (wider FPs) in Meniere's patients compared to Control ones. This may talk about possible slower conductivity of the stimulus in the vestibular organ of Meniere's patients.

Discussion

Tilts cause angular (rotational) accelerations and changes in the direction of gravity. For these reasons EVestG testing involves a combination of head movement responses that may or may not be consistent among patients with Meniere's disease. Our long-term goal is to develop an objective test that is diagnostic and specific for Meniere's disease. Our current tests, electronystagmography, rotary chair, and others, are supportive or helpful, but have no features that are unique to Meniere's disease. We observed a distinct difference in the pre- and post-potential parts within the period time of the interest of the average FP curve of the Meniere's and control subjects. Our finding that the fractal dimensions showed more complexity in Meniere's patients than controls is consistent with the general physiologic literature regarding chaos theory in other organ systems – that abnormal systems lose their variability [20,21].

The results of this study show a new potential of EVestG signals toward generating an adequate set of bio-features as a diagnostic and monitoring aid for dizziness related diseases, especially Meniere's disease. We suspect, but cannot prove at this point, that our data identify features unique to Meniere's disease as opposed to some general findings of reduced vestibular function. If EVestG turns out to be a general method of quantifying vestibular function, it should be clinically useful. This is an ongoing study, and we hope to confirm these results with other populations. The results may lead to a simple, objective and non-invasive clinical assessment of Meniere's disease. We acknowledge that this small dataset is not adequate to recommend clinical use without further development. The method must be tested in larger populations in future studies, which is currently under investigation at the EVestG lab at Winnipeg, Canada.

Conclusion

Modern signal processing techniques such as EVestG may identify neural firing patterns that are diagnostic in patients with vestibular disorders but much more work needs to be done.

Additional file

Additional file 1: Appendix.

Competing interests
The authors declare that they have no competing interests.

Authors' contributions
ZAD is a PhD graduate student in Electrical Engineering. She performed many of the tests and wrote the initial draft of the paper. BL obtained funding, developed the EvestG technique, wrote the initial software and set-up the EvestG lab in Winnipeg. BB supervised the clinical testing and examined patients clinically and re-wrote the initial paper, hopefully making it more readable by physicians. ZM is the Director of the Riverview EvestG lab in Winnipeg. She supervised and trained ZAD, participated in writing of the paper. All authors read and approved the final manuscript.

Acknowledgement
This research has been supported by Neural Diagnostics Canada Ltd. and Mathematics of Information Technology and Complex Systems (MITACS).

Author details
[1]Department of Electrical & Computer Engineering, University of Manitoba, Room E3-512 Eng. Bldg., 75A Chancellor's Circle, Winnipeg, MB R3T 5V6, Canada. [2]EVestG Research Lab, Riverview Health Centre, Room PE446, 1 Morley Avenue, Winnipeg, MB R3L2P4, Canada. [3]Department of Otolaryngology - Head and Neck Surgery, University of Manitoba, GB421 - 820 Sherbrook Street, Winnipeg, Manitoba R3A 1R9, Canada. [4]Department of Electrical & Computer Engineering, University of Manitoba, 75A Chancellor's Circle, Winnipeg, MB R3T 5V6, Canada.

References
1. Ferraro JA. Electrocochleography: a review of recording approaches, clinical applications, and new findings in adults and children. J Am Acad Audiol. 2010;21:145–52.
2. Ferraro J, Best LG, Arenberg IK. The use of electrocochleography in the diagnosis, assessment, and monitoring of endolymphatic hydrops. Otolaryngol Clin North Am. 1983;16:69–82.
3. Kim HH, Kumar A, Battista RA, Wiet RJ. Electrocochleography in patients with Meniere's disease. Am J Otolaryngol. 2005;26(2):128–31.
4. Lithgow B. "A neural response system", Australia Patent WO/2008/144840. Government of Australia Patent Office. Patent (WO 2008/144840, priority date June 2007)
5. Lithgow B. A methodology for detecting field potentials from the external ear canal: NEER and EVestG. Ann Biomed Eng. 2012;40:1835–50.
6. Lithgow BJ, Garrett A, Heibert D. "EVestG: a measure for Meniere's Disease". Conf Proc IEEE Eng Med Biol Soc. 2008;2008:4162–5.
7. Dastgheib ZA, Lithgow B, Moussavi Z. Diagnosis of Parkinson's disease using electrovestibulography. Med Biol Eng Comput. 2012;50:483–91.
8. Garrett A, Heibert D, Lithgow B. "Electrovestibulography: the "DC" potential used to separate Meniere's disease and Benign Paroxysmal Positional Vertigo,". Conf Proc IEEE Eng Med Biol Soc. 2007;2007:2381–4.
9. Haghgooie S, Lithgow BJ, Winograd-Gurvich C, Kulkarni J. "EVestG: a diagnostic measure for schizophrenia,". Conf Proc IEEE Eng Med Biol Soc. 2008;2008:4142–5.
10. Kinsner W. A Unified Approach to Fractal Dimensions. 2009.
11. Phothisonothai M, Nakagawa M. EEG signal classification method based on fractal features and neural network. Conf Proc IEEE Eng Med Biol Soc. 2008;2008:3880–3.
12. Sullivan R, Holden T, Tremberger Jr E, Cheung E, Branch C, Burrero J, et al. "Fractal dimension of breast cancer cell migration in a wound healing assay". Int J Biol Life Sci. 2011;7(Issue 3):170.
13. Higuchi T. Approach to an irregular time series on the basis of the fractal theory. Physica D: Nonlinear Phenomena. 1988;31:277–83.
14. Gómez C, Mediavilla A, Hornero R, Abásolo D, Fernández A. Use of the Higuchi's fractal dimension for the analysis of MEG recordings from Alzheimer's disease patients. Med Eng Phys. 2009;31:306–13.
15. Kimcheng K, Sourina O, Kulish V, Nguyen M. An algorithm for fractal dimension calculation based on Renyi entropy for short time signal analysis. In: Information, Communications and Signal Processing, 2009. ICICS 2009. 7th International Conference on. 2009. p. 1–5.
16. Rényi A. On a new axiomatic theory of probability. Acta Math Acad Sci Hung. 1955;6:285–335.
17. Peng H, Long F, Ding C. Feature selection based on mutual information: criteria of max-dependency, max-relevance, and min-redundancy. IEEE Trans Pattern Anal Mach Intell. 2005;27:1226–38.
18. Duda RO, Hart PE, Stork DG. Pattern classification. New York: Wiley; 2001.
19. Ehtiati T, Kinsner W, Moussavi ZK. Multifractal characterization of the electromyogram signals in presence of fatigue. In: University and Industry - Partners in Success, Conference Proceedings Vols 1–2. 1998. p. 866–9.
20. Halley JM, Kunin VE. Extinction risk and the 1/f family of noise models. Theor Popul Biol. 1999;56:215–30.
21. Kinsner W. A unified approach to fractal and multifractal dimensions. Winnipeg, Manitoba, Canada DEL94-4: University of Manitoba; 1994.

4

Assessment of the current Canadian rhinology workforce

Kristine A Smith[1] , Doron D Sommer[2], Sean Grondin[3], Brian Rotenberg[4], Marc A Tewfik[5], Shaun Kilty[6], Erin Wright[7], Arif Janjua[8], John Lee[9], Chris Diamond[8] and Luke Rudmik[1*]

Abstract

Background: The Canadian Rhinologic workforce and future needs are not well defined. The objective of this study was to define the current demographics and practice patterns of the Canadian Rhinologic workforce. Outcomes from this study can be used to perform rhinologic workforce needs assessments.

Methods: A national survey was administered to all Canadian otolaryngologists who were identified to have a clinical practice composed of >50% rhinology.

Results: 42 surgeons participated in the survey (65% response rate). The mean age was 46 (SD 10.1) years and the average age of planned retirement was 66 (SD 4.0). Eighty three percent of respondents had completed a rhinology fellowship and 17% practiced exclusively rhinology. Thirty three percent hold advanced degrees. Forty two percent of surgeons felt their access to operative time was insufficient. Six percent of surgeons reported not having access to image guided surgery. Fourteen percent felt that there were too many practicing rhinologists in Canada while 17% believed there were too few practicing rhinologists. Seventeen percent have advised their residents to pursue other fields due to a perceived lack of future jobs. Overall, 66% of respondents were satisfied with their income, and 83% were satisfied with their careers.

Conclusions: This study has demonstrated that there is a perceived mismatch between the current supply of Rhinology labor and the capacity to treat patients in a timely manner. Outcomes from this study will begin to improve Rhinologic workforce planning in Canada and reduce the gap between patient demand and access to high quality care.

Keywords: Rhinology, Sinusitis, Rhinosinusitis, Workforce, Otolaryngology

Introduction

Workforce planning is a relatively new approach to identifying the supply and demand of labor [1]. The goal of workforce planning is to identify talent surpluses and shortages, and project future needs to avoid similar issues. It also facilitates matching training to societal needs. In Canada, the lack of jobs in surgical subspecialties is well known. In 2013, the Royal College of Physicians and Surgeons of Canada reported the unemployment rate of recently graduated specialists was approximately 16% [2]. More specifically, of newly graduated otolaryngologists, almost 30% were unable to find permanent employment, despite a declining otolaryngologist to population ratio [2,3]. However, even

with this apparent 'surplus' of surgeons, operative and consultation wait times continue to grow [4]. Deficiencies in the appropriate matching of workforce needs combined with reduced capacity to treat patients in a timely and accessible manner significantly reduces the quality of care and may adversely affect patients' health [4-7]. Some of these issues would likely be resolved by improving the concordance between societal health needs and labor capacity.

All previous attempts to define the otolaryngology workforce have focused on the overall population of otolaryngologists, not individual subspecialties [3,8-11]. With an increasing number of residents pursing fellowship training, characterizing the subspecialist populations is paramount to create accurate workforce planning projections and improving efficient allocation of scarce health care resources [2,8]. Rhinology is a growing subspecialty

* Correspondence: lukerudmik@gmail.com
[1]Division of Otolaryngology, Head and Neck Surgery, Department of Surgery; University of Calgary, Calgary, Alberta, Canada
Full list of author information is available at the end of the article

within otolaryngology and this population has not been previously defined.

The purpose of this national survey was to describe the contemporary demographics, medical education, practice patterns, and surgeons' attitudes towards workforce requirements and training of the current Canadian rhinologic workforce. Outcomes from this study will provide the necessary information required for physician workforce modeling and allow us to begin strategically planning for Canada's future rhinologic needs.

Methods
Study design
This was an online survey-based study that invited participants between June and Aug 2014.

Participant sample
Otolaryngologists with large volume rhinology practices (at least 50% rhinology) were selected for inclusion in the study. We chose a cut off of 50% rhinology since the practice patterns of these otolaryngologists would likely have the largest impact on the overall rhinology workforce. For this study we defined "rhinology" to include all endonasal surgery and excluded the practice of managing nasal conditions which require a rhinoplasty. In order to coordinate across all the provinces and territories in Canada, a representative rhinologist was selected from each province by the principal investigator (LR). Potential participants were identified through a review of the Canadian Society of Otolaryngology – Head and Neck Surgery (CSO) database by the provincial representatives. Email addresses were obtained from the CSO registry where available and otherwise were identified from the provincial representatives.

Survey
The rhinology workforce survey was developed from the validated 'Canadian thoracic surgery workforce survey' using a modified Delphi technique by a panel of experts [12]. Questions from their survey were altered to reflect rhinology as the surgical specialty of interest, versus thoracic surgery. Any questions modified more than changing the surgical field of interest were reviewed using the Delphi technique until all authors agreed on the proposed question. The final survey consisted of 54 questions and was designed to collect data regarding demographics, education, current practice patterns, income, job satisfaction and future planning, and a basic workforce assessment. The survey was distributed using an online survey host, "Survey Monkey", a web survey company located in the USA (http://www.surveymonkey.com/).

Ethics, consent and permissions
Institutional ethics review board approval was obtained (ID: # REB14-0970). An email containing a link to the survey and an invitation to participate in the workforce survey was sent to all the otolaryngologists identified to have large volume rhinology practices (>50% rhinology). Participation was entirely voluntary. Two reminder emails were sent, the first one week after the initial invitation and the second two weeks after the initial invitation. Submission of the completed survey was considered informed consent to participate. No identifying data was collected and all survey responses were completely anonymous.

Outcomes
The primary outcome was to define the demographics of the current rhinologist workforce in Canada. Secondary outcomes included: education, medical training, current practice patterns, scope of practice, income and job satisfaction with rhinology.

Statistical analysis
Data was exported into Excel (Microsoft, 2010) for analysis. Data was correlated to survey results for accuracy and logic by one of the authors (KS). Descriptive statistics were calculated where appropriate.

Results
A total of 65 otolaryngologists were identified as having large volume rhinology practices and were invited to participate in this study. Forty two (42) responded to the survey, representing a 65% response rate. Participants answered an average of 90% of questions, with participation decreasing towards the end of the survey.

Demographics and education
Table 1 summarizes the demographic data of the respondents, including gender, age, practice location, country of birth and society memberships. The majority of respondents were male (91%), with an average age of 46 (SD = 10.1). Only 29% of respondents were over 50 years of age.

The details of respondents' medical training are summarized in Table 2. All surgeons had completed residency in Canada. 83% of respondents reported completing a rhinology fellowship. Forty six percent (46%) of fellowship trained rhinologists completed fellowship training in Canada, while 31% had completed fellowships in the United States (US). For rhinologists with a fellowship, the average year for beginning practice was 2005. For those who had not pursued a fellowship, the average year for starting their rhinology practice was 1991. Thirty three percent (33%) of surgeons had completed advanced graduate degrees (MSc, MPH, or PhD), with an additional 5% currently pursing post-graduate education.

Table 1 Demographics

Gender	
Male	91%
Female	9%
Age (years) (SD)	
Average	46 (10.1)
<40	40%
40-50	31%
50-60	21%
>60	8%
Practice Location	
British Columbia	14%
Alberta	24%
Quebec	17%
Ontario	43%
Nova Scotia	2%
Country of Birth	
Canada	72%
USA	0%
Other*	28%
Memberships	
CSO	97%
ARS	52%
ERS	24%

*Egypt, China, Kenya, Ireland, England, Iran, Israel, Scotland and Austria.
SD - Standard Deviation.
USA – United States of America.
ARS – American Rhinologic Society.
ERS – European Rhinologic Society.
CSO – Canadian Society of Otolaryngology – Head and Neck Surgery.

Table 2 Education

Year of completion of (SD)	
Medical School	1995 (10.3)
Residency	2001 (9.9)
Fellowship Training	2005 (8.2)
Fellowship training	
Rhinology	83%
None	17%
Location of Fellowship Training	
Canada	46%
USA	31%
Other*	23%
Advanced Degrees	
Masters degree	33%
Masters degree (in progress)	5%

*Australia, Egypt, France, New Zealand, Belgium, Armenia.
SD – Standard Deviation.
USA – United States of America.

Current practice patterns

The practice patterns of the respondents are outlined in Table 3. Surgeons reported dedicating over 75% of working hours to clinical and operative time, with the remaining quarter split between research, administrative duties and teaching. Approximately half (54%) were affiliated with a university, with the remainder in community practices. Seventy eight percent (78%) of respondents were involved in some form of research, with 32% involved in multiple types of research including educational, basic sciences, clinical outcomes, and health economics research. Eighty five percent (85%) reported at least one other surgeon performing rhinologic surgeries at their institutions.

Work hour requirements are outlined in Table 4. The majority of surgeons work 41-60 hours per week (61%), with 25% working over 60 hours per week. Forty four percent (44%) of respondents reported on-call requirements of 1 in 4 - 6 and an additional 44% reported call requirements of 1 in 7 -10. A majority, 66% of respondents, reported taking at least 3 to 5 weeks of vacation time and 98% of surgeons reported taking at least 3 to 7 days for continued medical education in the last year.

Table 3 Practice Patterns

Language of Practice	
English	90%
French	20%
Cantonese	2%
Scope of Practice	
Exclusively Rhinology	17%
>75% Rhinology	30%
<75% Rhinology	53%
Distribution of work hours	
Clinical Work	76%
Research	8%
Administration	9%
Teaching	7%
Participation in Research	
Clinical	78%
Educational	32%
Basic Science	24%
Health Economics	5%
None	22%
Hospital Setting	
Community Hospital, no residents	22%
Community Hospital, residents	24%
University Hospital, residents	35%
University Hospital, residents and fellows	19%

Table 4 Work Hours and Vacation Time

Work hours per week	
≤40	12%
41-50	27%
51-60	34%
61-70	12%
71-80	9%
81-90	2%
>90	2%
On call frequency	
1:1 to 1:3	2%
1:4 to 1:6	44%
1:7 to 1:10	44%
>1:10	10%
Weeks of personal vacation per year	
<1	2%
1-2	7%
3-4	49%
5-6	17%
7-8	22%
≥9	3%
Days away from practice for continuing education	
0	2%
<3	0%
3-7	24%
8-14	51%
15-21	15%
22-28	5%
>28	3%

Scope of practice and resources

At the time of the survey, only 17% of surgeons reported practicing exclusively rhinology, dedicating 100% of their operative time to rhinology. An additional 31% focused at least 75% of available time and resources on rhinologic cases. Most surgeons (81%) operate 1 or 2 days a week. Overall, 42% felt their operating room (OR) resources were insufficient to meet their patient care need. No surgeons described an excess of operative resources.

When evaluating endonasal surgical approaches, 63% reported using endoscopic approaches in greater than 80% of cases. Ninety four percent (94%) of surgeons had access to image guidance systems (IGS). Fifty eight percent (58%) of surgeons reported performing in office procedures, with 14% performing over 60 in-office cases per year.

In an effort to quantify the case load of a rhinologic surgeon, surgeons were asked to quantify the number of new rhinology consults and operative cases. Surgeons

reported an average of 58 new inpatient consults per year, with an average of 818 in office consults per year. The average number of new operative cases is described in Table 5. Respondents reported an average of 73 primary endoscopic sinus surgeries (ESS) per year and an average of 59 revision ESS cases per year.

Job satisfaction, income, and future practice plans

Overall physician wellbeing and satisfaction is being increasingly emphasized as poor physician health has been suggested to adversely affect health care systems [13,14]. The majority of surgeons surveyed were satisfied with their careers (83%). Sixty six percent (66%)of surgeons reported being satisfied with their current income. The reported incomes and overhead costs are reported in Table 6.

Eighty three percent (83%) of respondents reported no plan to relocate their practice. The average planned retirement age was 66 (SD = 4.0) years of age, which was 20 years from the average age of surveyed physicians. Eighty six percent (86%) of physicians planned to retire at an age greater than 60.

Waiting times and workforce assessment

Surgeons were asked to state the maximal acceptable waiting time and percentage of patients who receive surgery by the maximum acceptable wait time. Results are described in Table 7. Surgeons reported only 56% (range =44% to 63%) of patients receiving surgery within the maximum acceptable wait time, regardless of the procedure.

Table 8 summarizes the respondents' opinions regarding the current rhinologic workforce and factors influencing the delivery of care. When asked what factors affected delivery of timely care, 54% of surgeons reported that insufficient OR time was often or always a factor. 63% felt that prolonged surgical waitlists was a significant factor in reducing the quality of care to patients.

Currently, 68% and 71% of the respondents feel the number of surgeons practicing rhinology and the number of fellowship-trained rhinologists is appropriate, respectively. However, 23% feel there is a shortage of fellowship-trained rhinologists. Only 6% felt there were too many fellowship-trained rhinologists. Regarding training patterns, 42% felt too many rhinologists were being trained in North America. In contrast, only 19% felt too many rhinologists were being trained in Canada. Seventeen percent (17%) of surgeons reported advising residents not to pursue rhinology due to perceived lack of jobs. Overall, there appears to be diverse opinions regarding the current rhinologic workforce and the perceived need for future rhinologists in Canada.

Respondents suggested an appropriate rhinologist to population ratio would be 1:500,000. Currently, only 2 respondents reported that their institution was seeking an additional rhinologist. Thirty one percent (31%) believe

Table 5 Scope of Practice

OR days per week	
<1/week	17%
1/week	42%
2/week	39%
3/week	2%
% of OR time dedicated to rhinology	
<25%	2%
26%-50%	25%
51%-75%	25%
75%-99%	31%
100%	17%
Current OR time	
Too much	0%
Appropriate	58%
Too little	42%
% of cases performed endoscopically	
1-20%	9%
21-40%	6%
41-60%	11%
61-80%	11%
81-100%	63%
% of cases performed with IGS	
0%	11%
1-20%	20%
21-40%	17%
41-60%	11%
61-80%	9%
81-100%	26%
No IGS available	6%
Number of in office procedures per year	
None	42%
1 to 20	20%
20 to 40	16%
40 to 60	8%
Greater than 60	14%
Number of new rhinology consults per year (SD)	
Inpatient/ER	58 (22.3)
In office	818 (152.3)
Number of operative procedures per year (SD)	
Primary Endoscopic Sinus Surgery (CRS)	73 (24.1)
Revision Endoscopic Sinus Surgery (CRS)	59 (18.1)
Endoscopic resection of benign sinonasal neoplasms	14 (3.9)

Table 5 Scope of Practice *(Continued)*

Septoplasty	125 (40.4)
Endoscopic pituitary adenoma resection	14 (5.1)
Anterior Skull Base resection (benign)	4 (1.5)
Anterior Skull base resection (malignant)	3 (1.3)
Orbital Decompression (Grave's)	2 (1.0)

CRS - Chronic Rhinosinusitis.
SD - Standard Deviation.
IGS - Image Guidance System.

their institution will recruit an additional rhinologist in the next 2-5 years.

Discussion

The objective of this study was to define the demographics and current practice patterns of the Canadian Rhinologic Workforce. Of the otolaryngologists identified as having a practice comprised of at least 50% rhinology, 65% responded to the invitation to participate in the survey. Generally, a 40% response rate represents an average survey response rate – greater than 60% response is considered excellent in email and online surveys [15-17].

Table 6 Job Satisfaction, Income, Future Practice Plans

Satisfaction	
Very dissatisfied	8%
Somewhat dissatisfied	6%
Neutral	3%
Somewhat satisfied	33%
Very satisfied	50%
Income	
< $200,000	8%
$200,000 to $400,000	24%
$400,001 to $600,000	37%
$600,001 to $800,000	16%
> $800,000	5%
Undisclosed	10%
Income Satisfaction	
Satisfied	66%
Neutral	26%
Dissatisfied	8%
Relocation	
Definitely not moving	46%
Unlikely to move	37%
Not sure	14%
Probably moving	3%
Definitely moving	0%
Average Planned retirement age (SD)	66 (4.0)

SD – Standard Deviation.

Table 7 Waiting Times Assessment

	Maximal acceptable waiting time (weeks) (SD)	Percent of patients who receive surgery within maximal acceptable waiting times (SD)
Primary Endoscopic Sinus Surgery (CRS)	15 (8.5)	45% (38.9)
Revision Endoscopic Sinus Surgery (CRS)	16 (14.2)	44% (36.7)
Endoscopic resection of benign sinonasal neoplasms	11 (9.7)	63% (33.9)
Septoplasty	30 (31.7)	53% (37.7)
Endoscopic pituitary adenoma resection	10 (10.1)	55% (35.4)
Anterior Skull Base resection (benign)	10 (9.9)	60% (37.8)
Anterior Skull base resection (malignant)	4 (5.1)	66% (39.9)
Orbital Decompression (Grave's)	8 (10.4)	60% (34.4)

CRS - Chronic Rhinosinusitis.
SD - Standard Deviation.

Table 8 Workforce Assessment

Factors affecting delivery of care*	
Prolonged clinic wait times	57%
Delay in investigations	16%
Prolonged surgical waitlists	63%
Insufficient OR time	54%
# of Surgeons practicing rhinology	
Too Few	18%
Appropriate	68%
Too Many	14%
# of fellowship-trained Rhinologists	
Too Few	23%
Appropriate	71%
Too Many	6%
Training too many Rhinologists in North America	
Yes	42%
No	19%
Unsure	39%
Too many Rhinology fellowships in Canada?	
Yes	19%
No	53%
Unsure	28%
Advised residents not to pursue rhinology due to perceived lack of jobs	
Yes	17%
No	83%
Appropriate ratio of Rhinologists to population (median, mode)	1:500,000
Average additional required Rhinologists per region	1
Institutions currently seeking Rhinologist	6%
Institutions planning on recruiting in the next 2-5 years	31%

*often or always.

Given the excellent response rate, the outcomes from this survey are likely representative of the Canadian rhinologist population.

Supplying society with the appropriate health care in a timely and accessible manner requires accurate matching of societal needs with labor capacity. Therefore, workforce planning is a challenging but important component to improving the overall quality of health care delivery in Canada. Although several contributing factors to the current surgical labor inefficiencies have been proposed, such as increasing female surgeon workforce or generational differences in lifestyle demands, the first step toward improving workforce planning is to define the current labor characteristics [8,12,18,19]. The results of this survey demonstrate that the majority of rhinologists are male with an average age of 46. This reflects a persistent male prevalence in the surgical workforce [12,20,21]. There is a perception that female surgeons will be less productive than their male counterparts, thus contributing to a potential workforce shortage [8,22]. There is little doubt that the younger generations of surgeons are placing more emphasis on lifestyle than previous generations, however, the authors agree with Pillsbury who states: "any difference in proposed productivity based on gender is inappropriate" [18]. There is no current evidence to support this opinion, and previous literature that suggested a difference is outdated [19]. If there is a significant difference in the output of men and women, it more likely reflects society norms, and is unlikely to significantly affect workforce projections [19,23].

The age of the respondents is similar to that reported in the thoracic surgery workforce assessment, which echoes a somewhat younger surgeon workforce population [12]. The planned average age of retirement is 66. While this represents an older age of retirement than the general population, it is similar to that of US surgeons [10]. This delay in retirement may be linked to variations in the economic market over recent years and certainly affects workforce planning. As surgeons continue to work longer, the creation of new opportunities is delayed and this contributes to the perceived and actual lack of employment.

The majority of respondents completed a fellowship in rhinology (83%). The average year of beginning practice for non-fellowship trained rhinologists was 1991 while the average year of fellowship-trained rhinologists was 2005. This is in line with an increasing trend for residents to pursue additional training after residency and may be related to a number of factors. First, the Royal College of Physicians and Surgeons employment survey suggests that this may be due to trainees' perceptions that additional training will make them more employable. Second, it is also possible that residents are pursing fellowships as an alternative to unemployment [2]. Lastly, it may

be related to the fact that rhinology is a relatively young subspecialty with opportunities significantly increasing over the last 20 years. A recent survey study of Canadian otolaryngology residents had similar findings - 78% of respondents planned to pursue a fellowship and 90% stated this decision was moderately influenced by limited job options. Only 22% of graduating residents had confirmed employment. This study was performed several months prior to graduation and as some residents may have found positions closer to graduation, this may overestimate the degree of unemployment of Canadian otolaryngology residents [11].

Rhinologists appear to have reasonable work hour requirements compared to other surgical specialties. Only 25% of respondents work more than 60 hours per week, compared to 82% of thoracic surgeons [12]. Only 2% of surgeons reported a call frequency of more than 1 in 4. The current division of work responsibilities seems to be reasonably balanced, creating optimal conditions to prevent physician burnout [24]. Along these lines, rates of physician satisfaction both with careers and remuneration were high (>80%). These high rates of physician satisfaction are higher than those found in general surgery, orthopedic surgery and even ophthalmology [25].

Canada's relatively long waitlists for medical care is a well known issue [4]. More specifically, wait times for elective endoscopic sinus surgery for refractory chronic rhinosinusitis are among the longest with patients waiting between 6 to 12 months for surgery [26]. Prolonged waitlists are associated with tremendous costs, as well as adverse patient effects [6,7,27-29]. The survey respondents echoed these concerns. Surgical resources were thought to be a major limiting factor in providing timely care. Forty two percent felt their current OR time was inadequate and 63% suggested prolonged surgical waitlists often delayed care. Surgeons reported only 56% of patients received care within their maximal acceptable waiting time for common rhinologic procedures. Of note, the second most common reason for untimely care was prolonged clinical wait lists. This is consistent with reports of increasing referral wait times and emphasizes that while increasing operative time would shorten surgical waitlists, it may not improve Canadian's access to specialist consultations [4,7]. An increasing number of surgeons are performing in office procedures (58%), which may be a direct result of these waitlists. What procedures may be performed safely, their outcomes, and how this will affect surgical waitlists, are areas of ongoing study.

Assessments of the US otolaryngology workforce suggest an impending workforce crisis, projecting a deficit of over 2,000 otolaryngologists by 2025 [8,9]. Although we cannot accurately extrapolate and apply US-based workforce data toward Canadian workforce projections, why is there a perceived 'job crisis' for Canadian otolaryngologists given the well-documented issue of prolonged patient waitlists? This, unfortunately, would seem to be a result of a mismatch between the workforce needs and the Canadian health care system capacity/prioritization of resources. Increasing capacity is a complex and costly problem that is the focus of health services research but it undeniably needs to be addressed, and hopefully soon. The deficits in the accessibility and timeliness of care result in a significant decrease in the quality of care patients receive [5]. A formal workforce assessment, which is the next step in this analysis, will help define societal needs and provide a guide for capacity planning and resource allocation.

There are several limitations of this study that must be considered when interpreting the results. First, this study involved the use of a non-validated survey. Currently, there is no validated survey available for assessing surgical demographics for the use in future workforce planning. However, this survey has been used previously for surgical workforce planning and is therefore consistent with other studies in this area. Additionally, the modification via the Delphi method strengthens the rhinology related questions ensuring important topics specific to rhinologists are discussed. Second, data collection was performed using an electronic platform with online responses. While a 65% response rate is considered excellent for any electronically administered survey, the respondents are potentially biased to a more technologically inclined generation and therefore a potentially younger cohort. Third, while the results of the study may be valid for the country as a whole, they may not be generalizable to specific high or low demand regions. Fourth, several of the questions pertaining to surgical waitlist and regional need for another rhinologist are opinion-based rather then being objectively measured, which may result in a reporting bias. Finally, this study was limited to surgeons practicing >50% rhinology and thus does not capture all rhinologic practices in Canada, for example general otolaryngologists performing rhinologic procedures. However, surveying this population captures the demographics and practice patterns of surgeons that will have the most influence on workforce needs. Despite these limitations, this is the most robust attempt to define to Canadian Rhinologic workforce and provides valuable data for future workforce modeling.

Conclusion
This nationwide survey study defined the demographics, education, practice patterns, and surgeons attitudes toward workforce requirements and training of the current Canadian Rhinologic workforce. The rhinology workforce does not appear to be saturated, and combined with the current state of prolonged waitlists and poor timeliness of care, suggests that there is a potential need for more rhinology subspecialists in certain regions of Canada. This data will facilitate future rhinologic workforce planning to define population needs and identify possible solutions to these deficits.

Abbreviations
CSO: Canadian Society of Otolaryngology-Head and Neck Surgery; OR: Operating room; IGS: Image guidance systems; ESS: Endoscopic sinus surgery; SD: Standard deviation; USA/US: United States of America; ARS: American Rhinologic Society; ERS: European Rhinologic Society; CRS: Chronic Rhinosinusitis..

Competing interests
The authors declare that they have no competing interests.

Authors' contributions
KAS: contributed through study conception development, study design, survey development, distribution of survey, acquisition, analysis and interpretation of data, drafting and revising the manuscript, approving the manuscript in its final form and is accountable for all aspects of accuracy and integrity of the work. DDS: contributed through study conception development, study design, survey development, distribution of survey, acquisition, analysis and interpretation of data, revising the manuscript, approving the manuscript in its final form and is accountable for all aspects of accuracy and integrity of the work. SG: contributed through study conception development and design, survey development, the interpretation of data, revising the manuscript, approving the manuscript in its final form and is accountable for all aspects of accuracy and integrity of the work. BR: contributed through the interpretation of data, revising the manuscript, approving the manuscript in its final form and is accountable for all aspects of accuracy and integrity of the work. MAT: contributed through the interpretation of data, revising the manuscript, approving the manuscript in its final form and is accountable for all aspects of accuracy and integrity of the work. SK: contributed through the interpretation of data, revising the manuscript, approving the manuscript in its final form and is accountable for all aspects of accuracy and integrity of the work. EW: contributed through the interpretation of data, revising the manuscript, approving the manuscript in its final form and is accountable for all aspects of accuracy and integrity of the work. AJ: contributed through the interpretation of data, revising the manuscript, approving the manuscript in its final form and is accountable for all aspects of accuracy and integrity of the work. JL: contributed through the interpretation of data, revising the manuscript, approving the manuscript in its final form and is accountable for all aspects of accuracy and integrity of the work. CD: contributed through the interpretation of data, revising the manuscript, approving the manuscript in its final form and is accountable for all aspects of accuracy and integrity of the work. LR: contributed through study conception development, study design, survey development, distribution of survey, acquisition, analysis and interpretation of data, revising the manuscript, approving the manuscript in its final form and is accountable for all aspects of accuracy and integrity of the work.

Author details
¹Division of Otolaryngology, Head and Neck Surgery, Department of Surgery; University of Calgary, Calgary, Alberta, Canada. ²Division of Otolaryngology, Head and Neck Surgery, Department of Surgery, McMaster University, Hamilton, Ontario, Canada. ³Division of Thoracic Surgery, Department of Surgery, University of Calgary, Calgary, Alberta, Canada. ⁴Department of Otolaryngology, Head and Neck Surgery, University of Western Ontario, London, Ontario, Canada. ⁵Department of Otolaryngology, Head and Neck Surgery; McGill University, Jewish General Hospital, Montreal, Quebec, Canada. ⁶Department of Otolaryngology, Head and Neck Surgery, University of Ottawa, Ottawa, Ontario, Canada. ⁷Division of Otolaryngology-Head & Neck Surgery, University of Alberta, Edmonton, Alberta, Canada ⁸Division of Otolaryngology, Head and Neck Surgery, Department of Surgery, University of British Columbia, Vancouver, BC, Canada. ⁹Department of Otolaryngology, Head and Neck Surgery, University of Toronto, Toronto, Ontario, Canada.

References

1. Sinclair A. Workforce Planning: a literature review. IES Research Networks, Institute for Employment Studies; 2004. p. 1–20.
2. Frechette D, Hollenberg D, Shrichand C, Jacob C, Datta I. What's really behind Canada's unemployed specialists? Too many, too few doctors? Findings from the Royal College's employment study. The Royal College of Physicians and Surgeons; 2013. p. 1–59.
3. Gooden E, Brown D, Carr M. Otolaryngology manpower in Canada: a crisis in the making? J Otolaryngol. 2004;33:93–7.
4. Bacchus B, Esmail N. Waiting your turn: Wait times for health care in Canada, 2013 Report. Fraser Institute; 2013. p. 1–96.
5. Committee on Quality of Health Care in America; Institute of Medicine. In Crossing the Quality Chasm: A New Health System for the 21st Century. Washington (DC): The National Academies Press; 2001.
6. Esmail N. The private cost of public queues, 2013 edition. Fraser Alert, Fraser Institute; 2013. p. 1–9.
7. Institute. F: Waiting Your Turn: Hospital Waiting Lists in Canada. Fraser Institute 1993-2012. p. 1–96.
8. Kim JS, Cooper RA, Kennedy DW. Otolaryngology-head and neck surgery physician work force issues: an analysis for future specialty planning. Otolaryngol Head Neck Surg. 2012;146:196–202.
9. Williams Jr TE, Satiani B, Thomas A, Ellison EC. The impending shortage and the estimated cost of training the future surgical workforce. Ann Surg. 2009;250:590–7.
10. Pillsbury 3rd HC, Cannon CR, Sedory Holzer SE, Jacoby I, Nielsen DR, Benninger MS, et al. The workforce in otolaryngology-head and neck surgery: moving into the next millennium. Otolaryngol Head Neck Surg. 2000;123:341–56.
11. Brandt MG, Scott GM, Doyle PC, Ballagh RH. Otolaryngology – Head and Neck Surgeon unemployment in Canada: a cross-sectional survey of graduating Otolaryngology – Head and Neck Surgery residents. J Otolaryngol Head Neck Surg. 2014;43: doi: 10.1186/s40463-014-0037-3.
12. Grondin SC, Schieman C, Kelly E, Darling G, Maziak D, Mackay MP, et al. A look at the thoracic surgery workforce in Canada: how demographics and scope of practice may impact future workforce needs. Can J Surg. 2013;56:E75–81.
13. Frank E. STUDENTJAMA. Physician health and patient care. JAMA. 2004;291:637.
14. Wallace JE, Lemaire JB, Ghali WA. Physician wellness: a missing quality indicator. Lancet. 2009;374:1714–21.
15. Punch K. Survey Research: The basics. London: Sage Publications Ltd; 2003.
16. Hamilton M. Online survery response rates and times: background and guidance for industry. Ipathia, Inc. SuperSurvey; 2003
17. Sheehan K. Emailed survey response rates: a review. J Comput Mediated Commun. 2001;6: doi: 10.1111/j.1083-6101.2001.tb00117.x.
18. Pillsbury 3rd HC. Analysis of the workforce and otolaryngology specialty planning. Otolaryngol Head Neck Surg. 2012;146:340. author reply 340-341.
19. Pryor SP, Brodsky L, Chandrasekhar SS, Zaretsky L, Taylor DJ, Yaremchuk KL, et al. Commentary on "Otolaryngology-head and neck surgery physician workforce issues an analysis for future specialty planning" by Kim, Cooper, and Kennedy. Otolaryngol Head Neck Surg. 2012;146:203–5.
20. Schroen AT, Brownstein MR, Sheldon GF. Women in academic general surgery. Acad Med. 2004;79:310–8.
21. Ferguson BJ, Grandis JR. Women in otolaryngology: closing the gender gap. Curr Opin Otolaryngol Head Neck Surg. 2006;14:159–63.
22. Troppmann KM, Palis BE, Goodnight Jr JE, Ho HS, Troppmann C. Women surgeons in the new millennium. Arch Surg. 2009;144:635–42.
23. Kennedy DW. Otolaryngology workforce planning: why we cannot wait for perfect data. Otolaryngol Head Neck Surg. 2012;147:399.
24. Shanafelt TD. Enhancing meaning in work: a prescription for preventing physician burnout and promoting patient-centered care. JAMA. 2009;302:1338–40.
25. Wai PY, Dandar V, Radosevich DM, Brubaker L, Kuo PC. Engagement, workplace satisfaction, and retention of surgical specialists in academic medicine in the United States. J Am Coll Surg. 2014;219:31–42.
26. Smith KA, Rudmik L. Impact of continued medical therapy in patients with refractory chronic rhinosinusitis. Int Forum Allergy Rhinol. 2014;4:34–8.
27. Rudmik L, Smith TL, Schlosser RJ, Hwang PH, Mace JC, Soler ZM. Productivity costs in patients with refractory chronic rhinosinusitis. Laryngoscope. 2014;124:2007–12.
28. Stokes E, Somerville R. The economic cost of wait time in Canada. Centre for Spatial Economics; 2008. p. 1–57.
29. Smith KA, Smith TL, Mace JC, Rudmik L. Endoscopic sinus surgery compared to continued medical therapy for patients with refractory chronic rhinosinusitis. Int Forum Allergy Rhinol. 2014;4:823–7.

5

Optimal site for facial nerve transection and neurorrhaphy: a randomized prospective animal study

Adrian I. Mendez, Hadi Seikaly, Vincent Biron, Lin-fu Zhu and David W. J. Côté[*]

Abstract

Background: Since the first facial allograft transplantation was performed, several institutions have performed the procedure with the main objectives being restoration of the aesthetic appearance and expressive function of the face. The optimal location to transect the facial nerve during flap harvest in transplantation to preserve facial movement function is currently unknown. There are currently two primary methods to perform facial nerve neurorrhaphy between the donor and recipient-one protocol involves transection and repair of the facial nerve at the main trunk while the another protocol advocates for the neurorrhaphy to be performed distally at the main branches. The purpose of this study is to establish the optimal location for transection and repair of the facial nerve to optimize functional recovery of facial movement.

Methods: A prospective randomized controlled trial using a rat model was performed. Two groups of 12 rats underwent facial nerve transection and subsequent repair either at the main trunk of the nerve (group 1) or 2 cm distally, at the main bifurcation (group 2). Primary outcome of nerve functional recovery was measured using a previously validated laser curtain model, which measured amplitude of whisking at 2, 4, and 6 post-operatively. The deflection of the laser curtain sent a digital signal that was interpreted by central computer software.

Results: At week 2 post-nerve surgery, the average amplitude observed for group 1 and 2 was 4.4 and 10.8 degrees, respectively. At week 4, group 1 showed improvement with an average amplitude of 9.7 degrees, while group 2 displayed an average of 10.2 degrees. The week 6 results showed the greatest improvement from baseline for group 1. Group 1 and 2 had average amplitudes of 17.2 and 6.9 degrees, respectively. There was no statistically significant difference between the two groups at 2, 4, and 6 weeks after facial nerve surgery ($p > 0.05$).

Conclusions: We found no statistical difference between these two locations of nerve repair using identical methods. Therefore, the authors recommend a single versus multiple nerve repair technique. This finding has potential implications for future facial allograft transplantations and at minimum necessitates further study with long-term follow-up data.

Introduction

Since the first facial allograft transplantation was performed in Amiens, France, in 2005, several institutions have performed the procedure with the main objectives being restoration of the aesthetic appearance and expressive function of the face. An essential component of this procedure involves the neurorrhaphy of the donor facial nerve to the corresponding recipient patient's facial nerve. The optimal location to transect the facial nerve during flap harvest in transplantation to preserve facial movement function is currently unknown. There are presently two primary methods to perform facial nerve neurorrhaphy between the donor and recipient-one protocol involves transection and repair of the facial nerve at the main trunk while another protocol advocates for the neurorrhaphy to be performed just distally to the main trunk at the main upper and lower branches.

There are several known clinical factors that have an effect on peripheral nerve function recovery after nerve repair including time interval between trauma and repair, type of lesion and repair, and the age of the patient

* Correspondence: drdavidcote@me.com
Division of Otolaryngology, Head and Neck Surgery, University of Alberta, 8440-112 Street, Room 1E4, WMC, Edmonton T6G 2B7, AB, Canada

[1]. Furthermore, in order to optimize nerve function, there are certain techniques of nerve repair that have been shown to be vital for outcome. The basic requirement is to appose the cut ends of the nerve in such a fashion as to minimize scar formation and preserve the optimal blood supply [2]. In cases of sharp nerve division with minimal gap, as is the case with facial allograft transplantation, direct end-to-end nerve repair is indicated [3]. Furthermore, tension-free suture repair remains the preferred treatment option as tension will result in scaring and poor regeneration [2, 3].

Despite an abundance of knowledge regarding nerve regeneration physiology and nerve repair techniques, little is known about optimal *sites* of transection and repair along a peripheral nerve. Some literature has suggested that more proximal peripheral nerve injuries are associated with worse outcomes. In their 2009 study of upper extremity nerve injuries, Lohmeyer et al. found that increasing distance between nerve lesion and fingertip correlated significantly with decreasing fingertip sensibility [4]. The reason for this is complex and not fully understood but it is felt that the more proximal the nerve injury, the lower the chances for the axons to re-innervate adequate terminal receptors and organs because possible misdirection increase [4]. Also, in the time needed to reach the end organ, it is felt that multiple irreversible changes take place, which can negatively affect outcome [1].

In regards to peripheral nerve recovery, it is also well recognized that the functional outcome following repair of different individual nerves, in otherwise comparable circumstances, are not the same [1]. Although there is no widely accepted explanation, it is felt the intrinsic complexity of the function of the nerve plays a role [1].

Unfortunately, literature regarding optimal sites for transection and repair specifically of the facial nerve is exceedingly scarce. In their 2006 study, Liu et al. compared lesions of the central nervous system to those of the peripheral nervous system along the facial nerve. The authors found that axonal injuries of central facial motoneurons caused greater nerve damage than injuries along the axons of the peripheral facial nerve [5]. A recent study by Hadlock et al. did attempt to compare injuries along different lengths of the facial nerve [6]. The authors found no significant difference in recovery using similar repair techniques [6].

The technique of facial nerve transection and subsequent neurorrhaphy between donor and recipient during facial allograft transplantation proposed by the Amiens group specifies transecting the nerve at the main upper and lower bifurcation. That of the Cleveland group specifies transecting and repairing the nerve at the main trunk. There currently exists no literature comparing these two types of transection and repair.

Our objective in completing this study was to directly compare these two methods in an established animal model to better predict the ideal location of facial nerve transection to optimize facial nerve regeneration and functional recovery following repair.

Methods

Study design
This was a prospective randomized control animal trial conducted at the Surgical Medical Research Institute (SMRI) at the University of Alberta. A previously validated rat facial nerve model was used. Ethics approval was obtained from the Animal Care and Use Committee (ACUC) overseen by the University Animal Policy and Welfare Committee (UAPWC) at the University of Alberta in Edmonton, Alberta [AUP00000785].

Study subjects
24 female Wistar rats (Charles River Laboratories, Canada) weighing 200–220 g were used for this study. Sample size was based on the study by Heaton et al. which employed a similar outcome measure [7]. All rats were housed in pairs in cages at the Health Sciences Laboratory Animal Services (HSLAS) at the University of Alberta. Rats were weighed and handled daily 2 weeks prior to the commencement of the study to reduce animal stress during the study. The 24 rats were block randomized into two groups of 12. Each animal underwent unilateral facial nerve transection and repair at either the main trunk of nerve or at the main upper and lower bifurcation of the nerve. Facial nerve functional outcome assessment was collected at 2, 4, and 6 weeks post-operatively.

Facial nerve functional outcome assessment
The facial nerve functional outcome assessment model we employed in this study was based on the model described and validated by Heaton et al. in their 2008 study [7]. This model employs a head fixation device, body restraint, and bilateral photoelectric sensors to detect precise whisker movements as an objective measure for facial nerve function.

Head implant
In order to ensure proper head fixation during whisker movement measurement, an implantable head fixation device was required. In conjunction with the biomedical engineering department at the University of Alberta, we designed a unique head implant adequate for our purposes. The implant itself was composed of acrylic and long threaded screws. The exact procedure is described below in section 7 of the materials and methods.

Body restraint

Based on the design described by Heaten et al., we developed a custom body restraint device for the rat subjects in conjunction with the Metalworks Engineering Shop at the University of Alberta. Our body restraint apparatus consisted of a half-pipe (ABS-DWV IPEX Drainway) measuring 7.6 cm in diameter and 30 cm in length. Three Velcro® straps were then fastened across the top of the half-pipe for added restraint. A steel bar spanning across the half pipe provided a fixation point for the head implant as well as functioned to support the laser micrometers. Along the anterior portion of the half-pipe we added a circular platform to support the weight of the rat's head while placed in the apparatus (Fig. 1).

Tracking whisker movement

Two pairs of photoelectric sensors (Rx-Laser Micrometer, Metralight Inc., San Mateo, Ca) were placed along each side of the subject's face in order to track whisker movement (Fig. 2). Thin tubing 1.5 mm in diameter was placed over a midline whisker on either side of the subject's face to facilitate tracking by the laser micrometer. The laser micrometers were placed at exactly 17 degrees from the midline along each side of the face and this was considered parallel to the lateral surface of the face. The lasers were also positioned approximately 10 mm from the origin of the tracked whisker on each side of the face.

The laser micrometer itself was comprised of an emitter, which produced a 780 nm wavelength light curtain, and a detector composed of a 28 mm linear array of 4000 charge-coupled devices (CCD scanline). The emitter and detector were separated by a 5 cm vertical distance,

producing a laser curtain. Movement detected within the laser curtain sent a digital signal that could then be recorded. The laser micrometers themselves were calibrated to not detect objects less than 1 mm in size to avoid tracing multiple whiskers. Instead the laser curtain detected only the marked whisker.

Data acquisition

Whisker movement was elicited in each subject by providing a scented stimulus (chocolate milk). The laser micrometers themselves were connected to a 32-Channel Digital I/O Module (NI 9403, National Instruments, Dallas, Tx), which received digital output from the laser micrometers (Fig. 3). The I/O module was connected to a PC through a CompactDAQ chassis (cDAQ-9174, National Instruments, Dallas, Tx). The I/O module acquired the laser micrometer signal at a sampling rate of 1 kHz. LabVIEW (LabVIEW Full Development System, National Instruments, Dallas, Tx) software was used as the interface for data acquisition.

Surgical procedure

All subjects underwent both head implantation surgery as well as facial nerve surgery during the same anesthetic. All rats were first anesthetized with 3–4 % isoflurane. Subjects were then maintained under general anesthesia using 1.5 % isoflurane. Hair was then removed from the right side of the face and the top of the head using an electric shaver.

Facial nerve surgery

All facial nerve surgery was completed on the right side of the face on all subjects. A small incision was made just inferior to the right ear bony prominence. Under microscopic visualization, the parotid glad was visualized

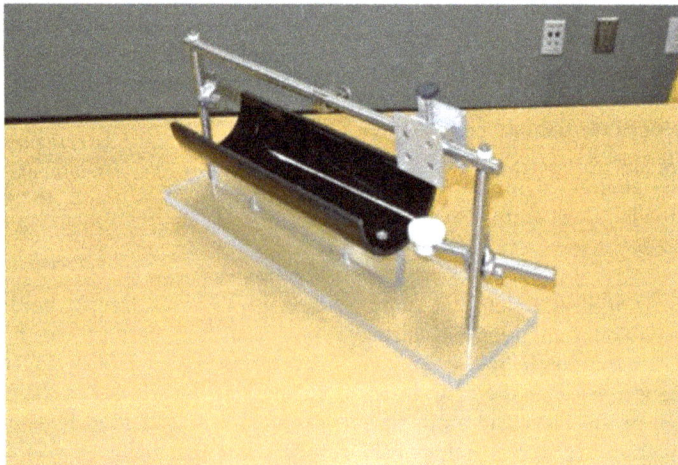

Fig. 1 Custom built rat body restraint apparatus

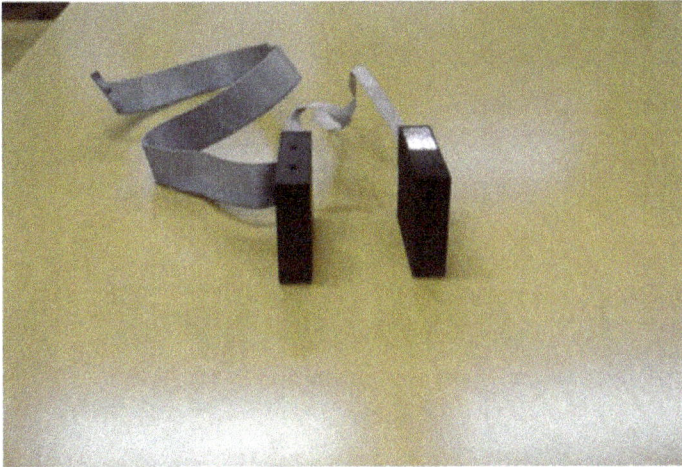

Fig. 2 Photoelectric sensors used in detecting rat whisking

and everted and retracted out of the surgical field, without removing it completely. Subsequently, distal branches of the facial nerve were identified just inferior to the parotid bed. These were followed proximally until the main trunk of the facial nerve was identified. Once identified, the main trunk and upper and lower bifurcation of the facial nerve were carefully dissected. If the subject was randomized to group 1 (main trunk), a single transection of the main trunk of the facial nerve was made using straight microscopic scissors. If the subject was randomized to group 2 (bifurcation), two nerve transections were completed: one at the upper bifurcation and one at the lower bifurcation of the nerve. These transections were similarly completed using straight microscopic scissors. In both groups, the cut nerve ends were immediately repaired using a direct end-to-end technique. Using 9–0 sutures, four simple interrupted sutures were made within the proximal and distal epineural nerve endings. Care was taken to ensure proper nerve alignment. In group 1 subjects, only one nerve repair was necessary while group 2 subjects underwent two nerve repair techniques in this fashion. The parotid gland was then reflected back into the surgical field. Skin was approximated using 3–0 vicryl sutures.

Head implant surgery

Following the facial nerve procedure, head implant surgery was then completed without reversing the general anesthetic. A small incision was made using a 15-blade

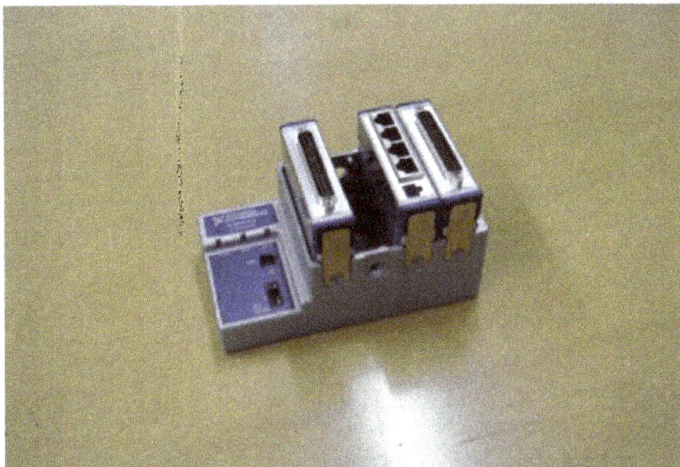

Fig. 3 32-channel digital I/O module

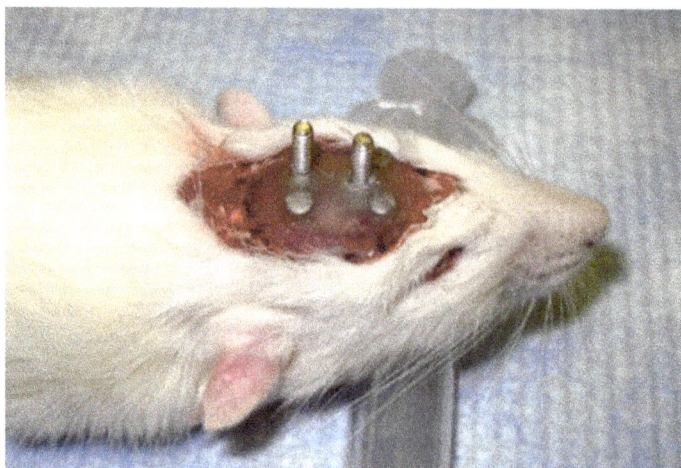

Fig. 4 Rat cadaver depicting custom built head implantation device made from dry acrylic resin

scalpel from the anterior to posterior margin of the cranium. Blunt dissection was employed to fully expose the underlying bony cranium. Using an electric drill, 4 holes were made in each quadrant of the skull approximately 15 mm apart from each other. 1.6 mm screws were then placed within each drill site. (Fig. 4) Dry acrylic resin was then liquefied and placed onto the skull, covering the placed screws. Two larger 5 mm threaded screws were then inverted with the threads directed upwards into the acrylic before it solidified. Once the acrylic completely solidified, the skin was then re-approximated overtop of the acrylic with interrupted 3–0 vicryl sutures, leaving the two larger threaded screws exposed through the incision (Fig. 5 and Fig. 6).

Head fixation and body restraint
Two weeks prior to surgery, all animal subject were handled daily for conditioning. After surgery, all subjects were placed in body restraints daily for a week. At postoperative day 14, whisker measurements were started. Subjects were initially given an injection of low dose ketamine and transported to the body restraint apparatus described in Body restraint. Here they underwent head fixation with bolts applied across the exposed threaded screws (Fig. 7). Whisker markers were then placed on either side of the rat's face as described in Tracking whisker movement.

Once this was completed, a scented stimulus was introduced and recording started usually for a period of

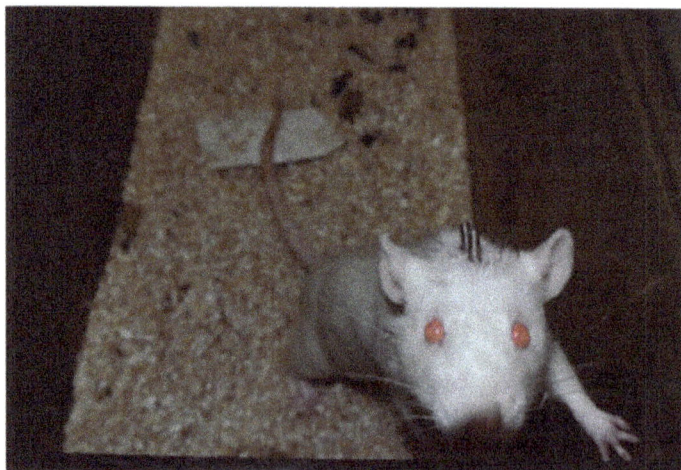

Fig. 5 Study rat 1 week post-op from head implantation surgery

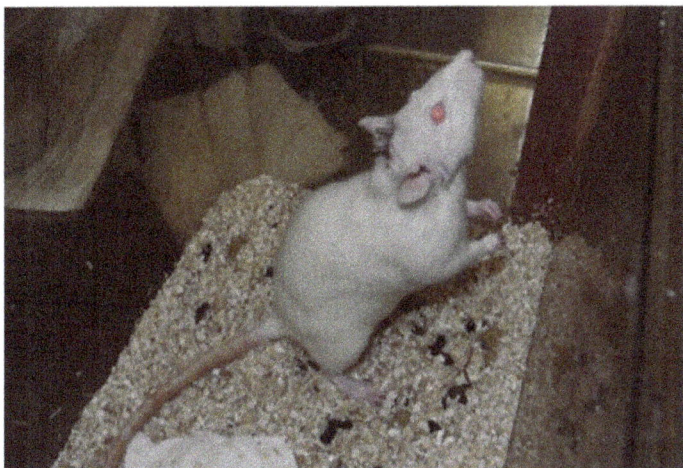

Fig. 6 Study rat 1 week post-op from head implantation surgery

5 min. The non-operative left side was used as the control for each subject. This procedure was completed for each rat at 2, 4, and 6 weeks post-operatively.

Results

All animals tolerated the surgical procedure very well. They exhibited normal cage behavior and did not lose weight. Three animals had problems with suture break down post-operatively. This occurred in all 3 animals within 5 days of the surgical procedure. For these animals, we re-anesthetized them with isoflurane and were able to re-approximate the incision edges with 3–0 vicryl sutures. No animals had to be removed from the study.

All animals experienced complete ipsilateral loss of whisking amplitude post-operatively. At week 2 the average amplitude observed for group 1 was 4.4 degrees (Table 1).

Similarly, the group 2 average was 10.8 degrees at 2 weeks post-operatively. At week 4, group 1 showed improvement having an average of 9.7 degrees, while group 2 remained relatively unchanged with an average of 10.2 degrees. The week 6 results showed the greatest improvement from baseline for group 1. Group 1 had an average amplitudes of 17.2 degrees at 6-weeks from surgery (Fig. 8). However, group 2 showed a slight decrease in amplitude with an average of 5.9 degrees. There was no statistically significant difference between the two groups at 2, 4 and 6 weeks after facial nerve surgery ($p > 0.05$).

Discussion

Since 2005, facial allograft transplantation has rapidly started becoming a more commonly employed surgical procedure, indicated for individuals disfigured from

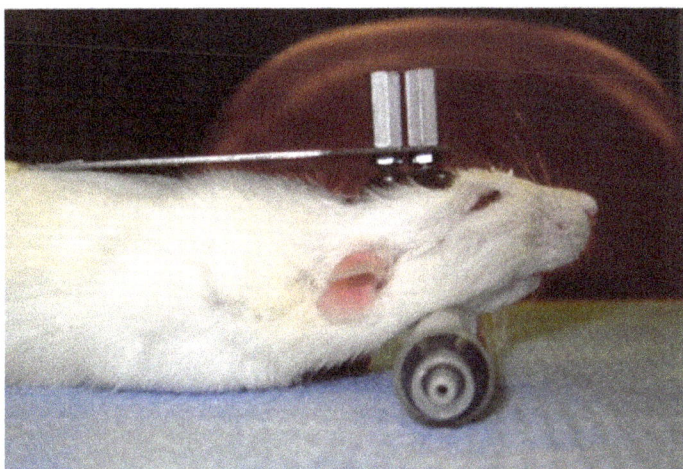

Fig. 7 Rat cadaver depicting fixation bolts applied to head implant for rat head stability

Table 1 Post-operative whisking amplitudes at week 2, 4, and 6

	Week 2 amplitude (degrees)	Week 4 amplitude (degrees)	Week 6 amplitude (degrees)
MAIN TRUNK (group 1) Right side (operated)	4.4	9.7	17.2
MAIN TRUNK (group 1) Left side (control)	72.1	66.6	71.8
MAIN BIFURCATION (group 2) Right side (operated)	10.8	10.2	5.9
MAIN BIFURCATION (group 2) Left side (control)	74.9	70.9	67.5

trauma, burns, and birth defects among other entities. As the procedure has become more commonly employed, knowing the exact location of where to transect and repair the facial nerve has become that much more vital.

The most significant study attempting to answer the question of the location to transect and repair the facial nerve for optimal functional outcome was published by Hadlock et al. in 2010 [6]. The authors studied a variety of different types of facial nerve injuries and injury locations in the rat model. When comparing proximal facial nerve lesions of the main trunk to peripheral facial nerve lesions of distal branches, the authors found no statistically significant difference in whisking amplitude [6].

In our study, we specifically compared the two locations employed by the Cleveland and Amiens groups to transect and repair the facial nerve in facial allograft transplantation (main trunk and main nerve bifurcation, respectively). Our literature search found that these two methods had never been compared in a randomized study. Similar to Hadlock et al., we found that there was no statistically significant difference between injuries at the main trunk and more distal injuries, which in our

study was specifically at the main bifurcation of the nerve. However, we did find a non-statistically significant improvement in whisking amplitude for group 1 (main trunk) as compared to group 2. The whisking amplitude of group 1 was consistently greater at week 6 postoperatively. Although the whisking amplitude difference is relatively small, it does raise the possibility that a greater follow-up time may reveal a larger, statistically significant difference between the two groups. This notion is further supported by the observation that the whisking amplitude difference between the two groups consistently became greater the further out from nerve surgery.

However, given that our study showed only a minimal, non-statistically significant difference in whisking amplitude between the two groups, it seems logical with the given evidence to favor the Cleveland facial nerve protocol. The Cleveland protocol, as previously mentioned, entails only a single nerve transection and repair (group 1), minimizing operative time.

Overall, facial nerve functional recovery remained fairly limited in both groups. This may be due to several reasons, including peripheral misrouting of axons and reduction of brainstem synaptic connection with facial motoneurons. A potential limitation of our study was our follow up time. A more protracted follow-up time may have elucidated a more significant difference between the two groups.

Our study has important findings to guide future facial allograft transplantations. Given the minimal difference in whisking amplitude between the two groups, single nerve repair is more advisable as it has the added benefit of less required operative time and potential cost savings.

Conclusion

Our study directly compared, in a rat model, the transection and subsequent neurorrhaphy of the facial nerve

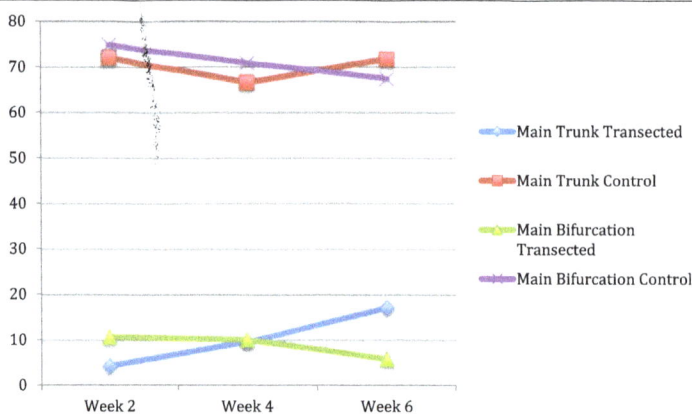

Fig. 8 Whisking amplitude in degrees at 2, 4, and 6 weeks postoperatively

at two distinct locations commonly used during facial allograft transplantation; the main trunk (group 1) and main bifurcation (group 2). We found no statistical difference between these two locations of nerve repair using identical methods. Therefore, the authors recommend the protocol outlined by the Cleveland group, which requires only single nerve repair as opposed to that described by the Amiens group. This finding has potential implications for future facial allograft transplantations and at minimum necessitates further study with long-term follow-up data.

Competing interests
The authors declare that they have no competing interests.

Authors' contributions
AM carried out the rat surgery, whisking testing, study design, data analysis, and drafted the manuscript. HS participated in the study design and helped revise the manuscript. VB participated in the rat surgery and statistical analysis. LZ participated in rat surgery, animal care, and whisking testing. DC participated in study design, data analysis, and manuscript revision. All authors read and approved the final manuscript.

References
1. Post R, de Boer KS, Malessy MJ. Outcome following nerve repair of high isolated clean sharp injuries of the ulnar nerve. PLoS One. 2012;7(10):e47928. doi:10.1371/journal.pone.0047928.
2. Fawcett JWKR. Peripheral nerve regenration. Annu Rev Neurosci. 1990;13:43.
3. Griffin JW, Hogan MV, Chhabra AB, Deal DN. Peripheral nerve repair and reconstruction. J Bone Joint Surg Am. 2013;95(23):2144–51. doi:10.2106/JBJS.L.00704.
4. Lohmeyer JA, Sommer B, Siemers F, Mailander P. Nerve injuries of the upper extremity-expected outcome and clinical examination. Plast Surg Nurs. 2009;29(2):88–93. doi:10.1097/01.PSN.0000356867.18220.73. quiz 94–5.
5. Liu PH, Yang LH, Wang TY, Wang YJ, Tseng GF. Proximity of lesioning determines response of facial motoneurons to peripheral axotomy. J Neurotrauma. 2006;23(12):1857–73. doi:10.1089/neu.2006.23.1857.
6. Hadlock TA, Kowaleski J, Lo D, Mackinnon SE, Heaton JT. Rodent facial nerve recovery after selected lesions and repair techniques. Plast Reconstr Surg. 2010;125(1):99–109. doi:10.1097/PRS.0b013e3181c2a5ea.
7. Heaton JT, Kowaleski JM, Bermejo R, Zeigler HP, Ahlgren DJ, Hadlock TA. A system for studying facial nerve function in rats through simultaneous bilateral monitoring of eyelid and whisker movements. J Neurosci Methods. 2008;171(2):197–206. doi:10.1016/j.jneumeth.2008.02.023.

6

Olfactory testing in children using objective tools: comparison of Sniffin' Sticks and University of Pennsylvania Smell Identification Test (UPSIT)

Sarah C Hugh[1], Jennifer Siu[2], Thomas Hummel[3], Vito Forte[1,4], Paolo Campisi[1,4], Blake C Papsin[1,4] and Evan J Propst[1,4]*

Abstract

Background: Detection of olfactory dysfunction is important for fire and food safety. Clinical tests of olfaction have been developed for adults but their use in children has been limited because they were felt to be unreliable in children under six years of age. We therefore administered two olfactory tests to children and compared results across tests.

Methods: Two olfactory tests (Sniffin' Sticks and University of Pennsylvania Smell Identification Test (UPSIT)) were administered to 78 healthy children ages 3 to 12 years. Children were randomized to one of two groups: Group 1 performed the UPSIT first and Sniffin' Sticks second, and Group 2 performed Sniffin' Sticks first and UPSIT second.

Results: All children were able to complete both olfactory tests. Performance on both tests was similar for children 5 and 6 years of age. There was an age-dependent increase in score on both tests (p < .01). Children performed better on the Sniffin' Sticks than the UPSIT (65.3% versus 59.7%, p < .01). There was no difference in performance due to order of test presentation.

Conclusions: The Sniffin' Sticks and UPSIT olfactory tests can both be completed by children as young as 5 years of age. Performance on both tests increased with increasing age. Better performance on the Sniffin' Sticks than the UPSIT may be due to a decreased number of test items, better ability to maintain attention, or decreased olfactory fatigue. The ability to reuse Sniffin' Sticks on multiple children may make it more practical for clinical use.

Keywords: Children, Olfactory testing, Smell

Background

Olfaction plays an important role in maintaining awareness of one's surroundings through detection of pleasant and noxious odors and contributes to the perception of flavor. Structural pathology preventing odorants from binding to olfactory receptors or any lesion along the olfactory pathway from the olfactory epithelium to the olfactory cortex may affect a person's ability to perceive odors. Olfactory impairment has been described in patients with congenital syndromes, head trauma, chronic rhinosinusitis, nasal masses, and neurodegenerative and autoimmune diseases. Various medications and smoking have also been implicated as causes of olfactory dysfunction [1]. Poor olfactory function has been associated with a decreased quality of life [2].

Approximately 19% of adults have some form of olfactory dysfunction (13% hyposmia, 6% anosmia) [3]. The prevalence of olfactory dysfunction in children is unknown. Unfortunately, diagnosing olfactory disorders based on history alone underestimates true prevalence rates in adults [4]. This underestimation is likely much greater in children. Since it is important for people with olfactory dysfunction to obtain counselling regarding fire safety and food inspection, proper diagnosis of this condition with objective testing is paramount.

There are a number of objective psychophysical olfactory tests commercially available for clinical use in adults,

* Correspondence: evan.propst@utoronto.ca
[1]Department of Otolaryngology – Head & Neck Surgery, University of Toronto, Toronto, ON, Canada
[4]The Hospital for Sick Children, Toronto, ON, Canada
Full list of author information is available at the end of the article

Table 1 Demographic and olfactory testing data for study participants

	Group 1 (UPSIT performed first)	Group 2 (Sniffin' Sticks performed first)	p-value
Age (SD)	8.1 years (2.5)	8.6 years (2.4)	.34
Sex			
Male	18	25	
Female	19	16	
Score			
UPSIT	57.2%	61.3%	.32
Sniffin' Sticks	60.1%	70.0%	.06

and normative data have been collected and thresholds determined for hyposmia and anosmia [5]. In general, various odors are presented to participants who are required to identify each odor from a defined list in a forced choice paradigm. The two most commonly employed tests in adults are the Sniffin' Sticks (Burghart Messtechnik, Wedel, Germany) and the University of Pennsylvania Smell Identification Test (UPSIT) (Sensonics Inc., Haddon Heights, New Jersey, USA) [6,7]. Sniffin' Sticks constitutes a 12-item test whereby odors are presented via reusable odor-dispensing pens. The UPSIT is a 40-item test whereby odors are presented on one-time-use scratch-and-sniff paper. Normative data for Sniffin' Sticks, based on a cohort of 201 healthy children aged 6 to 11 years, has been published [8]. Normative data for combined age categories of 5 to 9 years and 10 to 14 years are available for UPSIT [9,10]. Similarly, in adults, normal ranges of scores for olfactory tests vary according to age [6,7,11]. There has been limited use of these tests in younger children. Previous authors have found olfactory testing to be difficult and unreliable in children less than six years of age, due to lack of motivation to complete the test or difficulty in understanding test instructions [12]. Testing in young children is further complicated by their lack of familiarity with test odors [13]. Olfactory test batteries have been created for children, however, they are more difficult to obtain and are not widely used [13,14]. To date, there have been no studies comparing Sniffin' Sticks to the UPSIT in children.

The purpose of this study was to obtain data for normal healthy children ages 3 to 12 years on both the Sniffin' Sticks and the UPSIT and to compare performance on the two tests. We hypothesized that children less than six years of age would be able to complete olfactory testing, that scores on both tests would increase with increasing age, that performance would be better using Sniffin' Sticks than the UPSIT given that Sniffin' Sticks contains fewer test items, and that performance would drop off over time due to physical and olfactory fatigue.

Methods

This project was approved by The Hospital for Sick Children Ethics Review Board, which adheres to the "Tri-Council Policy Statement: Ethical Conduct for Research Involving humans." Healthy children aged 3 to 12 years were recruited through an ambulatory tertiary care Pediatric Otolaryngology clinic from May to August, 2013. Exclusion criteria included the following: 1) syndromic patients including craniofacial anomalies and developmental delay; 2) nasal obstruction or sinus complaints such as allergy or nasal polyposis; 3) symptoms or signs of recent (within prior 4 weeks) respiratory tract infection such as congestion, rhinorrhea, fever, sore throat, acute otitis media or otitis media with effusion; 4) sleep disordered breathing; 5) prior upper aerodigestive tract surgery within preceding year (including tonsillectomy and/or adenoidectomy); 6) comorbidity such as cardiovascular, endocrine, autoimmune or pulmonary disease; 7) head trauma. The majority of participants were

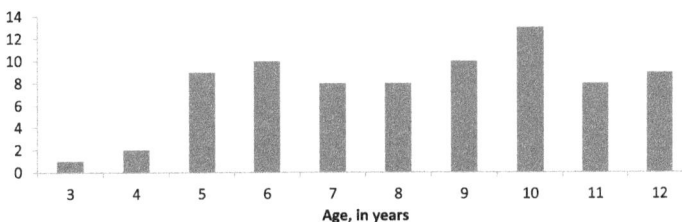

Figure 1 Distribution of study participants by age in years.

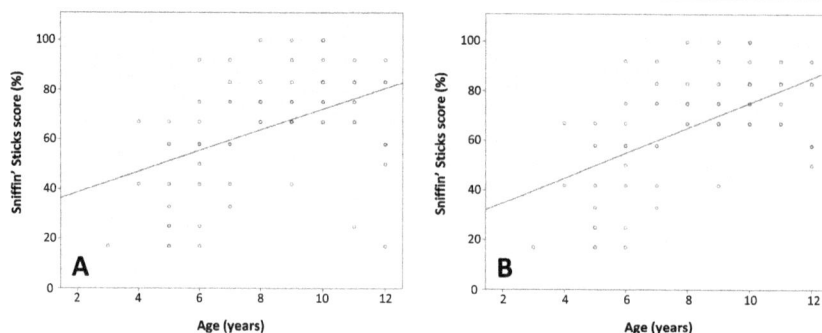

Figure 2 Scatter plot of Sniffin' Sticks scores, by age of participant, with line of best fit. **A**, All participants included ($R^2 = 0.20$; line of best fit: score = 4.17 x age + 30.4). **B**, Two outliers removed ($R^2 = 0.31$; line of best fit: score = 5.1 x age + 24.5).

healthy siblings who accompanied their sibling to their appointment or patients referred for otologic complaints.

Prior to enrolment in the study, children were screened for bilateral nasal patency using a mirror to detect condensation from each nostril. Children were randomized, using a computerized random number generator, to one of two groups: Group 1 performed the UPSIT first and Sniffin' Sticks second, and Group 2 performed Sniffin' Sticks first and UPSIT second. Randomization was performed to control for attentional or olfactory fatigue. To control for differences in reading comprehension, multiple choice answers were provided in written format and read aloud to children by the test administrator. Participants were forced to choose an answer for every odor presented. Answers were recorded by one of two administrators (SCH, JS) and there was no time limit for completion of either test. Statistical analysis (paired samples t-test and linear regression) were performed using IBM SPSS Statistics Version 22.0 (IBM, Armonk, New York), with significance set at a $p < .05$. A sample size calculation using numbers from van Spronson (2013) (p value of .05, power of .80, clinically significant difference of 1.86 and standard deviation of 1.63) revealed that 8 participants were required per age group.

Results

Seventy-eight children (43 male, 35 female) with a mean age of 8.4 ± 2.4 years (range 3 to 12 years) were included in this study (Table 1, Figure 1). Thirty-seven children were randomized to Group 1 and 41 children were randomized to Group 2. All participants completed both olfactory tests.

Children under the age of 6 years were able to complete both olfactory tests. Statistical analysis was not performed on children in age category of 3 years (N = 1) and 4 years (N = 2). Statistics were obtained from children as young as 5 years of age (N = 9) and there was no difference in Sniffin' Sticks or UPSIT scores compared with scores from children 6 years of age (p = 0.11 and 0.80, respectively). Scores on Sniffin' Sticks and UPSIT increased with increasing age in a linear fashion as demonstrated by regression analysis (performed between score and age, yielding $R^2 = 0.20$ and 0.36, respectively, $p < .01$) (Figures 2 and 3). Removal of two outlying values for Sniffin' Sticks scores (lowest Sniffin' Sticks score for children of age 11 and 12 years, each lying more than two SD below the mean for their age category) resulted in an increase in R^2 to 0.31. Effect size for analysis of variance (ANOVA) between age groups

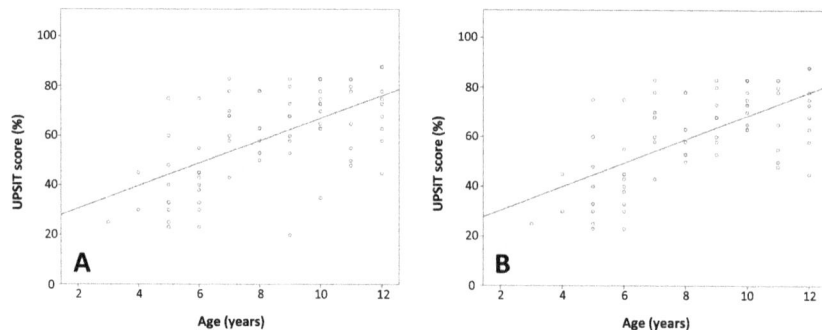

Figure 3 Scatter plot of UPSIT scores, by age of participant, with line of best fit. **A**, All participants included ($R^2 = 0.36$; line of best fit: score = 4.57 x age + 21.4). **B**, Two outliers removed ($R^2 = 0.42$; line of best fit: score = 4.76 x age + 20.9).

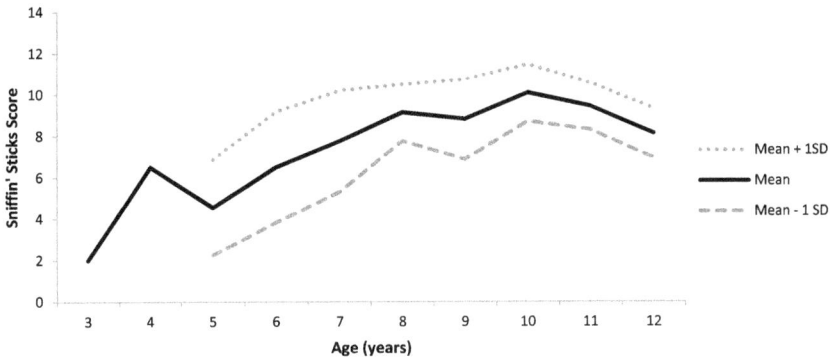

Figure 4 Descriptive statistics of values for Sniffin' Sticks, by age.

for Sniffin' Sticks scores was large ($n^2 = 0.47$, outliers removed from analysis). Removal of two outlying values for UPSIT scores (lowest UPSIT score for children of age 9 and 10 years, each lying more than two SD below the mean for their age category) resulted in an increase in R^2 to 0.42. Effect size for ANOVA between age groups for UPSIT scores was large ($n^2 = 0.55$, outliers removed from analysis).

The overall mean score (SD) for Sniffin' Sticks was 65.3% (22.6) and for the UPSIT was 59.7% (18.6). Paired t-test to compare the two means demonstrated a significant difference between participants' scores (p < .01) with children performing better on Sniffin' Sticks than on the UPSIT. There was no difference in Sniffin' Sticks or UPSIT scores between Group 1 and Group 2 (Table 1). Descriptive statistics for values of Sniffin' Sticks scores and UPSIT score by age (with outliers removed as described above) are shown in Figures 4 and 5, respectively.

Discussion

The Sniffin' Sticks and UPSIT olfactory tests were successfully administered to 78 children aged 3 to 12 years

and data for this normal healthy population were obtained. All children, including those aged 3 to 5 years, were able to complete both tests. Children 5 years of age were capable of completing olfactory tests and did not score differently than children 6 years of age. Unfortunately, statistical analysis was precluded for age categories 3 and 4 years due to an insufficient number of participants. Contrary to previous findings, results suggest that testing may be extended to children 5 years of age.

Performance on both Sniffin' Sticks and UPSIT increased with age. Effect size for ANOVA was large when analysed between age groups for scores on both tests. This is in keeping with previously demonstrated age-related increases in children's performance on various olfactory tests [8,10,12,14,15]. However, we are unable to tell if this is due to development of the olfactory system over time, exposure to a wider variety of odors over time or simply due to broadening of the child's lexicon. Thresholds for odor detection are similar in children and young adults, suggesting that performance on clinical olfactory tests depends not only on olfactory but also cognitive ability.

Overall mean scores for Sniffin' Sticks were higher than on the UPSIT. This is in keeping with our hypothesis

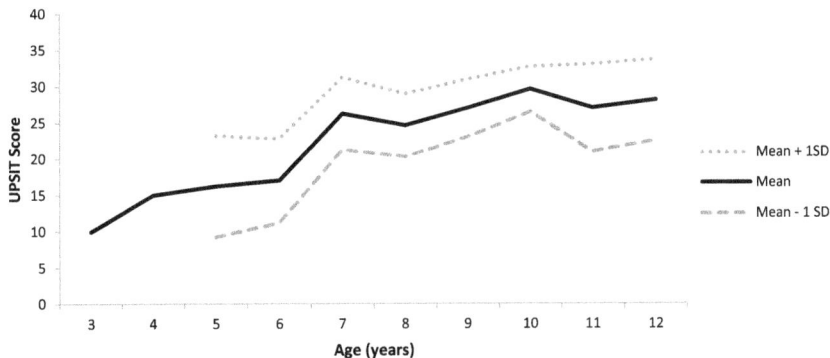

Figure 5 Descriptive statistics of values for UPSIT, by age.

that children would perform better on the shorter 12-item Sniffin' Sticks test than on the 40-item UPSIT. Better performance on the test with fewer items may have resulted from a faster administration time, greater ability to pay attention, or less olfactory fatigue. This may have practical implications whereby a shorter test battery may be more desirable in a busy clinical setting. However, the absolute difference between Sniffin' Sticks and UPSIT scores should be interpreted with caution, as there is insufficient evidence to conclude that this difference is clinically significant. Further research in this area is warranted.

The order of test presentation was randomized to control for attentional or olfactory fatigue. Interestingly, there was no difference in Sniffin' Sticks or UPSIT scores regardless of the order of test presentation. We conclude that differences in performance across tests were more likely due to inherent features of the tests themselves rather than the experimental condition.

A limitation of this study is the small sample size and limited number of participants under the age of 5 years. A larger sample size may elucidate the utility of these tests amongst younger children and perhaps even differences across sexes. Future studies comparing performance on these tests with other tests of olfactory function designed specifically for children are warranted. It would also be interesting to compare these perceptive tests of olfactory function to objective measures of olfaction.

Conclusions
The Sniffin' Sticks and UPSIT olfactory tests can both be completed by children as young as 5 years of age. Performance on both tests increased with increasing age. Children performed better on the Sniffin' Sticks than on UPSIT, which may be due to a decreased number of test items, resulting in better ability to maintain attention or decreased olfactory fatigue. The ability to reuse Sniffin' Sticks on multiple patients may make it more practical for clinical use.

Abbreviations
SD: Standard deviation; UPSIT: University of Pennsylvania Smell Identification Test; ANOVA: Analysis of variance.

Competing interests
The authors declare that they have no competing interests.

Authors' contributions
SCH designed the study, performed the clinical tests on participants, analysed the data and prepared the manuscript. JS performed clinical tests on participants. EJP, TH, VF, PC, BCP conceptualized the study, participated in study design, and reviewed and revised the manuscript. All authors read and reviewed the final manuscript.

Acknowledgements
We thank the participants and their families for their time.

Author details
¹Department of Otolaryngology – Head & Neck Surgery, University of Toronto, Toronto, ON, Canada. ²School of Medicine, Queen's University, Kingston, ON, Canada. ³Department of Otorhinolaryngology, Interdisciplinary Center Smell & Taste, Technische Universitat Dresden, Dresden, Germany. ⁴The Hospital for Sick Children, Toronto, ON, Canada.

References
1. Malaty J, Malaty IAC. Smell and taste disorders in primary care. Am Fam Physician. 2013;88:852–9.
2. Croy I, Nordin S, Hummel T. Olfactory disorders and quality of life – an updated review. Chem Senses. 2014;39:185–94.
3. Bramerson A, Johansson L, Ek L, Nordon S, Bende M. Prevalence of olfactory dysfunction: the Skovde population-based study. Laryngoscope. 2004;114:733–7.
4. Murphy C, Schubert CR, Cruickshanks CJ, Klein BE, Klein R, Nondahl DM. Prevalence of olfactory impairment in older adults. JAMA. 2002;288:2307–12.
5. Doty RL, Shaman P, Dann M. Development of the University of Pennsylvania Smell Identification Test: a standardized microencapsulated test of olfactory function. Physiol Behav. 1984;32:489–502.
6. Hummel T, Kobal G, Gudziol H, Mackay-Sim A. Normative data for the "Sniffin' Sticks" including tests of odor identification, odor discrimination, and olfactory thresholds: an upgrade based on a group of more than 3,000 subjects. Eur Arch Otorhinolaryngol. 2007;264:237–43.
7. Doty RL, Shaman P, Kimmelman CP, Dann MS. University of Pennsylvania Smell Identification Test: a rapid quantitative olfactory function test for the clinic. Laryngoscope. 1984;94(2 Pt 1):176–8.
8. van Spronsen E, Ebbens FA, Fokken WJ. Olfactory function in healthy children: Normative data for odor identification. Am J Rhinol Allergy. 2013;27:197–201.
9. Christopher HH, Richard LD. Clinical evaluation. In: The Neurology of Olfaction. 1st ed. Cambridge: Cambridge University Press; 2009. p. 59–110.
10. Doty RL, Shaman P, Applebaum SL, Giberson R, Siksorski L, Rosenberg L. Smell identification ability: changes with age. Science. 1984;226:1441–3.
11. Ship JA, Weiffenbach JM. Age, gender, medical treatment, and medication effects on smell identification. J Gerontol. 1993;48:26–32.
12. Hummel T, Bensafi M, Nikolaus J, Knecht M, Laing DG, Schall B. Olfactory function in children assessed with psychophysical and electrophysiological techniques. Behav Brain Res. 2007;180:133–8.
13. Dalton P, Mennella JA, Maute C, Castor SM, Silva-Garcia A, Slotkin J, et al. Development of a test to evaluate olfactory function in a pediatric population. Laryngoscope. 2011;121:1843–50.
14. Cameron EL, Doty RL. Odor identification testing in children and young adults using the smell wheel. Int J Pediatr Otorhinolaryngol. 2013;77:346–50.
15. Richman RA, Post EM, Sheehe PR, Wright HN. Olfactory performance during childhood. I. Development of an odorant identification test for children. J Pediatr. 1992;121:908–11.

7

Nasal Chondromesenchymal Hamartoma (NCMH): a systematic review of the literature with a new case report

Katrina Anna Mason[1*] , Annakan Navaratnam[2], Evgenia Theodorakopoulou[1] and Perumal Gounder Chokkalingam[2]

Abstract

Background: Nasal chondromesenchymal hamartoma (NCMH) is a very rare, benign tumour of the sinonasal tract usually presenting in infants. We present a systematic review of NCMH cases alongside a case report of an adult with asymptomatic NCMH.

Methods: A systematic review was conducted in accordance with PRISMA guidelines. A PubMed, EMBASE and manual search through references of relevant publications was used to identify all published case-reports of NCMH. Data was collected from each case-report on: patient demographics, laterality, size and location of NCMH, presentation, co-morbidities, investigations, treatment and follow-up.

Results: The systematic review identified 48 patients (including ours): 33 male, 15 female. Mean age was 9.6 years (range: 1 day–69 years) with the majority aged 1 year or younger at presentation ($n = 18$). Presentations included: nasal congestion ($n = 17$), nasal mass ($n = 15$) and eye signs ($n = 12$). NCMH also involved the paranasal sinuses ($n = 26$), orbit ($n = 16$) and skull-base ($n = 14$). All patients underwent operative resection of NCMH. A small 2014 case-series found DICER1 mutations in 6 NCMH patients, establishing a link to the DICER1 tumour spectrum.

Conclusions: NCMH is a rare cause of nasal masses in young children and adults. In light of the newly established link between NCMH and DICER1 mutations surgeons should be vigilant for associated DICER1 tumours, as NCMH may be the 'herald tumour' of this disease spectrum.

Keywords: Nasal neoplasms, Hamartoma, DICER1 protein human, Review

Background

Nasal chondromesenchymal hamartoma (NCMH) is a very rare, benign tumour of the sinonasal tract. Forty-seven cases have been reported in the English literature and the vast majority of these presentations are in infants and young children often below the age of one. NCMHs have a mixed morphological structure comprised of predominantly mesenchymal and cartilaginous components. NCMH patients present with symptoms that are dependent on the location of the tumour in the nasal cavity or paranasal sinuses and their compression of local structures. These symptoms range from nasal obstruction to visual impairment and facial and dental pain. To date there have only been 6 cases of adult presentation of NCMH. Here we present the first systematic review of NCMH cases published in the literature to assess the patient demographics, presentation, management and prognosis of NCMH alongside a new and unusual case in an adult.

Case report

A 49-year-old man was referred to our outpatient clinic presenting with a small mass in his right nasal cavity. The lump, which the patient first noticed 5 years ago, had been growing insidiously over time and by the time of presentation had become visible at the right anterior naris. The patient did not complain of any symptoms but sought consultation as his wife was concerned by the cosmetic appearance of the mass.

* Correspondence: katrina.a.mason@gmail.com
[1]Barts and The London School of Medicine and Dentistry, The Blizard Institute of Cell and Molecular Science, 4 Newark Street, Whitechapel, E1 2AT London, UK
Full list of author information is available at the end of the article

Examination revealed a large firm mass arising from the right side of the anterior nasal septum with approximately 0.5 cm attachment to the anterior cartilage of the septum. The left and right nasal cavities were otherwise unremarkable. Clinically, the mass had the appearance of a papilloma confined to the nasal cavity with an attachment to the septum only and therefore further imaging was not undertaken. The differential diagnoses considered at the time of presentation were: nasal polyp, squamous papilloma or inverted papilloma.

The patient subsequently underwent excisional biopsy of the right nostril mass under general anaesthetic using a circumferential subperichondrial incision with a small margin. Intraoperatively, the mass had the macroscopic appearance of a 0.5 cm × 2 cm × 2 cm calcified nodule. Due to a small 0.5 cm base, subsequent healing was achieved by secondary intention aided by the routine application of topical antibacterial cream. Histopathological analysis showed the nodule to contain cartilage and aneurysmal bone covered in stratified squamous epithelium with keratinisation (Figs. 1 and 2). Histopathological diagnosis was made using a haematoxylin & eosin stain. These findings were consistent with a diagnosis of a nasal chondromesenchymal hamartoma.

The patient was followed up in clinic and was discharged after 2 years having shown no signs of recurrence. Furthermore, a telephone interview was conducted 4 years post operation and the patient reported no recurrence of the nasal mass. He confirmed that he had no postoperative complications and was happy with the outcome of the operation.

Methods

A systematic review was undertaken in accordance with PRISMA guidelines [1]. No systematic review protocol was used, however our systematic review methodology is described below and a four-phase flow diagram is represented in Fig. 3. All published case-reports of NCMH were included in the review. A PubMed search (MEDLINE) (1975 to May Week 2, 2015) was carried out using the following terms [(chondromesenchymal hamartoma) AND (nasal OR sinus OR maxillary OR ethmoid OR sphenoid OR frontal OR orbit OR cranial)]. An EMBASE search (1975 to May Week 2, 2015) was carried out using a best sensitivity-combination strategy. The PubMed search resulted in 32 citations of which 24 were relevant, 6 were not NCMH case-reports, one was a Chinese language case-report, and one case was a duplicate case-report publication [2]. An EMBASE search and a manual search through references of relevant publications yielded 11 further relevant citations. Of these only 6 were included in the analysis; one case was found to have been a duplicate case report [3, 4] and four other possible cases of NCMH were found through publication citation search, but were labelled as "Mesenchymal chondrosarcoma" [5] "nasal hamartoma" [6], "nasopharyngeal hamartoma" [7], and "congenital mesenchymoma" [8], and were therefore not included. Thirty-one publications that report 47 cases of NCMH were included in this systematic review. Data was collected on patient demographics (age, gender), laterality, size and site of NCMH, presentation, co-morbidities, investigations, treatment and follow-up. These were also the principle summary measures. Two

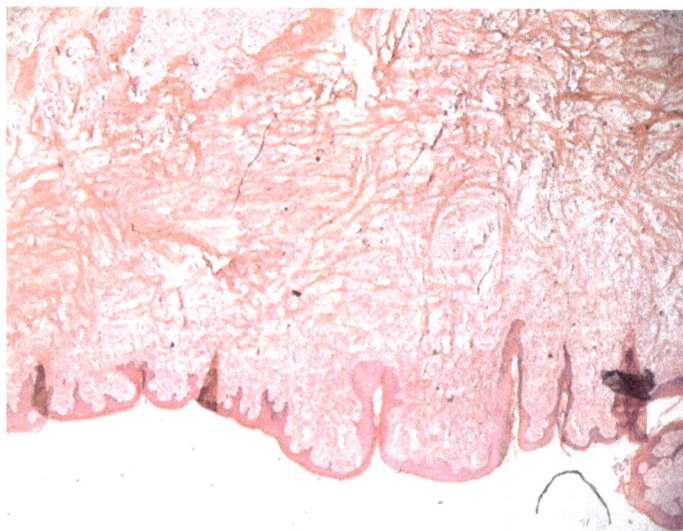

Fig. 1 Nodule containing cartilage and aneurysmal bone and covered by stratified squamous epithelium with keratinisation (magnification ×25, haematoxylin & eosin stain)

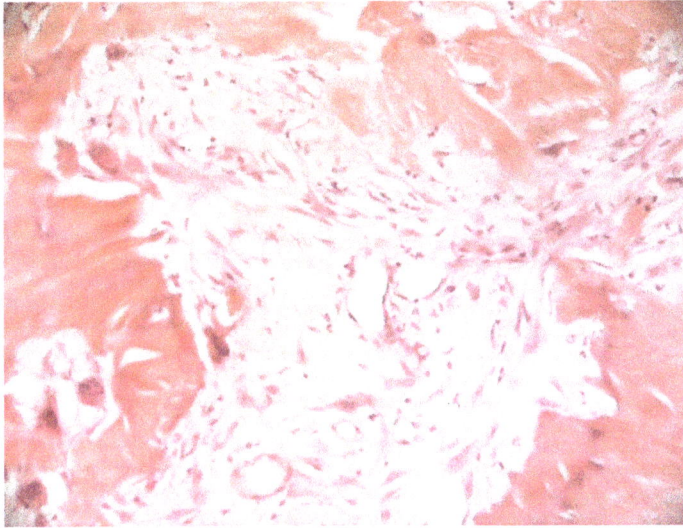

Fig. 2 Areas of osteoid formation (magnification ×200, haematoxylin & eosin stain)

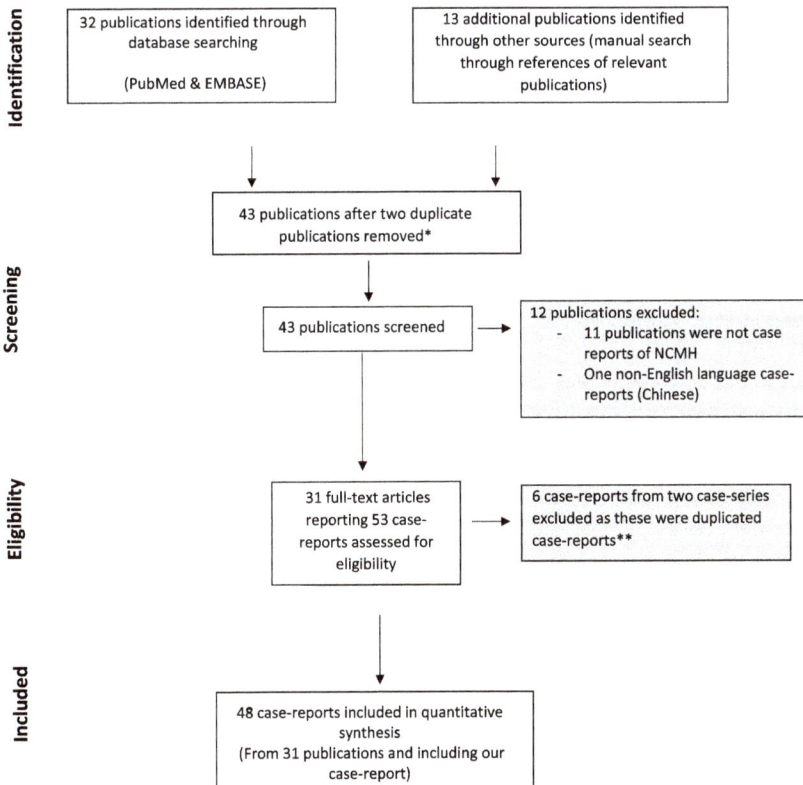

Fig. 3 Four-phase flow diagram of systematic review in accordance with PRISMA guidelines * Two individual publications of single case-reports were excluded from analysis as these had previously been published, Schultz et al. [2] and Kang et al. [3].** See Table 1

authors performed the database search, the manual search through references of relevant publications, and extracted the relevant data from the case-reports. Data was entered into an Excel 2013 Microsoft Office™ database which was used to carry out basic statistical analysis.

Results of systematic review

Forty-Eight NCMH patients (including our case) have been reported in the English literature (Fig. 3). Most cases presented in males; 33 male and 15 female, with a male to female ratio of 2.2:1 ratio. The mean age was 9.6 years (range: 1 day–69 years). A large proportion of these patients were aged 1 year or younger at presentation ($n = 18$) and only 8 adult patients (including our case) have been described. Site of pathology was limited to the nasal cavity only in 10 patients, and involved the paranasal sinuses (maxillary, ethmoid, sphenoid) in 26 patients, the orbit in 16 patients, extending to the skull base in 14 patients, had intracranial extension in 8 cases, involved the nasopharynx in 3 patients and the oropharynx in 2 patients (see Table 1).

Clinical presentations of NCMH patients included: nasal congestion or obstruction ($n = 17$), nasal mass ($n = 15$), eye signs (proptosis, hypotropia, enopthalmos, strabismus, exotropia etc.) ($n = 12$), facial swelling ($n = 8$), headaches or facial pain ($n = 6$), stertor or respiratory distress ($n = 8$), ophthalmoplegia ($n = 4$), recurrent sinusitis ($n = 4$), rhinorrhoea ($n = 3$), otitis media ($n = 2$), epistaxis ($n = 2$), toothache ($n = 1$), hyposmia ($n = 1$), hydrocephalus ($n = 1$) and 4 patients were asymptomatic or had no signs and symptoms documented (see Table 1).

All patients underwent operative resection of NCMH and the surgical approach was dependent on disease location. One patient had pre-operative chemotherapy due to initial misdiagnosis on biopsy as spindle cell sarcoma. One patient had pre-operative embolization to reduce operative blood loss. Follow up times were included for 24 patients, mean time for follow-up was 24 months, (range 2–156 months). Eleven patients were found to have persistent disease or disease recurrence on follow up, seven required further surgery, three patients were described as stable, and no further information was given on the other patient. Li et al. described the first and only reported case of malignant transformation of NCMH [9].

Thirty-six patients had no documented past medical problems. One adult patient had a history of multiple vascular aneurysms. Eleven of the patients had been diagnosed with pleuropulmonary blastoma (PPB) prior to NCMH detection. Of these 11 patients, 5 had other co-morbidities including three with Sertoli-Lleydig cell ovarian tumours, two with pulmonary cysts, one jejunal polyps, one papillary thyroid carcinoma, one cystic nephroma and one multinodular goitre.

A potential weakness of this systematic review is the possibility of reporting bias through publication bias both within individual case reports and across the review. This reporting bias is three-fold: firstly in the incomplete publication of all the clinical aspects of the case-reports by the original authors, for example not reporting follow-up times or co-morbidities etc. Secondly it is possible that there have been cases of NCMH that have not been reported in the literature and can therefore not be included in the systematic review. Thirdly the exclusion of case-reports of "Mesenchymal chondrosarcoma" [5] "nasal hamartoma" [6], "nasopharyngeal hamartoma" [7], and "congenital mesenchymoma" [8] alongside others, which are published prior to the first description of NCMH by McDermot et al. in 1998, may have resulted in an underreporting of true NCMH cases. However without being able to retrospectively assess and re-classify the histology of these cases we feel it is appropriate to have excluded them from our analysis and conclusions. These sources of reporting biases could potentially reduce the validity of conclusions drawn in terms of not fully representing or capturing all possible cases of NCMH.

Discussion

NCMHs are predominantly benign lesions that are locally destructive and because of their aggressive appearance can be mistaken for a malignant tumour. However NCMHs can be slow growing and therefore have a delayed presentation. Histopathologically these lesions are analogous to other mesenchymal hamartomas, and consist of islands of chondroid tissue such as hyaline cartilage, areas of calcification, and mesenchymal cellular elements such as spindle cells and myxoid stroma.

McDermott et al. were the first to recognise NCMH as a distinct clinic-pathological entity in 1998 when they described a case series of seven patients with a tumefactive process of the nasal passages and contiguous paranasal sinuses with a detectable mass in the nose [10]. In this case series, six of the seven patients were infants under the age of 3 months. As our systematic review demonstrates NCMH predominantly presents in young children and infants under the age of one, but there have now been seven case reports, including ours, of adults with NCMH up to the age of 69 [9, 11–14]. In 2013 the first and only reported case of malignant transformation of an NCMH was described in the literature [9].

In our case, the NCMH was initially thought to be a papilloma confined to the nasal septal wall and therefore further imaging was not undertaken prior to resection. However pre-operative imaging of these lesions provides valuable information regarding involvement of adjacent structures such as the paranasal sinuses, orbit and intracranial cavity. On computed tomography (CT) imaging,

Table 1 Summary table of systematic review of NCMH cases reported in the literature

Author, Publication date	Case No	Age D/M/Y	Sex	Side & Size	Site	Symptoms	Co-morbidity	Investigations	Treatment	Follow Up/
(1) McDermot, 1998 [10] USA	1	5 D	M	ND	1. Nasal cavity	1. Nasal Mass 2. Respiratory Difficulties	ND	CT	Surgical excision	No recurrence at 2 years
	2	3 M	F	ND	1. Nasal cavity 2. Ethmoid Sinus 3. Intracranial extension	1. Nasal Mass 2. Otitis Media	ND	MRI	Surgical excision	No recurrence at 2 years
	3	3 M	M	ND	1. Nasal cavity	1. Choanal Mass 2. Respiratory distress	ND	ND	Biopsy then surgical excision Subsequent chemotherapy	No recurrence at 4 years
	4	2 M	M	ND	1. Nasal cavity 2. Intracranial extension	1. Nasal Mass	ND	ND	Surgical excision	No recurrence at 18 months
	5	12 D	F	ND	1. Nasal cavity 2. Intracranial extension	1. Nasal Mass	ND	CT	Surgical excision & further re-excision after 16 months	Unchanged persistent tumour in superior nasal cavity at 12 months
	6	14 D	M	ND	1. Nasal cavity 2. Ethmoid sinus 3. Intracranial extension	1. Nasal Mass 2. Hydrocephalus & agenesis of corpus callosum	ND	CT	Surgical excision VP shunt for hydrocephalus	Residual tumour in anterior cranial fossa at 9 months
	7	7 Y	M	ND	1. Nasal cavity 2. Sphenoid sinus	1. Nasal Mass 2. Nasal Congestion	PPB	ND	Surgical excision	No recurrence at 2 months NB later reported by Priest et al. 2010 [27]- showed with multiple recurrences in first 3 years
(2) Chae 1999 Korea [30] *abstract only, Korean paper	8	3 M	F	Right Size: 3.5 × 7.5 × 2.5 cm	1. Nasal cavity 2. Ethmoid sinus 3. Cribriform plate	1. Epistaxis 2. Obstruction	ND	CT	Surgical excision	ND
(3) Kim D 1999 [31] USA	9	3 M	F	Right Size: ND	1. Nasal cavity 2. Intracranial extension 3. Ethmoid sinus	1. Nasal mass 2. Otitis media	None stated	CT MRI	Surgical excision with mid-facial de-gloving and bi-frontal craniotomy	No recurrence at 18 months
(4) Kato, 1999 [17] Japan	10	4 M	M	Left Size: ND	1. Nasal cavity 2. Intracranial extension	1. Nasal Mass 2. Respiratory distress with cyanosis when feeding	None stated	CT	Two stage surgical excision 1st intracranial/sinus	No recurrence at 13 years

Table 1 Summary table of systematic review of NCMH cases reported in the literature (Continued)

#	Age	Sex	Side/Size	Location	Symptoms		Imaging	Treatment	Outcome
11	0 D	M	Left Size: ND	1. Nasal cavity 1. Sphenoid sinus 3. Ethmoid sinus 4. Compression of left orbit	3. Opthalmoplegia left eye 1. Left facial swelling 2. Left nasal mass 3. Respiratory distress & cyanosis when feeding 4. Proptosis on recurrence	None stated	CT MRI	Excision biopsy then subsequent surgical excision with lateral rhinotomy and craniofacial approach	Recurrence after excision biopsy No recurrence at 5 years after second surgery
12	9 M	M	Right ND	1. Nasal cavity 2. Maxillary sinus	1. Asymmetric face 2. Right opthalmoplegia, enopthalmos and hypotropia	None stated	CT MRI	Surgical resection	No recurrence at 9 months
13	16 Y	M	Left 1.5 × 1.5 cm	1. Nasal cavity	1. Nasal swelling	None stated	CT MRI	Surgical resection with delayed reconstruction with forehead flap	No recurrence at 8 months
14	1 Y	M	Left Size: ND	1. Nasal cavity 2. Extension into left orbit 3. Ethmoid sinus 4. Sphenoid sinus	1. Proptosis of left eye 2. Left facial swelling	Non stated	CT	Chemotherapy (VID) as biopsy suggested spindle cell sarcoma- 30 % reduction in tumour size Then Left maxillectomy and surgical excision	Residual tumour at 1.5 years near eye but no further re-growth & stable
15	5 M	M	Left Size: ND	1. Nasal cavity 2. Compression of left orbit 3. Defect left ethmoidal bone 4. Defects anterior cranial fossa	1. Left eye ptosis	None stated	CT	Frontal craniotomy & trans-nasal surgical resection	ND
16	11 Y	M	Left Size: ND	1. Nasal cavity 2. Displacement left orbital wall	1. Headaches left sided	None stated	CT	Endoscopic biopsy and anterior craniofacial resection	ND
17	11 Y	M	Left Size: ND	1. Nasal cavity 2. Ethmoid sinus 3. Extension into left orbit	1. Nasal mass	None stated	ND	Surgery and care undertaken in another hospital	ND Surgery and care undertaken in another hospital

(5) Hsueh 2001 [3] Taiwan (2 cases)

(6) A rawi 2003 [14] Ireland

(7) Shet, 2004 [21] India

(8) Kim B, 2004 [22] Korea

(9) Norman, 2004 [15] USA

(10) Ozolek, 2005 [11] USA (4 cases)

Table 1 Summary table of systematic review of NCMH cases reported in the literature (Continued)

Case	Reference	Age	Sex	Side/Size	Location	Symptoms	Associated	Imaging	Treatment	Outcome
18		17 Y	F	ND Size: ND	1. Nasal cavity	1. Nasal obstruction 2. Facial pain	None stated	ND	Surgical excision	ND
19		25 Y	M	Bilateral 8 × 5 × 3.5 cm	1. Nasal cavity 2. Maxillary sinus 3. Nasopharynx 2. Oropharynx	1. Respiratory distress from obstructing oropharyngeal tumour requiring emergency tracheostomy 2. Chronic sinusitis	1. Multiple intracranial vascular aneurysms 2. Longstanding nasopharyngeal tumour- biopsy aged 13 'chronic inflamed polyp'	CT	Multiple surgical resections within one year including, tracheostomy and initial surgical resection, further surgical resection of bulbar mass and nasal tumour, then Le-Fort osteotomy and further surgical resection	ND
20		69 Y	F	Right Size: ND	1. Nasal cavity 2. Ethmoid sinus	ND	None stated	ND	Surgical excision	ND
21	(11) Low 2006 [33] UK	11 Y	M	Right Size: ND	1. Nasal cavity	1. Nasal Obstruction 2. Epistaxis	None stated	CT	Surgical excision	No recurrence at 2 months
22	(12) Johnson, 2007 [29] USA	15 Y	F	Bilateral Size: ND	1. Nasal cavity 2. Nasopharynx	1. Nasal obstruction 2. Chronic sinusitis	1. PPB 2. Sertoli-Leydig cell Ovarian Tumour 3. Congenital phthisi bulbi	CT	Endoscopic surgical excision	No recurrence at 6 months
23	(13) Silkiss, 2007 [18] USA	7 M	M	Right 3.2 × 1.4 cm	1. Nasal cavity 2. Erosion of cribriform plate 3. Compression of right orbit	1. Ptosis 2. Extropia 3. Strabismus 4. Stertor	None stated	CT MRI	Surgical resection-right lateral rhinotomy	No recurrence at 18 months
24	(14) Nakagawa 2008 [34] Japan	12 Y	M	Left 1.5 cm	1. Nasal cavity 2. Sphenoid sinus 3. Ethmoid sinus 4. Maxillary sinus	1. Nasal obstruction	None stated	CT	Endoscopic surgical resection and further endoscopic surgical resection after recurrence	Recurrence at 2 months No recurrence at 5 months post second surgery
25	(15) Finitsis, 2009 [35] Greece	12 M	M	Left 4 cm × 4.2 cm	1. Nasal cavity 2. Compression of left orbit 3. Maxillary sinus compression	1. Respiratory distress	None stated	CT MRI	Pre-operative embolization Then Surgical resection with midface de-gloving	ND

Table 1 Summary table of systematic review of NCMH cases reported in the literature (Continued)

Study	No.	Age	Sex	Size / Laterality	Location	Symptoms	Associated	Imaging	Treatment	Outcome
(16) Kim J, 2009 [23] Korea	26	19 M	M	Left 2.7 × 3.5 cm	1. Nasal cavity 2. Orbital extension 3. Intracranial extension 4. Nasopharynx	1. Watery rhinorrhoea 2. Nasal Obstruction	None stated	CT MRI	Endoscopic surgical resection ×2	Recurrence at one year; 2nd surgery. No recurrence 10 months after second surgery
(17) Priest, 2010 [27] USA *case previously reported by McDermot et al. 1998 **case previously reported by Johnson et al. 2007 (2 new cases)	-	7 Y *	M	Initially unilateral, then bilateral	1. Sphenoid sinus 2. Left Nasal cavity	1. Nasal Congestion 2. Nasal mass	1. PPB type II-III 2. Lung cysts		Four resections over 3 years	Followed up for 13 years with multiple recurrences in first 3 years
	-	15 Y **	F	Bilateral	1. Bilateral nasal cavities 2. Bony erosion of posterior septum 2. Extending into nasopharynx	1. Chronic Sinusitis 2. Facial Pain 3. Nasal Congestion 4. Nasal obstruction	1. PPB Type II 2. Sertoli-Leydig Cell Ovarian Tumour 3. Congenital phthisi bulbi Stickler syndrome		Surgical resection	No recurrence at 51 months
	27	10 Y	F	Bilateral Size: ND	1. Bilateral nasal cavities	1. Nasal obstruction	1. PPB Type III	CT	Surgical resection	No recurrence at 21 months
	28	11 Y	M	Right Size: ND	1. Nasal cavity 2. Extension to anterior skull base	1. Nasal obstruction	1. PPB Type III	ND	Surgical resection	No recurrence at 4 months
(18) Sarin, 2010 [24] India	29	2.5 Y	M	Right Size: ND	1. Nasal cavity 2. Maxillary, ethmoid and sphenoid sinus 3. Erosion of middle wall of orbit	1. Right eye oculomotor impairment	ND	MRI	Biopsy and then lateral rhinotomy for excision	ND
(19) Eloy 2011 [25] Belgium	30	18 M*	M	Right 0.5 × 0.4 cm	1. Nasal cavity 2. Ethmoid sinus 3. Extension into right orbit 4. Intracranial extension	1. Nasal obstruction 2. Nasal mass 3. Hypertelorism, proptosis, diplopia 4. Nasal swelling *symptoms 1st noticed at 2 months- delayed referral from Algeria to Brussels	None stated	CT MRI	Endoscopic surgical resection	ND
(20) Jayakumar 2011 [26] USA	31	7 D	F	Right Size: ND	1. Nasal cavity	1. Nasal Mass 2. Stertor	None stated	CT MRI	Endoscopic surgical excision	ND

Table 1 Summary table of systematic review of NCMH cases reported in the literature (Continued)

Case / Reference	Age	Sex	Size	Location	Symptoms	Associated	Imaging	Treatment	Outcome
(21) Mattos 2011 [20] USA	3 Y	M	Left Size : ND	1. Nasal cavity 2. Ethmoid sinus 3. Extension into right orbit 4. Left maxilla	3. Proptosis right eye 1. Eye infections 2. Eye congestion 3. Nasal obstruction 4. Cheek fullness 5. Intermitted left eye/face pain	None stated	CT MRI	Endoscopic excision the further surgical excision	Recurrence at 21 months required further resection
(22) Behery, 2012 [36] USA	11 Y	M	ND	ND	Nasal Obstruction	1. PPB		Surgical resection	ND
(23) Uzomefuna, 2012 [37] Ireland	8 Y	M	ND	1. Sphenoid sinus 2. Ethmoid sinus	1. Frontal Headache	ND	CT MRI	Endoscopic surgical resection	No recurrence at 6 months
(24) Cho, 2013 [4] Korea	14 Y	M	Left 5 cm × 5.3 cm × 4 cm	1. Nasal cavity 2. Maxillary sinus 3. Intraoral 4. Orbital floor destruction	1. Swelling and pain to left face 2. Tooth mobility	None stated	CT	Subtotal maxillectomy, removal or orbital floor, removal of medial nasal mucous membrane. Reconstruction with iliac crest bone block	No recurrence at 4 years
(25) Li Y, 2013 [12] China	40 Y	F	Bilateral Size: ND	1. Nasal Cavity 2. Maxillary sinus 3. Ethmoid sinus	1. Nasal Obstruction 2. Bloody rhinorrhoea	None stated	CT MRI	Complete radical resection	Recurrence at 3 months *Malignant transformation seen on histology
(26) Li GY 2013 [9] China	23 Y	M	Left 3.2 × 2.5 cm	1. Naval cavity 2. Extension to lacrimal sac & left orbit 3. Ethmoid sinus	1. Left Lacrimal Sac 2. Proptosis 3. Lateral displacement of globe	None stated	ND	Endoscopic surgical excision	No recurrence at 3 months follow up
(27) Moon, 2014 [19] Korea	9 M	F	Right Size: ND	1. Nasal cavity 2. Maxillary sinus 3. Erosion of orbital wall 4. Erosion of cribriform plate	1. Incomitant esotropia of right eye (inability to abduct right eye) No nasal symptoms	None stated	CT MRI	Surgery and care undertaken in another hospital	ND Surgery and care undertaken in another hospital
(28) Wang T, 2014 [38] China (2 cases)	5 Y	M	Right 2.5 × 3.6 × 4.3 cm	1. Nasal cavity 2. Ethmoid sinus	1. Recurrent sinusitis	None stated	CT MRI	Surgical resection	No recurrence at 3 years

Table 1 Summary table of systematic review of NCMH cases reported in the literature (Continued)

Reference	Case	Age	Sex	Laterality/Size	3. Intracranial extension	2. Nasal Obstruction (Symptoms)	Associated conditions	CT MRI	Treatment	Recurrence
[29] Obidan, 2014 [39] Saudi Arabia	40	6 W	F	Left 2.6 × 3.4 × 3.9 cm	1. Nasal cavity 2. Pressure remodelling of adjacent bones	1. Nasal obstruction 2. Watery rhinorrhoea	None stated	CT MRI	Surgical resection	No recurrence at 10 months
	41	14 Y Size: ND	M	Bilateral	1. Bilateral nasal cavities	1. Nasal Obstruction 2. Decreased sense of smell	1. PPB	CT	Surgical endoscopic resection	ND
[30] Stewart, 2014 [13] USA **4 patients previously reported by Priest et al. 2010 [27] (4 new cases)	-	7 Y**	M	Initially unilateral, then bilateral	ND	1. Nasal Congestion	1. PPB 2. Lung cysts		Surgical resection	Multiple recurrences
	-	15 Y**	F	Bilateral	ND	1. Chronic Sinusitis 2. Facial Pain 3. Nasal Congestion	1. PPB 2. Sertoli-Leydig Cell Ovarian Tumour		Surgical resection	No recurrence
	-	10 Y**	F	Bilateral	ND	1. Nasal congestion	1. PPB		Surgical resection	No recurrence
	-	11 Y**	M	Right	ND	1. Nasal Congestion	1. PPB		Surgical resection	No recurrence
	42	8 Y	M	ND Size: ND	ND	1. ND	1. PPB 2. Pulmonary cysts in utero 3. Jejunal Polyps	ND	Surgical resection	No recurrence
	43	13 Y	F	Bilateral Size: ND	ND	1. ND	1. PPB 2. Thyroid Papillary carcinoma 3. Sertoli-Leydig tumour	ND	Surgical resection	No recurrence
	44	8 Y	M	Bilateral Size: ND	ND	1. Chronic Sinusitis	1. PPB	ND	Surgical resection	No recurrence
	45	6 Y	F	ND Size: ND	ND	ND	1. PPB 2. Left cystic nephroma 3. Small bowel loop	ND	Surgical resection	No recurrence
	46	21 Y	F	Right Size: ND	ND	1. Nasal Congestion 2. Septal deviation	1. PPB 2. Sertoli-Leydig Tumour	ND	Surgical resection	Recurrence at 4 years

Table 1 Summary table of systematic review of NCMH cases reported in the literature (Continued)

					3. Nasal Obstruction (at recurrence)	3. Multi-nodular goitre			
(31) Chandra 2014 [40] India	47	12 Y	M	Right Size: ND	1. Nasal cavity 2. Ethmoid sinus 3. Extension into right orbit	1. Nasal Obstruction 2. Proptosis 3. Right facial pain	None stated	CT MRI	Surgical excision	No recurrence at 5 months
(32) Mason 2015 UK	48	49 Y	M	Right 0.5 × 2 × 2 cm	1. Nasal cavity	1. Nasal mass	None stated	None	Surgical excision	No recurrence at 4 years

Y Years, *M* Months, *D* Days, *M* Male, *F* Female, *ND* not documented, *PPB* Pleuropulmonary blastoma, *CT* Computed Tomography, *MRI* Magnetic Resonance Imaging

NCMH are typically seen as non-encapsulated, poorly defined masses often with cystic components [15]. Magnetic resonance imaging (MRI) of NCMH demonstrates a heterogeneous mass on T1 weighted images and T2 weighted images show the presence of cystic components. MRI also has the advantage of superior tissue characterisation and delineation of invasion of adjacent structures in comparison to CT [16]. Due to rarity of NCMH, even after thorough clinical and radiographic examination NCMH can be misdiagnosed, and differential diagnoses include: inverted papilloma, aneurysmal bone cysts or ossifying fibromas, nasoethmoidal encephalocoele, chondrosarcoma, nasal lymphoma, nasal glioma and rhabdomyosarcoma. Histopathological analysis following surgical resection is therefore needed for accurate diagnosis.

Patients with NCMH most commonly present with symptoms of nasal obstruction, nasal mass, or eye signs, which reflects the involvement of NCMH in the nasal passages and orbit. Ophthalmic signs include signs of globe displacement such as strabismus, extropia, hypertelorism, proptosis, enophthalmus and ophthlmoplegia, direct results of the intra-ocular extension of NCMH or ocular compression by NCMH [17–26]. There has also been a report of a patient presenting with intra-oral symptoms due to involvement of the oral cavity [4]. Patients can therefore present to otolaryngology, ophthalmology or maxillo-facial departments and doctors in these specialties should be aware of this rare pathology. In our case, the patient did not complain of any cranial, ophthalmic or nasal symptoms but was aware of a slowly enlarging nasal mass. This is most likely due to the relatively small size of the tumour at the anterior nasal septum which did not obstruct the nasal passage.

The aetiology of NCMH is thought to be due to an underlying genetic predisposition therefore accounting for the early presentation in the majority of cases. Priest et al. and Stewart et al. investigated patients with both NCMH and the rare paediatric dysembryonic sarcoma of the lung and pleura: pleuropulmonary blastoma (PPB) [13, 27]. In patients with NCMH and PPB Stewart et al. found germline *DICER1* mutations in 6 out of 8 evaluated patients, and somatic *DICER1* mutations in 2 out of those 6 patients with germline mutations [13]. This recent finding has established genetic proof of NCMH tumour association with *DICER1* mutations and Stewart et al. therefore feel that NCMH should be considered part of the *DICER1* tumour spectrum. The *DICER1* familial tumour susceptibility syndrome confers an increased risk most commonly for pleuropulmonary blastoma (PPB) but also ovarian sex cord-stromal tumours; Sertoli-Leydig cell tumor [SLCT], juvenile granulosa cell tumour [JGCT] and gynandroblastomas. Less commonly the *DICER1* tumour spectrum includes: cystic nephroma (CN), and thyroid gland neoplasia,

multinodular goitres [MNG], adenomas, or differentiated thyroid cancers. The rarest observed tumours in this spectrum, alongside NCMHs, are ciliary body medulloepithelioma (CBME), botryoid-type embryonal rhabdomyosarcoma (ERMS) of the cervix or other sites, renal sarcomas, pituitary blastomas, and pineoblastomas [28]. Eleven patients in our systematic review had previous PPB and five of these also had other *DIECR1* tumours. Surgeons and physicians should therefore be aware of these disease associations and should be vigilant of a diagnosis of NCMH in patients presenting with sino-nasal or orbital symptoms who have a history of any of these tumours. Johnson et al. importantly also point out that due to its location, NCMH is more likely to present early in life than the other *DICER1* tumours [29]. Surgeons and physicians should therefore either offer *DICER1* mutation analysis if available, or ensure long-term follow up of these patients and be vigilant for associated tumours, as NCMH may be the 'herald tumour' of this disease spectrum.

There are also cases in the literature of children, adolescents and adults with NCMH who have had an asymptomatic infancy [9, 11, 12, 14]. This may imply that there are non-genetic components to NCMH pathogenesis. Alternatively it may simply reflect the insidious growth of the tumour or that some NCMH patients may only exhibit the phenotype later in life. However as this is an extremely rare pathology with only very recent formal association with the *DICER1* mutation, the majority of the 42 reported cases have not had formal *DICER1* mutation analysis. Therefore an association or lack thereof in the non-tested cases cannot be inferred.

Successful management of NCMH entails complete resection in order to prevent recurrence. A complete excision however is not always technically feasible, especially in cases of intracranial extension of NCMH. An incomplete resection poses the risk of recurrence as well as the possibility of continued tumour growth and progressive symptoms. Nine patients in this systematic review were found to have disease recurrence, most likely from incomplete surgical excision.

Conclusions

We present an unusual case of NCMH in an adult without nasal obstructive symptoms due to the anatomical location of the NCMH attached to the nasal septum. A systematic review of the literature has highlighted that presentation is mostly related to tumour location, with nasal mass, nasal obstruction and ophthalmic signs being the most common forms of presentation. The majority of patients presenting with NCMH are children and infants below the age of one, but there have now been a few adult cases of presentation. Surgical resection is the treatment of choice with low recurrence rates in the majority of cases. There has only been one reported case of malignant transformation and NCMH is still considered a benign tumour. NCMH's association with the *DIECR1* mutation has very recently been established and therefore in light of this any patient with a *DICER1*-related tumour spectrum and new nasal or orbital symptoms should raise the suspicion of NCMH. Furthermore surgeons should subsequently be vigilant for associated *DICER1* related tumours, as due to their location NCMHs may be the 'herald tumour' for this disease spectrum. This case and systematic review highlights the fact that NCMH can mimic other benign and malignant lesions and that surgeons and physicians should be aware of rare pathologies accounting for nasal masses.

Consent

Written consent was obtained from the patient for publication of this case report and accompanying images. A copy of the written consent is available for review by the editor-in-chief of this journal.

Abbreviations

NCMH: Nasal chondromesenchymal hamartoma; EMBASE: Excerpta medica database; CT: Computed tomography; MRI: Magnetic resonance imaging; PPB: Pleuropulmonary blastoma; SLCT: Sertoli-leydig cell tumour; JGCT: Juvenile granulosa cell tumour; CN: Cystic nephroma; MNG: Multinodular goitres; CBME: Ciliary body medulloepithelioma; ERMS: Embryonal rhabdomyosarcoma; DICER1: is not an abbreviation, but the name of gene located on chromosome 14 at position q32.13.

Competing interests

The authors declare that they have no competing interests.

Authors' contributions

Contribution to conception and design: KM, AN, PC. Contribution to acquisition of data, analysis and interpretation: KM, AN, ET. Involved in drafting the manuscript & revising it critically: KM, AN, ET, PC. All authors read and approved the final manuscript.

Authors' information

KM is a clinical teaching fellow with Barts and The London School of Medicine and Dentistry. ET is a clinical teaching fellow with Barts and The London School of Medicine and Dentistry AN is a junior registrar in ENT surgery in the London Deanery. PC is a locum consultant at a regional teaching hospital where the case was encountered.

Acknowledgements

Thanks to Dr Ian Seddon (Consultant Histopathologist, Colchester Hospital University NHS Foundation Trust) for providing the histopathology images.

Author details

[1]Barts and The London School of Medicine and Dentistry, The Blizard Institute of Cell and Molecular Science, 4 Newark Street, Whitechapel, E1 2AT London, UK. [2]Colchester Hospital University NHS Foundation Trust, Colchester, UK.

References

1. Moher D, Liberati A, Tetzlaff J, Altman DG, Group P. Preferred reporting items for systematic reviews and meta-analyses: the PRISMA statement. J Clin Epidemiol. 2009;62(10):1006–12.

2. Schultz KA, Yang J, Doros L, Williams GM, Harris A, Stewart DR, et al. pleuropulmonary blastoma familial tumor predisposition syndrome: a unique constellation of neoplastic conditions. Pathology Case Rev. 2014;19(2):90–100.

3. Kang Jun HYO, Ahn Gueng H, Kim Young M, Cha Hee J, Choi H-J. Nasal Chondromesenchymal Hamartoma a case report. Korean J Pathol. 2007;41:258–62.

4. Cho YC, Sung IY, Son JH, Ord R. Nasal chondromesenchymal hamartoma: report of a case presenting with intraoral signs. J Oral Maxillofac Surg. 2013;71(1):72–6.

5. Roland NJ, Khine MM, Clarke R, Van Velzen D. A rare congenital intranasal polyp: mesenchymal chondrosarcoma of the nasal region. J Laryngol Otol. 1992;106(12):1081–3.

6. Terris MH, Billman GF, Pransky SM. Nasal hamartoma: case report and review of the literature. Int J Pediatr Otorhinolaryngol. 1993;28(1):83–8.

7. Zarbo RJ, McClatchey KD. Nasopharyngeal hamartoma: report of a case and review of the literature. Laryngoscope. 1983;93(4):494–7.

8. Ludemann JP, Tewfik TL, Meagher-Villemure K, Bernard C. Congenital mesenchymoma transgressing the cribriform plate. J Otolaryngol. 1997;26(4):270–2.

9. Li Y, Yang QX, Tian XT, Li B, Li Z. Malignant transformation of nasal chondromesenchymal hamartoma in adult: a case report and review of the literature. Histol Histopathol. 2013;28(3):337–44.

10. McDermott MB, Ponder TB, Dehner LP. Nasal chondromesenchymal hamartoma: an upper respiratory tract analogue of the chest wall mesenchymal hamartoma. Am J Surg Pathol. 1998;22(4):425–33.

11. Ozolek JA, Carrau R, Barnes EL, Hunt JL. Nasal chondromesenchymal hamartoma in older children and adults: series and immunohistochemical analysis. Arch Pathol Lab Med. 2005;129(11):1444–50.

12. Li GY, Fan B, Jiao YY. Endonasal endoscopy for removing nasal chondromesenchymal hamartoma extending from the lacrimal sac region. Can J Ophthalmol. 2013;48(2):e22–3.

13. Stewart DR, Messinger Y, Williams GM, Yang J, Field A, Schultz KA, et al. Nasal chondromesenchymal hamartomas arise secondary to germline and somatic mutations of DICER1 in the pleuropulmonary blastoma tumor predisposition disorder. Hum Genet. 2014;133(11):1443–50.

14. Alrawi M, McDermott M, Orr D, Russell J. Nasal chondromesynchymal hamartoma presenting in an adolescent. Int J Pediatr Otorhinolaryngol. 2003;67(6):669–72.

15. Norman ES, Bergman S, Trupiano JK. Nasal chondromesenchymal hamartoma: report of a case and review of the literature. Pediatr Dev Pathol. 2004;7(5):517–20.

16. Yao-Lee A, Ryan M, Rajaram V. Nasal chondromesenchymal hamartoma: correlation of typical MR, CT and pathological findings. Pediatr Radiol. 2011;41(5):675–7.

17. Kato K, Ijiri R, Tanaka Y, Hara M, Sekido K. Nasal chondromesenchymal hamartoma of infancy: the first Japanese case report. Pathol Int. 1999;49(8):731–6.

18. Silkiss RZ, Mudvari SS, Shetlar D. Ophthalmologic presentation of nasal chondromesenchymal hamartoma in an infant. Ophthal Plast Reconstr Surg. 2007;23(3):243–4.

19. Moon SH, Kim MM. Nasal chondromesenchymal hamartoma with incomitant esotropia in an infant: a case report. Can J Ophthalmol. 2014;49(1):e30–2.

20. Mattos JL, Early SV. Nasal chondromesenchymal hamartoma: a case report and literature review. Int J Pediatric Otorhinolaryngology Extra. 2011;6(4):215–9.

21. Shet T, Borges A, Nair C, Desai S, Mistry R. Two unusual lesions in the nasal cavity of infants–a nasal chondromesenchymal hamartoma and an aneurysmal bone cyst like lesion. More closely related than we think? Int J Pediatr Otorhinolaryngol. 2004;68(3):359–64.

22. Kim B, Park SH, Min HS, Rhee JS, Wang KC. Nasal chondromesenchymal hamartoma of infancy clinically mimicking meningoencephalocele. Pediatr Neurosurg. 2004;40(3):136–40.

23. Kim JE, Kim HJ, Kim JH, Ko YH, Chung SK. Nasal chondromesenchymal hamartoma: CT and MR imaging findings. Korean J Radiol. 2009;10(4):416–9.

24. Sarin V, Singh B, Prasher P. A silent nasal mass with ophthalmic presentation. Orbit. 2010;29(6):367–9.

25. Eloy P, Trigaux H, Nassogne MC, Weynand B, Rombaux P. Nasal chondromesenchymal hamartoma: case report. Int J Pediatric Otorhinolaryngology Extra. 2010;6(4):300–3.

26. Jeyakumar A, McEvoy T, Fettman N. Neonatal nasal mass: Chondromesenchymal hamartoma. Int J Pediatric Otorhinolaryngology Extra. 2011;6(4):223–5.

27. Priest JR, Williams GM, Mize WA, Dehner LP, McDermott MB. Nasal chondromesenchymal hamartoma in children with pleuropulmonary blastoma–A report from the International Pleuropulmonary Blastoma Registry registry. Int J Pediatr Otorhinolaryngol. 2010;74(11):1240–4.
28. Doros L, Schultz KA, Stewart DR, Bauer AJ, Williams G, Rossi CT, et al. DICER1-Related Disorders. In: Pagon RA, Adam MP, Ardinger HH, Bird TD, Dolan CR, Fong CT, et al., editors. GeneReviews(R) Seattle (WA). 1993.
29. Johnson C, Nagaraj U, Esguerra J, Wasdahl D, Wurzbach D. Nasal chondromesenchymal hamartoma: radiographic and histopathologic analysis of a rare pediatric tumor. Pediatr Radiol. 2007;37(1):101–4.
30. Chae HJ SJ, Lee SK. Nasal Chondromesenchymal Hamartoma. Korean J Pathol. 1999;33:225–7.
31. Kim DW, Low W, Billman G, Wickersham J, Kearns D. Chondroid hamartoma presenting as a neonatal nasal mass. Int J Pediatr Otorhinolaryngol. 1999;47(3):253–9.
32. Hsueh C, Hsueh S, Gonzalez-Crussi F, Lee T, Su J. Nasal chondromesenchymal hamartoma in children: report of 2 cases with review of the literature. Arch Pathol Lab Med. 2001;125(3):400–3.
33. Low SE, Sethi RK, Davies E, Stafford JS. Nasal chondromesenchymal hamartoma in an adolescent. Histopathology. 2006;49(3):321–3.
34. Nakagawa T, Sakamoto T, Ito J. Nasal chondromesenchymal hamartoma in an adolescent. Int J Pediatr Otorhinolaryngology Extra. 2008;4(3):111–3.
35. Finitsis S, Giavroglou C, Potsi S, Constantinidis I, Mpaltatzidis A, Rachovitsas D, et al. Nasal chondromesenchymal hamartoma in a child. Cardiovasc Intervent Radiol. 2009;32(3):593–7.
36. Behery RE, Bedrnicek J, Lazenby A, Nelson M, Grove J, Huang D, et al. Translocation t(12;17) (q24.1;q21) as the sole anomaly in a nasal chondromesenchymal hamartoma arising in a patient with pleuropulmonary blastoma. Pediatr Dev Pathol. 2012;15(3):249–53.
37. Uzomefuna V, Glynn F, Russell J, McDermott M. Nasal chondromesenchymal hamartoma with no nasal symptoms. BMJ Case Rep. 2012;2012.
38. Wang T, Li W, Wu X, Li Q, Cui Y, Chu C, et al. Nasal chondromesenchymal hamartoma in young children: CT and MRI findings and review of the literature. World J Surg Oncol. 2014;12(1):257.
39. Obidan AA, Ashoor MM. Nasal chondromesenchymal hamartoma in an adolescent with pleuropulmonary blastoma. Saudi Med J. 2014;35(8):876–8.
40. Chandra Manis SN, Venkatahalam VP. Nasal Chondormesenchymal Hamartoma: a case report and review of literature. JK-Practitioner. 2014;19:1–2.

8

Immunoglobulin G4-related diseases in the head and neck: a systematic review

Graeme B. Mulholland* ⓘ, Caroline C. Jeffery, Paras Satija and David W. J. Côté

Abstract

Background: Immunoglobulin G4 related disease (IgG4-RD) is a poorly understood chronic inflammatory disorder affecting the middle-aged and elderly that can present to the otolaryngologist. We aim to summarize the current literature regarding the manifestations and management of IgG4-RD in the head and neck.

Methods: Pubmed and EMBASE were searched using the term relevant search algorithm utilizing keywords such as: IgG4 related disease, head and neck, orbit, salivary glands, sialadenitis, Kuttner, angiocentric eosinophilic fibrosis, submandibular, lacrimal, thyroid, dacryoadenitis, nasal, sinus, and Mikulicz's. Reference lists were searched for identification of relevant studies.

Case reports, original research and review articles published in English from 1964 to 2014 whose major topic was IgG4-RD affecting the head and neck were included. Data regarding patient demographics, presentation, histopathology, management and treatment outcomes of IgG4-RD were extracted. Level of evidence was also assessed and data were pooled where possible. Three independent reviewers screened eligible studies; extracted relevant data and discrepancies were resolved by consensus, where applicable. Descriptive and comparative statistics were performed.

Results: Fourty-three articles met our inclusion criteria. IgG4-RD most often presents as a mass lesion in the head and neck region. Common diagnostic features include: 1) elevated serum IgG4 level, 2) marked infiltration of exocrine glands by IgG4-positive plasma cells with fibrosis, and 3) marked improvement with corticosteroid therapy and additional immunosuppressive therapy in corticosteroid refractory cases. Early diagnosis and involvement of rheumatology is important in management.

Conclusions: IgG4-RD is a challenging non-surgical disease that has multiple manifestations in the head and neck. It must be distinguished from various mimics including malignancy, systemic diseases, and infectious. Otolaryngology-Head and Neck surgeons should be aware of this condition and its management.

Keywords: IgG4-RD, Head and neck, Systematic review, Salivary glands, Lacrimal glands, Lymphandenopathy

Introduction

Immunoglobulin G4 – related disease (IgG4-RD) is a newly described fibroinflammatory condition that often presents as a tumefactive lesion that can affect nearly every organ system. IgG4-RD was first recognized after a connection between elevated serum IgG4 levels and inflammatory mass lesions in the pancreas causing autoimmune pancreatitis was made by Hamano *et al.* in 2001 [1]. An initial consensus statement regarding diagnosis of IgG4-RD was developed by Deshpande *et al.* at the first international symposium for IgG4-RD held in October of 2011 [2]. After the pancreas, the head and neck region is second most common site for presentation of IgG4-RD. More, a number of historically perplexing pseudotumor disorders have been attributed to IgG4-RD; these include Mikulicz's disease, Küttner's tumor and Reidel's thyroiditis [3].

The exact etiology of IgG4-RD is unknown and no known role of the IgG4 molecule itself has been identified. It is postulated that the inflammatory and fibrotic processes that drives IgG4-RD are propagated by a combination of Th2 cells and regulatory T cells (Treg cells) [4]. This is contrary to most autoimmune disorders where

* Correspondence: graemem@ualberta.ca
Division of Otolaryngology-Head and Neck Surgery, 1E4 Walter MacKenzie Centre, University of Alberta, 8440 112 Street, Edmonton, AB T6G 2B7, Canada

polarized T helper 1 (Th1) and/or Th17 subsets are responsible for the inflammatory process [5]. Histologically, the hallmark findings for IgG4-RD include lymphoplasmacytic infiltration, storiform fibrosis, obliterative phlebitis, and mild to moderate tissue eosinophilia [6]. However, the exact histological findings vary greatly depending on the tissue affected and clinical presentation. Currently, the histologic diagnosis of IgG4-RD is based primarily on IgG4 positive to IgG containing cell ratio and the number of IgG4 positive cells per high powered field, a ratio of IgG4 to IgG that is higher than 50 % and 30 IgG4-positive cells per high-power field is considered to be highly suggestive of IgG4-RD [6].

Currently, the literature proposes that IgG4-RD could be both over and under recognised [7]. This study aims to examine the various presentations of IgG4-RD in the head and neck, and present the management and outcomes reported in the literature.

Material and methods
This systematic review was performed using the following search strategy and study selection criteria.

Literature search strategy
The databases PubMed (1966-December 2014) and Embase (1988-December 2014) were searched using an

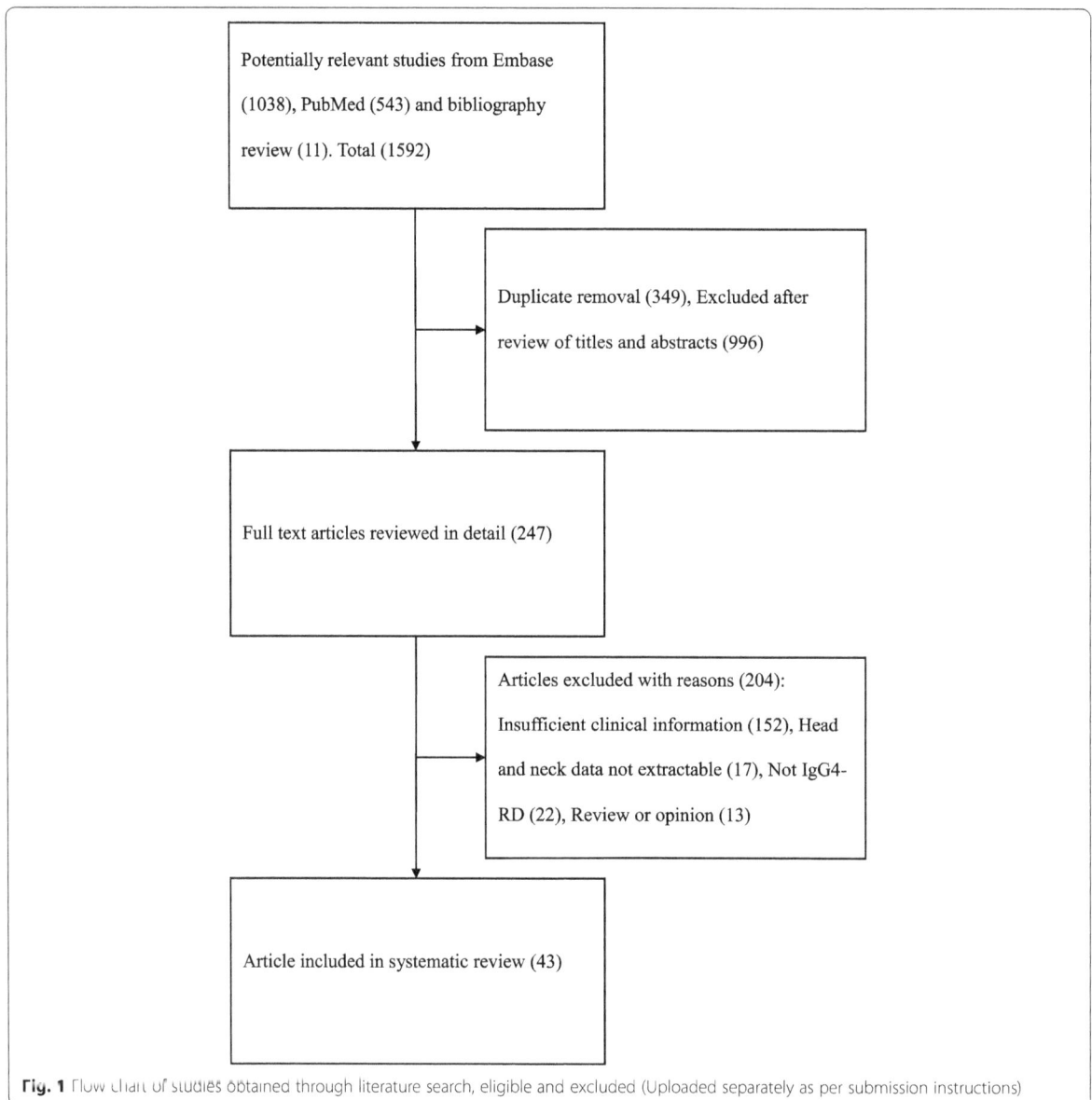

Fig. 1 Flow chart of studies obtained through literature search, eligible and excluded (Uploaded separately as per submission instructions)

algorithm designed from an extensive list of relevant search terms (see Appendix A for Pubmed and Embase search algorithms).

We included all original studies, case reports, case series, and reviews. Relevant articles and abstracts were selected and reviewed and the reference lists from these sources and recent review articles were also reviewed for additional publications.

Study selection

Three independent reviewers screened the identified articles (GBM, CCJ and PS). Relevant articles were obtained and reviewed in full. Discrepancies were resolved by consensus amongst the reviewers. The inclusion criteria comprised of all original clinical studies, case series and case reports of histologically confirmed IgG4-RD in the head and neck. Histologic diagnosis of IgG4-RD required identification of >10 IgG4 positive plasma cells per high powered field, IgG4 + plasma cell to IgG containing cell ratio 40 % or greater, and characteristic finding of fibrosis, sclerosis and phlebitis. Articles were excluded on the basis of biopsy information not being from a head and neck site, insufficient histologic

information, inability to extract head and neck specific information and narrative review and expert opinions.

Data extraction

The information gathered for each study included study design, country of publication and number of patients. Where possible, patient-specific data was extracted, including age at presentation, duration and nature of symptoms. Specifically, we collected data regarding head and neck manifestations, laboratory and histologic findings as well as specific treatments and outcome information.

Statistical analysis

Basic statistical analysis, including descriptive statistics was performed using Excel (Version 19.0, Microsoft ®).

Results

We initially identified 1592 articles through a combination of literature search and citation review. After reviewing abstracts, 247 articles of interest were identified. Three authors independently reviewed the articles and 43 articles met inclusion criteria (Fig. 1). Of the 43 articles, 21 case reports and 5 large case series (greater than 15 patients) were included (Table 1). A large

Table 1 Country of origin and characteristics of included articles

			N (Articles)	%	N (Individual Cases)	%
Total number of studies			43		484	
	Case Reports		21	48.8	21	4.3
	Small Case Series		17	39.5	107	22.1
	Large Case Series		5	11.6	356	73.6
Country of Origin	North America		10	23.3	27	5.6
		Canada	1	2.3	1	0.2
		USA	9	20.9	26	5.4
	Asia		22	51.2	429	88.6
		Japan	18	41.9	419	86.6
		Hong Kong	2	4.7	8	1.7
		Taiwan	1	2.3	1	0.2
		Singapore	1	2.3	1	0.2
	Oceania		6	14.0	7	1.4
		Australia	5	11.6	6	1.2
		New Zealand	1	2.3	1	0.2
	Europe		4	9.3	20	4.1
		United Kingdom	1	2.3	1	0.2
		Netherlands	1	2.3	12	2.5
		Czech Republic	1	2.3	6	1.2
		Switzerland	1	2.3	1	0.2
	South America		1	2.3	1	0.2
		Brazil	1	2.3	1	0.2

Table 2 Basic patient demographics

Total number of Patients	484
Average Age (years)	60.4
Percent Males	47.5 %

proportion of articles were from Japan (41.9 %), contributing 86.6 % of the total individual cases (Table 1).

Four hundred and eighty-four patients were identified with an average patient age of 60.4 years (Table 2). Table 3 shows the proportion of patients presenting by various sites in the head and neck. Cervical lymphadenopathy was document in 22 cases. Many of the patients also had involvement of other organ systems at the time of presentation, including 56 patients with lymphadenopathy outside of the head and neck (see Table 3). All patients had tissue biopsy from head and neck sites confirming the diagnosis of IgG4-RD. Confirmatory laboratory investigations was included where documented. The laboratory and histologic findings of patients indentified in the literature are summarized in Table 4.

Treatment information was available for 26.7 % of patients. Patients were treated with surgical excision, radiotherapy, corticosteroids with or without adjunct medical

Table 3 Systemic and head and neck manifestations

Head & Neck Manifestations	Site	Subsite	n	%
	Total presentations		730	
	Orbit		384	52.6
		Lacrimal Gland	136	18.6
		Extra Ocular Muscles	9	1.2
		Optic Nerve	5	0.7
	Salivary Glands		162	22.2
		Submandibular Gland	107	14.7
		Parotid Gland	29	4.0
		Sublingual Gland	1	0.1
		Minor Salivary Gland	1	0.1
	Thyroid		31	4.2
	Facial Skin		6	0.8
	Trigeminal Nerve		1	0.1
	Cervical Lymphadenopathy		22	3.0
Non Head & Neck Manifestations	Site		n	%
	Other Organ Involvement		68	9.3
	Mediastinal/Pelvic Lymphadenopathy		56	7.7

Table 4 Laboratory and histologic findings

	Mean Values
Serum IgG4 (mg/dL)	702.9
Serum IgG (mg/dL)	2445.0
IgG4 + ve Plasma Cells / HPF	69.8
IgG4 + ve Cells / IgG Containing Cells	48.0 %

treatment, or some combination of treatment modalities. The distribution of patients in terms of treatment(s) received and their outcomes are summarized in Table 5. Treatment outcomes were known in 99 patients. Of these, full remission was seen in 90.0 % in response to medical treatment. Corticosteroids treatment alone was effective for 67 patients (67.7 %) in achieving full remission.

Discussion

This is the first systematic review of IgG4-RD presentation in the head and neck. Our study demonstrates a strong propensity for IgG4-RD to present in the head and neck region. We included 43 articles containing 484 patients. The most common site of presentation was the orbit, followed by the submandibular gland – with many patients having presentations in multiple head and neck and distant sites. Treatment information was also collected, showing that majority of patients receiving corticosteroids responded very well to treatment.

The vast majority of the included cases were from Asia (429 of 484 or 88.6 %) and more specifically Japan (419 of 484 or 86.6 %). Indeed, much of the literature on IgG4-RD originates from Japan [8]. This poses the question of whether IgG4-RD more prevalent in the Japanese population or simply better recognized? While IgG4-RD was first recognized in Japan, it is increasingly recognized throughout the rest of the world [7]. While cases have been reported on every continent and in most ethnic groups, reports from countries outside of Asia comprise smaller case series. This highlights the emerging status of IgG4-RD in the literature and likely an increase in reporting in the future.

While systemic presentations of IgG4-RD favor males over females with a reported ratio of 2.8-3.5:1, our study demonstrates an almost 1 to 1 ratio of head and neck manifestations [6, 9, 10]. Orbital involvement was most common subsite in the head and neck and the majority of the orbital presentations (219 cases) came from a single study [11]. Common orbital manifestations included periorbital swelling, eyelid swelling, and proptosis. Salivary gland and lacrimal gland involvement were very common and included submandibular, parotid gland, and lacrimal gland enlargement, infiltration, and formation of pseudotumours. Lymphadenopathy was a

Table 5 Treatment and progress

Treatments Received by Patients (N = 129)		n	%
Surgical Management Alone		15	11.6
Combined Surgical and Medical Management		4	3.1
Medical Management Alone		107	82.9
	Treatment with Corticosteroids[a] Alone	84	65.1
	Treatment with Corticosteroids and One Additional Immunosuppressive Agent[b]	16	12.4
	Treatment with Corticosteroids and Multiple Additional Immunosuppressive Agents	10	7.8
Treatment Outcomes (N = 99)		n	%
Full Remission with Medical Treatment		89	90.0
Full Remission with Corticosteroids Alone		67	67.7
	Intolerance, Relapse with Taper, or Treatment Failure with Corticosteroids as First Line	32	32.3
Full Remission with Addition of Single Immunosuppressive Agent to Corticosteroids		14	14.1
Full Remission with Addition of Multiple Immunosuppressive Agents to Corticosteroids		8	8.1
Remission Not Achieved		9	9.1

[a]Corticosteroids included: prednisolone, methylprednisone and triamcinolone injections
[b]Additional immunosuppressive agents included: rituximab, methotrexate, azathioprine, mycophenolate mofetil, tamoxifen, 6-mercaptopurine, chlorambucil, cyclosporine and cyclopohosphamide

particularly common presentation in the head and neck. This was often associated with lymphadenopathy elsewhere including the mediastinum and retroperitoneum. More rare forms of head and neck involvement included the thyroid gland in the form of Riedel's Thyroiditis as well as sinonasal and airway manifestations.

Few patients in our series received surgical excision alone. The majority cases received some form of medical management comprising of high-dose corticosteroids. Patients had excellent response to medical therapy alone with full remission rate of 90 %. A consensus statement from 17 referral centres in Japan developed a treatment regime of 0.6 mg/Kg prednisolone for 2 to 4 weeks with a taper over 3 to 6 months and a low daily dose for 3 years. Importantly, this regime was developed for treatment of autoimmune pancreatitis, where consequences of not treating are associated with significant morbidity and mortality [12]. However, other authors advocate watchful waiting with observation over a number of years as an acceptable treatment approach [13]. Based on our results, surgery remains most useful for obtaining histologic diagnosis.

Strict selection criteria was used in article selection. Histologic diagnosis was based on IgG4 + ve cells/ HPF and the IgG4 + ve/IgG ratio. This is considered the most rigorous definition of IgG4-RD [4, 6]. However, since biopsy from the head and neck was one of the criteria, there are likely many studies of IgG4-RD in the head and neck that were excluded as biopsies were obtained from other tissues. Unfortunately, there is a paucity of high quality publications on this topic. The majority of the information available exists in the form of case reports and small case series, which comprise of low level of evidence. There are also inconsistencies in reporting key information. Many studies were excluded due to insufficient information (152 or 74.5 %) or a lack of basic histologic information; articles lacking IgG4+ cell/HPF or the IgG4+/IgG ratio –items critical to confirming the presence of IgG4-RD-- were excluded.

Conclusions

Due to the numerous potential manifestations of IgG4-RD in the head and neck, it is crucial for otolaryngologists to be aware of this condition. A high index of suspicious is required particularly in the setting of patients who present with recurrent salivary and lacrimal gland swelling, lymphadenopathy, along with fibroinflammatory systemic involvement. This disease process remains under recognized and poorly understood. Future studies are necessary to better understand the pathophysiology and natural history of this disease.

Appendix A: search strategy
Ovid: Embase search:

1. exp salivary gland/
2. mouth disease/ or lip disease/ or exp mouth tumor/ or exp palate disease/ or exp pharynx disease/ or

exp salivary gland disease/ or exp tongue disease/ or xerostomia/
3. head/ or exp "face, nose and sinuses"/ or exp skull/
4. "head and neck disease"/ or exp "head and neck tumor"/
5. neck/
6. exp lacrimal apparatus/
7. exp lacrimal gland disease/
8. exp ear nose throat disease/
9. angiocentric eosinophilic fibrosis.mp.
10. (Facial or eyelid* or mouth or oral or gingival or lip or lips or palate or palatal or tonsil* or sinuses or sinus cavit* or salivary gland* or tongue or otorhinolaryngologic or ear or ears or larynx or laryngeal or nose or noses or paranasal or pharyngeal or parathyroid or thyroid or tracheal or sialadenitis or kuttner or submandibular or lacrimal or thyroid or dacryoadenitis or orbit or mikulicz*).ti,ab.
11. or/1-10
12. (immunoglobulin g4 or igg4).mp.
13. 11 and 12
14. limit 13 to english language
15. limit 14 to exclude medline journals
16. 14 not 15
17. limit 16 to (conference abstract or conference paper or conference proceeding or "conference review")
18. 14 not 17
19. limit 18 to embase

Ovid: Pubmed search:

1. exp Salivary Gland Diseases/
2. exp Head/
3. Neck/
4. exp Lacrimal Apparatus Diseases/ or exp Lacrimal Apparatus/ or exp Lacrimal Duct Obstruction/
5. angiocentric eosinophilic fibrosis.mp.
6. nose diseases/ or granuloma, lethal midline/ or nasal obstruction/ or exp nose neoplasms/ or exp paranasal sinus diseases/
7. orbital diseases/ or exp exophthalmos/ or orbital pseudotumor/
8. exp Frontal Sinus/ or exp Sphenoid Sinus/ or exp Maxillary Sinus/ or exp Pyriform Sinus/ or exp Ethmoid Sinus/
9. (Facial or eyelid* or mouth or oral or gingival or lip or lips or palate or palatal or tonsil* or sinuses or sinus cavit* or salivary gland* or tongue or otorhinolaryngologic or ear or ears or larynx or laryngeal or nose or noses or paranasal or pharyngeal or parathyroid or thyroid or tracheal or sialadenitis or kuttner or submandibular or

lacrimal or thyroid or dacryoadenitis or orbit* or mikulicz*).mp.
10. (immunoglobulin g4 or igg4).mp.
11. or/1-9
12. 10 and 11
13. limit 12 to english language
14. remove duplicates from 13

Competing interests
The authors declare that they have no competing interests.

Authors' contributions
GBM was involved in study design, carried out literature search, reviewed all articles, collected data, performed statistical analysis and drafted the manuscript. CCJ contributed to conception of idea for project and study design, reviewed articles critically, collected data and writing the manuscript. PS critically reviewed articles, collected data and assisted in with writing the manuscript. DWJC conceived of the study, and participated in its design and coordination and helped to draft the manuscript. All authors read and approved the final manuscript.

Acknowledgement
The authors would like to thank Dr. Hamdy El-Hakim MB, ChB, Associate Clinical Professor in the Department of Surgery and Research Director for the Division of Otolaryngology at the University of Alberta for direction in study design. As well as Mr. Dale Storie MA, MILS, Liaison librarian to the School of Public Health and Faculty of Medicine and Dentistry, University of Alberta for his kind and thorough assistance in developing search algorithm.

References
1. Hamano H, Kawa S, Horiuchi A. High serum IgG4 concentrations in patients with sclerosing pancreatitis. N Engl J Med. 2001;344(10):732–8.
2. Deshpande V, Zen Y, Chan JK. Consensus statement on the pathology of IgG4-related disease. Mod Pathol. 2012;25(9):1181–92.
3. Umehara H, Okazaki K, Masaki Y. A novel clinical entity, IgG4-related disease (IgG4RD): General concept and details. Mod Rheumatol. 2012;22(1):1–14.
4. Zen Y, Nakanuma Y. Pathogenesis of IgG4-related disease. Curr Opin Rheumatol. 2011;23(1):114–8.
5. Stromnes IM, Cerretti LM, Liggitt D, Harris RA, Goverman JM. Differential regulation of central nervous system autoimmunity by T(H)1 and T(H)17 cells. Nat Med. 2008;14(3):337–42.
6. Stone JH, Zen Y, Deshpande V. IgG4-related disease. N Engl J Med. 2012;366(6):539–51.
7. Cheuk W, Chan JK. Lymphadenopathy of IgG4-related disease: an underdiagnosed and overdiagnosed entity. Semin Diagn Pathol. 2012;29(4):226–34.
8. Brito-Zeron P, Ramos-Casals M, Bosch X, Stone JH. The clinical spectrum of IgG4-related disease. Autoimmun Rev. 2014;13(12):1203–10.
9. Mahajan VS, Mattoo H, Deshpande V, Pillai SS, Stone JH. IgG4-related disease. Annu Rev Pathol. 2014;9:315–47.
10. Kanno A, Nishimori I, Masamune A. Nationwide epidemiological survey of autoimmune pancreatitis in japan. Pancreas. 2012;41(6):835–9.
11. Japanese study group of IgG4-related ophthalmic disease. A prevalence study of IgG4-related ophthalmic disease in japan. Jpn J Ophthalmol. 2013;57(6):573–9.
12. Kamisawa T, Shimosegawa T, Okazaki K. Standard steroid treatment for autoimmune pancreatitis. Gut. 2009;58(11):1504–7.
13. Sato Y, Ohshima K, Ichimura K, et al. Ocular adnexal IgG4-related disease has uniform clinicopathology. Pathol Int. 2008;58(8):465–70.

Further reading
Abe T, Sato T, Tomaru Y, et al. Immunoglobulin G4-related sclerosing sialadenitis: Report of two cases and review of the literature. Oral Surg Oral Med Oral Pathol Oral Radiol Endod. 2009;108(4):544–50.
Aga M, Kondo S, Yamada K, et al. Warthin's tumor associated with IgG4-related disease. Auris Nasus Larynx. 2013;40(5):514–7.

Andrew N, Kearney D, Sladden N, Goss A, Selva D. Immunoglobulin G4-related disease of the hard palate. J Oral Maxillofac Surg. 2014;72(4):717–23.

Bosco JJ, Suan D, Varikatt W, Lin MW. Extra-pancreatic manifestations of IgG4-related systemic disease: A single-centre experience of treatment with combined immunosuppression. Intern Med J. 2013;43(4):417–23.

Caputo C, Bazargan A, McKelvie PA, Sutherland T, Su CS, Inder WJ. Hypophysitis due to IgG4-related disease responding to treatment with azathioprine: An alternative to corticosteroid therapy. Pituitary. 2014;17(3):251–6.

Chen TS, Figueira E, Lau OC, et al. Successful "medical" orbital decompression with adjunctive rituximab for severe visual loss in IgG4-related orbital inflammatory disease with orbital myositis. Ophthal Plast Reconstr Surg. 2014.

Cheuk W, Lee KC, Chong LY, Yuen ST, Chan JK. IgG4-related sclerosing disease: A potential new etiology of cutaneous pseudolymphoma. Am J Surg Pathol. 2009;33(11):1713–9.

Cheuk W, Yuen HK, Chan JK. Chronic sclerosing dacryoadenitis: Part of the spectrum of IgG4-related sclerosing disease? Am J Surg Pathol. 2007;31(4):643–5.

da Fonseca FL, Ramos Rde I, de Lima PP, Nogueira AB, Matayoshi S. Unilateral eyelid mass as an unusual presentation of ocular adnexal IgG4-related inflammation. Cornea. 2013;32(4):517–9.

Dahlgren M, Khosroshahi A, Nielsen GP, Deshpande V, Stone JH. Riedel's thyroiditis and multifocal fibrosclerosis are part of the IgG4-related systemic disease spectrum. Arthritis Care Res (Hoboken). 2010;62(9):1312–8.

Deshpande V, Khosroshahi A, Nielsen GP, Hamilos DL, Stone JH. Eosinophilic angiocentric fibrosis is a form of IgG4-related systemic disease. Am J Surg Pathol. 2011;35(5):701–6.

Geyer JT, Ferry JA, Harris NL, et al. Chronic sclerosing sialadenitis (kuttner tumor) is an IgG4-associated disease. Am J Surg Pathol. 2010;34(2):202–10.

Gill J, Angelo N, Yeong ML, McIvor N. Salivary duct carcinoma arising in IgG4-related autoimmune disease of the parotid gland. Hum Pathol. 2009;40(6):881–6.

Hagiya C, Tsuboi H, Yokosawa M, et al. Clinicopathological features of IgG4-related disease complicated with orbital involvement. Mod Rheumatol. 2014;24(3):471–6.

Higashiyama T, Nishida Y, Ugi S, Ishida M, Nishio Y, Ohji M. A case of extraocular muscle swelling due to IgG4-related sclerosing disease. Jpn J Ophthalmol. 2011;55(3):315–7.

Inaba H, Hayakawa T, Miyamoto W, et al. IgG4-related ocular adnexal disease mimicking thyroid-associated orbitopathy. Intern Med. 2013;52(22):2545–51.

Jalilian C, Prince HM, McCormack C, Lade S, Cheah CY. IgG4-related disease with cutaneous manifestations treated with rituximab: Case report and literature review. Australas J Dermatol. 2014;55(2):132–6.

Japanese study group of IgG4-related ophthalmic disease. A prevalence study of IgG4-related ophthalmic disease in japan. Jpn J Ophthalmol. 2013;57(6):573–9.

Kase S, Suzuki Y, Shinohara T, Kase M. IgG4-related lacrimal sac diverticulitis. Orbit. 2014;33(3):217–9.

Katsura M, Morita A, Horiuchi H, Ohtomo K, Machida T. IgG4-related inflammatory pseudotumor of the trigeminal nerve: Another component of IgG4-related sclerosing disease? AJNR Am J Neuroradiol. 2011;32(8):E150–2.

Khan TT, Halat SK, Al Hariri AB. Lacrimal gland sparing IgG4-related disease in the orbit. Ocul Immunol Inflamm. 2013;21(3):220–4.

Khosroshahi A, Carruthers MD, Deshpande V, Leb L, Reed JI, Stone JH. Cutaneous immunoglobulin G4-related systemic disease. Am J Med. 2011;124(10):e7–8.

Khosroshahi A, Carruthers MN, Deshpande V, Unizony S, Bloch DB, Stone JH. Rituximab for the treatment of IgG4-related disease: Lessons from 10 consecutive patients. Medicine (Baltimore). 2012;91(1):57–66.

Laco J, Ryska A, Celakovsky P, Dolezalova H, Mottl R, Tucek L. Chronic sclerosing sialadenitis as one of the immunoglobulin G4-related diseases: A clinicopathological study of six cases from central europe. Histopathology. 2011;58(7):1157–63.

Lee LY, Chen TC, Kuo TT. Simultaneous occurrence of IgG4-related chronic sclerosing dacryoadenitis and chronic sclerosing sialadenitis associated with lymph node involvement and warthin's tumor. Int J Surg Pathol. 2011;19(3):369–72.

Li Y, Zhou G, Ozaki T, et al. Distinct histopathological features of hashimoto's thyroiditis with respect to IgG4-related disease. Mod Pathol. 2012;25(8):1086–97.

Matsuo T, Ichimura K, Sato Y, et al. Immunoglobulin G4 (IgG4)-positive or -negative ocular adnexal benign lymphoid lesions in relation to systemic involvement. J Clin Exp Hematop. 2010;50(2):129–42.

Mudhar HS, Bhatt R, Sandramouli S. Xanthogranulomatous variant of immunoglobulin G4 sclerosing disease presenting as ptosis, proptosis and eyelid skin plaques. Int Ophthalmol. 2011;31(3):245–8.

Origuchi T, Yano H, Nakamura H, Hirano A, Kawakami A. Three cases of IgG4-related orbital inflammation presented as unilateral pseudotumor and review of the literature. Rheumatol Int. 2013;33(11):2931–6.

Paulus YM, Cockerham KP, Cockerham GC, Gratzinger D. IgG4-positive sclerosing orbital inflammation involving the conjunctiva: A case report. Ocul Immunol Inflamm. 2012;20(5):375–7.

Pusztaszeri M, Triponez F, Pache JC, Bongiovanni M. Riedel's thyroiditis with increased IgG4 plasma cells: Evidence for an underlying IgG4-related sclerosing disease? Thyroid. 2012;22(9):964–8.

Sato Y, Takeuchi M, Takata K, et al. Clinicopathologic analysis of IgG4-related skin disease. Mod Pathol. 2013;26(4):523–32.

Singh K, Rajan KD, Eberhart C. Orbital necrobiotic xanthogranuloma associated with systemic IgG4 disease. Ocul Immunol Inflamm. 2010;18(5):373–8.

Suzuki M, Nakamaru Y, Akazawa S, et al. Nasal manifestations of immunoglobulin G4-related disease. Laryngoscope. 2013;123(4):829–34.

Takahashi H, Yamamoto M, Tabeya T, et al. The immunobiology and clinical characteristics of IgG4 related diseases. J Autoimmun. 2012;39(1-2):93–6.

Takahashi Y, Kitamura A, Kakizaki H. Bilateral optic nerve involvement in immunoglobulin G4-related ophthalmic disease. J Neuroophthalmol. 2014;34(1):16–9.

Takahira M, Ozawa Y, Kawano M, et al. Clinical aspects of IgG4-related orbital inflammation in a case series of ocular adnexal lymphoproliferative disorders. Int J Rheumatol. 2012;2012:635473.

Tay SH, Thamboo TP, Teng GG. A case of multi-system IGG4-related disease. Int J Rheum Dis. 2013;16(5):599–601.

Teichman JC, Wu AY, El-Shinnawy I, Harvey JT. A case of orbital involvement in IgG4-related disease. Orbit. 2012;31(5):327–9.

Verdijk RM, Heidari P, Verschooten R, van Daele PL, Simonsz HJ, Paridaens D. Raised numbers of IgG4-positive plasma cells are a common histopathological finding in orbital xanthogranulomatous disease. Orbit. 2014;33(1):17–22.

Wallace ZS, Khosroshahi A, Jakobiec FA, et al. IgG4-related systemic disease as a cause of "idiopathic" orbital inflammation, including orbital myositis, and trigeminal nerve involvement. Surv Ophthalmol. 2012;57(1):26–33.

Yamamoto H, Yamaguchi H, Aishima S, et al. Inflammatory myofibroblastic tumor versus IgG4-related sclerosing disease and inflammatory pseudotumor: A comparative clinicopathologic study. Am J Surg Pathol. 2009;33(9):1330–40.

Zen Y, Nakanuma Y. IgG4-related disease: a cross-sectional study of 114 cases. Am J Surg Pathol. 2010;34(12):1812–9.

9

Methods considerations for nystagmography

Brian W. Blakley and Laura Chan[*] iD

Abstract

Objectives: 1. To assess the reproducibility of eye movement velocity measurement using two methods: traditional electro-oculography (EOG) and infrared video-oculography (VOG) and,
2. Determine whether the normal values for unilateral weakness and bilateral reduction of caloric responses vary according to method employed.

Background: Vestibular testing frequently involves measurement of eye movements. EOG has been the standard method for decades, but VOG and other methods have recently become popular. The assumption has been that all methods measure eye movements equally and accurately but this assumption has not been validated. In this paper we examine this assumption.

Methods: Eye movements were recorded simultaneously with commercially available EOG and VOG methods to evaluate differences in results for nineteen normal subjects undergoing caloric tests with warm and cold water. Examination of the records permitted identification and simultaneous measurement of 840 nystagmus beats.

Results: EOG and VOG measurements were correlated but the correlation was not strong (Spearman rho = 0.529, p < 0.01). Eye velocities recorded by the VOG system were greater than that for the EOG system. The mean VOG/EOG ratio was 1.71. Normal values used at our centre were adjusted to accommodate the use of video technology to account for the differences in sensitivity between EOG and VOG methods.

Conclusion: The traditional EOG-based normal value for bilateral reduction of caloric response, 30 degree per second (d/s) based on traditional EOG measurements should be revised to 50 d/s for modern VOG testing in our lab. Normal values for vestibular testing may need to be re-evaluated when new technology is introduced. Each lab should verify normal values for their own methods and equipment.

Introduction

New clinical testing techniques should be accompanied by re-evaluation of normal values. Recently developed eye movement measurement techniques include infrared, video technology and scleral search coil technology [1–3]. Of these, the scleral search coil technique is generally agreed to be the most accurate, but its use requires the patient to wear a contact lens and the equipment is expensive and prone to problems [2, 4].

The goal of this report is to assess the concurrence between electro-oculography (EOG) and video-oculography (VOG) measurements. For decades, the electrical difference between the cornea and the retina of the eye has been used to record eye movements. This electrical potential difference is small but with amplification and proper filtering it can be detected using surface electrodes. This is called electro-oculography. When EOG is used to record eye movements for caloric, saccade, pursuit and other tests, it is part of the electronystagmography (ENG) battery of tests. If video techniques are used, the test may be called videonystagmography and the eye movement recordings are video-oculography (VOG). EOG and/or VOG can be used to measure the response to caloric stimulation and is called nystagmography [5]. Some fundamental differences between EOG and VOG that could be clinically important have become apparent after experience and consideration of the recording technique [5–7]. Some of these are indicated in Table 1.

Normal values for clinical caloric testing have been based on traditional EOG measurements. The most important parameter is the unilateral weakness (UW) [3, 5, 6] which assesses the percent difference of the maximum slow phase velocity (SPEV) for warm and cool water stimuli in each ear. UW may be called reduced vestibular response or caloric weakness but is the same measure. Values are

* Correspondence: laurachan@mymts.net
Department of Otolaryngology, University of Manitoba, GB420-820 Sherbrook Street, Winnipeg, MB R3A 1RJ, Canada

Table 1 Some differences between EOG and VOG

	ELECTRO-oculography (EOG)	VIDEO-oculography (VOG)
Entity measured	Corneo-retinal electrical potential	Digitized position of a black circle presumed to be the pupil
Drift	Shift of baseline if DC recording used. Variable if AC recording	Theoretically no shift
Artifact	Eye blinks and muscle contraction are the most frequent artifacts	Dark features such as mascara, closed eyes, eye brows "fool" the system momentarily. Eye blinks, difficulty detecting the pupil causes large artifacts
Sampling rates	While most commercial units sample calorics at 30 Hz, much higher sampling rates are feasible. This is critical for accurate measurement of quick phases	Video sampling rates are usually 30–60 Hz. Sampling rates of 100 Hz requires specialized equipment.
Ease of use	Sticky electrodes are required with possible impedance problems, electrical drift and small signal	The patient wears goggles to mount the camera to, which limits eye displacement to approximately 20°
Determination of maximum slow phase velocity (SPEV)	Maximum average SPEV of the three greatest consecutive beats	Maximum average SPEV for a 10 s window of recording

considered abnormal for clinical purposes if the UW is greater than 25 % or the sum of the four caloric tests (right warm + right cool + left warm + left cool) is less than 30 d/s [5, 6]. We conducted this study to evaluate whether EOG and VOG methods provide equivalent results or whether some change in the values scale is needed according to the technique used.

Several methods of recording eye movements have emerged so it is important to compare established technique with newer ones as they are brought into practice. Fortunately, it is possible to use both the EOG and VOG systems at the same time to study exactly the same eye movements. As far as we are aware, this is the first paper in the literature to directly compare EOG and VOG results simultaneously recorded.

The number of ways that eye movement measurement techniques can be employed is large. Computer algorithms and their underlying assumptions, sampling rates, filtering, DC electrical shift, noise, and other factors may produce different results but consideration of the effects of different methods are not prominent in the literature [8, 9]. This project was performed using commercially available equipment that is assumed to represent valid general protocols for electro- and video- techniques. In deference to the possible sensitivity that manufacturers may have, the names of the companies are not included and are not considered important. Differences between the two techniques, EOG and VOG, are the focus of this paper.

Methods

We measured the slow phase velocity for the same nystagmus beats using both EOG and VOG techniques simultaneously. Preliminary data suggested that we could

expect to identify at least ten simultaneous slow-phase eye movements in each subject. We wished to have results with statistical power greater than 95 %. Using SYSTAT 3.5's power calculator and applying the standard deviation of 8 d/s and the mean difference of 3 d/s we calculated that 19 normal subjects would be required to detect a difference of 3 d/s with 95 % power at the $p = 0.05$ level. In fact, we were able to determine over 40 simultaneous SPEVs per subject.

The Human Research Ethics Committee of the University of Manitoba approved the protocol. Subjects were 19 normal volunteers who had no complaints of dizziness or ear dysfunction and who had normal otoscopic exams. EOG recording was carried out with electrocardiogram-type surface electrodes. These were applied posterior to the lateral canthus bilaterally, above and below the left eye and in the center of the forehead (reference electrode). Caloric irrigations were performed similar to ANSI standards [7] - the sampling rates were 30 Hz for EOG and 60 Hz for VOG caloric tests. Warm and cool water irrigations at 44 °C and 30 °C respectively for 20 s at 200 cm^3/min were administered in each ear with eye movement recording for 60 s. VOG recording was carried out with a camera mounted in the right eye of specially designed goggles as part of a commercially available system. Each eye was recorded with a different technique. Conjugate eye movements were assumed. The EOG electrodes were worn under the goggles, which helped stabilize the electrodes. Both systems were calibrated according to the manufacturer's directions using arrays of red diode lights. Examining the EOG and VOG records together allowed us to identify the two system's measurement of the same beats of nystagmus. The velocities measured with both methods were entered into a database.

Statistical analysis: Eye velocity data departed from a normal distribution so non-parametric tests were applied. The correlation between EOG and VOG recordings was calculated using Spearman's rho and the significance of differences assessed with the Wilcoxon signed ranks test. For UW scores, the Pearson correlation coefficient and paired t-tests were used because the UW data were normally distributed. Statistical calculations were performed using IBM SPSS v22.0.

The Jongkees formula [6] was used to calculate UW for the electro- and video recording systems for these normal subjects

$$UW = \frac{(RW + RC) - (LW + LC)}{RW + RC + LW + LC}$$

where RW, RC, LW and LC refer to the responses for right ear warm, right ear cool, left ear warm, and left ear cool, respectively. If abnormal values were obtained for these normal subjects, doubt would be cast on the validity of the technique used.

The two parameters that are most significant clinically are UW and the sum of the four caloric tests. Abnormal UW suggests that responses from the two ears are not symmetric so one ear is hypo-responsive. If the sum of the four caloric tests is less than a normal threshold value, bilateral reduction of caloric response is present which suggests significant dysfunction. Even if the two systems provide different values for eye movements, and the error is linear, the UW should still be meaningful because UW is a ratio or relative measure. This is not true for the sum of the four caloric tests. The sum of the caloric tests is an absolute measure so it will vary according to the magnitude of the measures.

Results

Eight hundred forty slow phases from the resulting nystagmus were identified on both records according to the time that they occurred. Spearman's rho for the measured velocity for EOG and VOG methods was only 0.529, departing significantly from perfect correlation of 1.0. EOG and VOG velocities were statistically significantly different ($p < 0.001$) and the correlation fell far short of our expectations, given that we were objectively measuring exactly the same quantity. Fig. 1 displays the bivariate relationship. Velocities for VOG recording were higher than for the same beats of nystagmus recorded with EOG. Fig. 2 illustrates the differences between EOG and VOG measures with box and whisker plots. The median velocities for VOG and EOG were 16 and 9.6 d/s respectively. The mean VOG/EOG ratio was 1.71.

Although the eye velocities were not normally distributed, the UW data were normally distributed so parametric tests were applied. The mean (+/-s.d.) unilateral

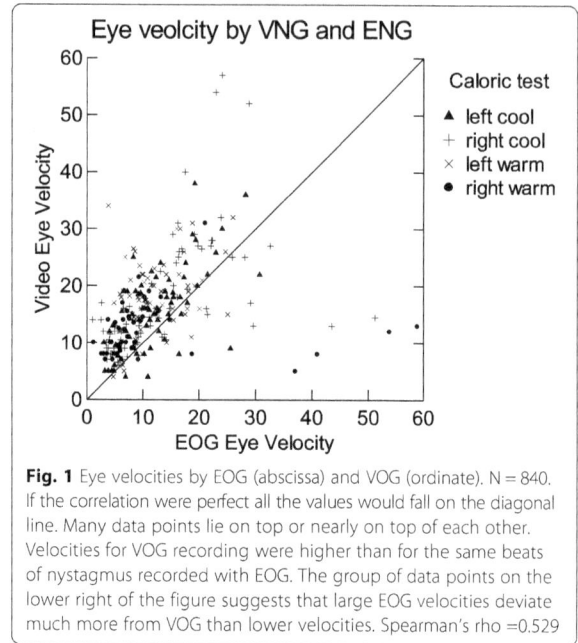

Fig. 1 Eye velocities by EOG (abscissa) and VOG (ordinate). N = 840. If the correlation were perfect all the values would fall on the diagonal line. Many data points lie on top or nearly on top of each other. Velocities for VOG recording were higher than for the same beats of nystagmus recorded with EOG. The group of data points on the lower right of the figure suggests that large EOG velocities deviate much more from VOG than lower velocities. Spearman's rho =0.529

weakness for EOG and VOG was 0.1 % (+/−22.3) and 9.3 % (+/−12.9) respectively. The Pearson correlation coefficient between unilateral weakness for EOG and VOG was 0.59, which is minimally better than the correlation for eye movement velocities.

UWs for EOG and VOG (mean +/−s.d.) were 14.69 +/−8.7 and 14.46 +/−8.48. Although these means and standard deviations were close they were statistically significantly different using the paired t-test ($p = 0.02$). Note that at the accepted threshold for normal UW (<25 %), two normal subjects would have been incorrectly labeled as abnormal whereas none of the VOG measures suggested abnormal results as shown in Fig. 3.

Discussion

For years, EOG measures have been based on the assumption that electrical potential difference between two surface electrodes is linearly dependent on degrees of rotation of the eye. This assumption must be violated because the change of corneoretinal potential occurs over a curved space but is detected between two points. As the eye displacement increases, the error under this assumption also increases. Even if the velocity measurements are inaccurate for EOG, they may still be clinically useful as long as the errors are made consistently. For these reasons, in the interest of quality, it seems important that each lab verify their own normal values using their own techniques and equipment.

New techniques of recording eye movements include scleral search coil techniques, infrared and video techniques. It is logical that the results from different

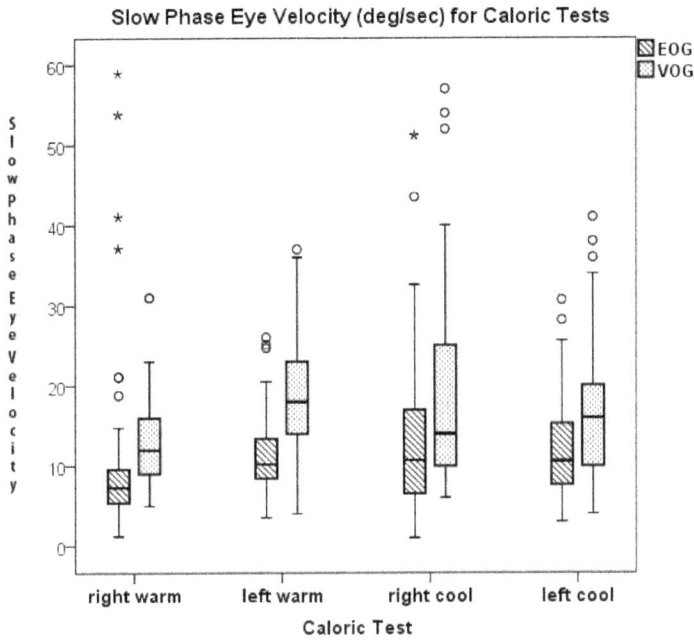

Fig. 2 Box and whisker plot of SPEV showing the median (horizontal line), interquartile range (limits of the box), outliers (o), and extreme cases (*) of the four types of caloric tests. Over all caloric tests, the median SPEV was 9.6 and 16 for EOG and VOG, respectively. The EOG measure for the same SPEV was greater suggesting greater sensitivity of the EOG technique

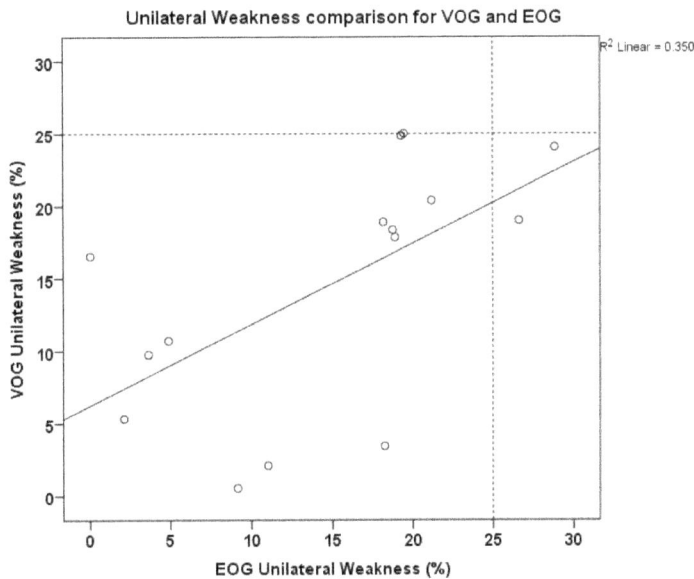

Fig. 3 Unilateral Weakness as determined by video-oculography (VOG) *versus* electro-oculography (EOG) techniques. The R [2] value suggests that 35 % of the variability of the data is explained by the two variables which is less than we expected. We suspect that the variability of the EOG measurements accounts for much of the reduced R [2]. Note that at the accepted threshold for normal UW (<25 %), two normal subjects would have been incorrectly labeled as abnormal whereas none of the VOG measures suggested abnormal results

techniques will vary to some extent but we were disappointed at how poorly EOG and VOG results correlated. EOG usually yielded lower velocities than VOG for the same slow phase eye movement. Based on these data, it appears that our normal values for the sum of four caloric tests should be reconsidered in our lab. The traditional upper limit of normal for the sum is 30 d/s using EOG methods. If VOG methods are used, this traditional normal limit should be multiplied by the ratio of the median magnitude of the velocities or 30 d/s × (16/9.6) = 50 d/s. For this reason 50 d/s is the normal value for our lab. Again, individual labs should verify these values.

For each technique, there is an infinite number of ways that the tests could be performed. Software development requires that certain assumptions be made about the data. These assumptions potentially affect results. Some of these include assumptions about optimal filtering, optimal digitization, and definition of slow phase, fast phase and artifact. The EOG system functioned properly but is old technology. While these assumptions may have accounted for some variability it seems likely that the nature of the technique (electro or video) was also a major source of error as suggested by the R [2] value of 0.35 in Fig. 3. The UW correlated a little better (R = 0.59) than absolute eye velocity measurements for the two methods. UW is a relative measure, so differences in eye velocity should give similar results assuming that measurements are accurate.

The finding that two normal subjects had an abnormal UW on EOG recording but not with VOG suggests that the lower velocities measured by EOG maybe more likely to give false results than VOG. This makes sense because variability in small velocities is more likely to result in apparent abnormal calculations for UW than larger velocities with smaller relative variability. For example, the sensitivity of EOG is approximately 2 d/s [6] or 21 % of the median EOG measure [6]. An error of the same magnitude would be only 12 % for VOG. All subjects in this study were asymptomatic normal subjects so we were reassured that UW measures were normal for VOG techniques. Since adopting the 50 d/s criteria for lower limit of normal for the sum of the four caloric tests, we have found that it seems reliable in explaining chronic, idiopathic imbalance in many patients. This will be the subject of another report on rotary chair testing.

This study has limitations. We could not assess all equipment by all manufacturers. It would also be interesting to see how the techniques differ across a range of abnormal subjects or those with eye problems.

Conclusion

EOG and VOG techniques do not provide equivalent results. Normal values should be adjusted depending on

technique used. When using video techniques, our upper limit for normal for the sum of the four caloric tests should be 50 d/s. VOG may provide more accurate caloric results but EOG can still be useful if normal values have been verified using consistent methods for the lab.

Competing interests
The authors declare that they have no competing interests.

Authors' contributions
Research performed by LC, research designed and paper written by BB. Both authors approved final manuscript prior to submission.

References
1. Gananca MM, Caovilla HH, Gananca FF. Electronystagmography *versus* videonystagmography. Braz J Otorhinolaryngol. 2010;76:399–403.
2. West PD, Sheppard ZA, King EV. Comparison of techniques for identification of peripheral vestibular nystagmus. J Laryngol Otol. 2012;126:1209–15.
3. Szirmai A, Keller B. Electronystagmographic analysis of caloric test parameters in vestibular disorders. Eur Arch Otorhinolaryngol. 2013;270:87–91.
4. MacDougall HG, Weber KP, McGarvie LA, Halmagyi GM, Curthoys IS. The video head impulse test: diagnostic accuracy in peripheral vestibulopathy. Neurology. 2009;73:1134–41.
5. Baloh RW, Honrubia V. Nystgmography Clinical Neurophysiology of the Vestibular System 4th edition. New York: Oxford University Press; 2011. p. 171–217.
6. Barber H, Stockwell C. Caloric Test. Manual of Electronystagmography. St. Louis: CV Mosby Co; 1980. p. 159–87.
7. ANSI. Procedures for testing basic vestibular function Acoustical Society of America. New York: American National Standard Institute; 1999.
8. Jalocha-Kaczka A, Pietkiewicz P, Zielinska-Blizniewska H, Milonski J, Olszewski J. Sensitivity evaluation in air and water caloric stimulation of the vestibular organs using videonystagmography. Otolaryngol Pol. 2014;68:227–32.
9. Bell SL, Barker F, Heselton H, MacKenzie E, Dewhurst D, Sanderson A. A study of the relationship between the video head impulse test and air calorics. Eur Arch Otorhinolaryngo. 2014;272(5):1287–94.

10

Postoperative abnormal response of C-reactive protein as an indicator for infectious complications after oral oncologic surgery with primary reconstruction

Masaya Akashi[1*], Shungo Furudoi[1], Kazunobu Hashikawa[2], Akiko Sakakibara[1], Takumi Hasegawa[1], Takashi Shigeta[1], Tsutomu Minamikawa[1] and Takahide Komori[1]

Abstract

Background: C-reactive protein (CRP) screening has been reported to be reliable for detection of infectious complications. Postoperative abnormal response of CRP can predict wound infection in colorectal surgery. This study aimed to determine the efficacy of CRP monitoring to detect infectious complications in oral oncologic surgery.

Methods: One hundred patients who underwent oral cancer resection with primary reconstruction were enrolled. Postoperative kinetics of CRP were classified into a normal or abnormal response.

Results: A normal CRP response after surgery was observed in 61 patients and an abnormal response was observed in 39. There were postoperative infectious complications in 21 patients, with surgical site infections in 13 patients (early onset in six and late onset in seven). Non-wound infections were found in nine patients. Sensitivity, specificity, the positive predictive value, and the negative predictive value for abnormal CRP response as a predictor for early infectious complications were 100%, 70.1%, 35.9%, and 100%, respectively.

Conclusion: Postoperative serial CRP screening is a useful test as an indicator of infectious complications in oral oncologic surgery. Normal CRP responses can rule out almost all early infectious complications.

Keywords: Oral cancer, Infectious complication, Surgical site infection, Non-wound infection, C-reactive protein

Background

Infectious complications after oral oncologic surgery with primary reconstruction are common, and associated with functional morbidity and prolonged hospitalization [1]. Because oral oncologic surgery is a clean-contaminated surgery, the postoperative surgical site infection (SSI) rate is high, occurring in approximately 20% of patients [2,3]. Severe SSI in oral oncologic surgery sometimes causes oro-cervical fistula, which can be a heavy burden for patients and medical staff. Significant morbidity in the immediate postoperative period is also caused by non-wound infections, with an incidence of 10% in patients who undergo

oral cancer surgery, with the majority being pulmonary [4]. Inadequate treatment of pulmonary complications can be life-threatening for patients. Prediction for infectious complications contributes to their appropriate management.

C-reactive protein (CRP) is an acute-phase reactant synthesized by hepatocytes, largely in response to pro-inflammatory cytokines [5]. CRP is not specific for a particular disease because a rise in CRP level is observed with inflammation, trauma, malignancy, and tissue infarction. CRP is present only in trace amounts in healthy subjects, and CRP levels increase within 6 hours after the onset of bacterial infection [6,7]. A rise in CRP levels may be earlier in a pathological process than other non-specific markers (e.g., fever), and falls rapidly on resolution of inflammation [8]. CRP is considered to be

* Correspondence: akashim@med.kobe-u.ac.jp
[1]Department of Oral and Maxillofacial Surgery, Kobe University Graduate School of Medicine, Kusunoki-cho 7-5-1, Chuo-ku, Kobe 650-0017, Japan
Full list of author information is available at the end of the article

useful for detection of an inflammatory response early in its course, and also for monitoring disease activity [5].

A rise in CRP level in acute-phase reactants has been successfully used as a marker of infection after surgical procedures [9,10]. In relation to surgery, the normal CRP response is rapid production of CRP until the peak level is reached, and this postsurgical response (i.e., an initial rise in CRP) is followed by reduction, and an eventual return to the normal range. CRP levels rise postoperatively to a maximum on the 3rd day, and then CRP levels returned to near normal levels on postoperative day 7 [7,11]. These characteristic kinetics of CRP levels after surgery are termed an "increase and decrease pattern". In eventful cases, "a steady rise or second rise" in CRP level tends to be seen [11]. These abnormal CRP responses are considered to be a predictor for incisional SSI in general surgery such as colorectal surgery, if pneumonia or anastomotic leakage are unlikely or excluded [11].

The purpose of this study was to determine the efficacy of CRP monitoring as a detector of infectious complications in oral oncologic surgery, as well as general surgery.

Methods

A total of 102 consecutive patients underwent oral cancer resection with primary reconstruction at Kobe University Hospital from May 2009 to October 2013. The criterion for enrollment in this study was 1 month or more of follow-up postoperatively without a loss. Two patients were excluded because of perioperative mortalities, with one patient with postoperative acute respiratory distress syndrome, and one multiorgan failure after surgery. Epidemiological data were retrospectively gathered from the medical charts as follows: age, sex, histological diagnosis, primary tumor sites, TNM classification, diabetes, preoperative radiotherapy, concurrent neck dissection, reconstructive procedures, postoperative infectious complications, including SSI and non-wound infections, estimated blood loss, and surgical time.

All of the patients received prophylactic antibiotic therapy for 3 days after surgery. Blood samples were taken preoperatively, and on postoperative days 1–7. The reference value of CRP was < 4.0 mg/L. The patterns of postoperative CRP kinetics were classified into three groups as follows: (1) CRP values at day 7 that were below 4.0 mg/L without an abnormal response were defined as "early decrease"; (2) an abnormal response included a "second rise" in either parameter at day 5 or 7, with an increase over 3.0 mg/L; and (3) CRP values at day 7 that were over 4.0 mg/L were defined as "delayed decrease".

The definition of SSI was purulent discharge either spontaneously or by incision, and drainage from the surgical region, including the flap donor site or the presence of an orocutaneous fistula, regardless of etiology within 30 days after surgery [12]. SSI within 14 days after surgery was defined as early onset, and other SSIs were late onset. Perioperative non-wound infections were defined as infections of the tracheobronchial tree, urinary tract, or blood, proven by the isolation of pathogenic organisms from appropriate sources in the clinical settings of fever, sputum, pyuria, or sepsis within 14 days after surgery [4]. Pneumonia was diagnosed with chest-X-ray or computed tomography (CT) suggestive of pneumonia and increased oxygen requirement. Sensitivity, specificity, the positive predictive value (PPV), and the negative predictive value (NPV) were determined based on the results.

Fisher's exact test was used to identify significant associations among categorical values. Statistical significance was accepted for p values of <0.05.

The Institutional Review Board of the Kobe University Hospital approved this retrospective study.

Results
Study population
At the time of surgery, the median age of the 100 patients was 68 years (range, 32–90 years), and there were 60 men and 40 women. Histological diagnosis was squamous cell carcinoma in 99 patients and mucoepidermoid carcinoma in one patient. Primary tumor sites were as follows: 35 in the tongue, 24 in the lower gingiva, 15 in the floor of the mouth, 13 in the buccal mucosa, nine in the upper gingiva, three in the mandible, and one in the lower lip. Clinical T-stages were as follows: T2 51, T3 16, and T4 19; N-stages N0 33, N1 24, and N2 29; M-stage M0 86; and recurrence in 14 patients. Twenty-six patients had diabetes. Eight patients underwent preoperative radiotherapy. Unilateral modified radical neck dissection (MRND) was performed in 61 patients, unilateral supraomohyoid neck dissection (SOHND) in 19, bilateral MRND in 11, unilateral MRND/SOHND in one, and neck dissection was not performed in eight. Reconstructive procedures were as follows: radial forearm free flap in 53 patients, rectus abdominis myocutaneous free flap in 25, fibula osteocutaneous free flap in 12, pedicled pectoralis major myocutaneous flap in seven, double free flap (combination of the radial forearm free flap and fibula osteocutaneous free flap) in two, and latissimus dorsi myocutaneous free flap in one. The median operation duration and blood loss were 724.3 minutes (range, 513–1057 minutes) and 891.2 ml (range, 96–4742 ml), respectively.

Postoperative infectious complications and pattern of CRP response
After surgery, CRP levels increased in all of the patients and the peak amplitude varied depending on the surgical stress. The median CRP levels in the "early decrease", "delayed decrease", and "second rise" groups are shown in Figure 1.

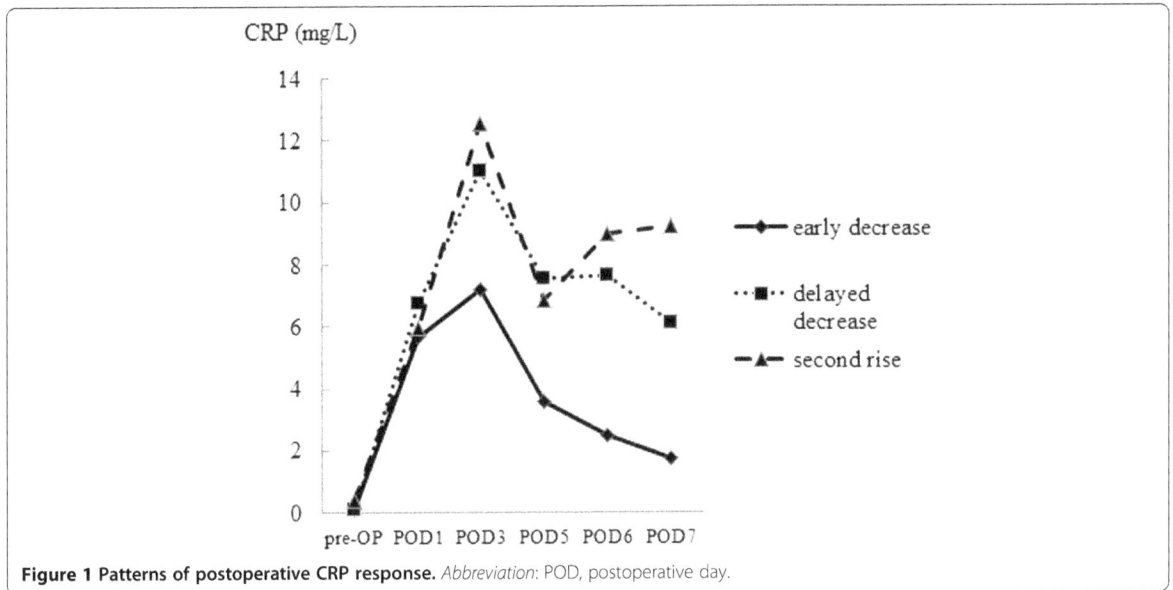

Figure 1 Patterns of postoperative CRP response. *Abbreviation*: POD, postoperative day.

There were postoperative infectious complications in 21 patients. Their characteristics are shown in Table 1. SSIs were found 13 in patients (early onset in six and late onset in seven). Eleven SSIs were in the orocervical region and two were in the donor site of the free fibula flap. Early onset SSIs occurred at a median of 7.5 postoperative days (range, 3–9 days). Late onset SSIs occurred at a median of 26 postoperative days (range, 19–30 days). Non-wound infections were as follows: pneumonia in six patients, catheter-related blood stream infection (CRBSI) in two, and sepsis of unknown cause with positive bacterial blood culture in one. The coincidence of early onset SSI and pneumonia was observed in one patient. Pneumonia, confirmed with chest CT in five patients and with chest X-ray in one patient, was treated with intravenous antibiotic therapy selected by the Division of Infectious Diseases Therapeutics in our hospital (tazobactam/piperacillin

[TAZ/PIPC] in two patients, SBT/ABPC in one, TAZ/PIPC and ciproxan in one, and azactam for pseudomonas pneumonia in one). CRBSI was found from an intra-arterial catheter (A-line) in one patient and from a central venous catheter in one patient. Bacteria isolated from blood cultures were Enterobacter species in an A-line case treated with meropenem, and Bacillus species in a central venous catheter case treated with vancomycin. There was no significant association between the occurrence of infectious complications and diabetes ($p = 0.78$) or preoperative radiotherapy ($p = 0.12$).

Six of eight patients with a second rise in CRP (75.0%) had postoperative infectious complications (pneumonia, four; CRBSI, one; sepsis of unknown cause, one). Eleven of 31 patients with a delayed decrease in CRP (35.5%) had postoperative infectious complications (early onset SSI, five; late onset SSI, three; pneumonia, one; CRBSI,

Table 1 Postoperative infectious complications and CRP response

Characteristic	No. of Patients (N = 100)	Pattern of CRP response (%)		
		Early decrease (N = 61)	Delayed decrease (N = 31)	Second rise (N = 8)
Infectious complications	21	4 (6.6)	11 (35.5)	6 (75.0)
SSI	13	4 (6.6)	9 (29.0)	–
Early onset	6	–	6 (19.4)	–
Late onset	7	4 (6.6)	3 (9.7)	–
Non-wound infections	9	–	3 (9.7)	6 (75.0)
Pneumonia	6	–	2 (6.5)	4 (50.0)
CRBSI	2	–	1 (3.7)	1 (12.5)
Unknown cause	1	–	–	1 (12.5)

Abbreviations: *SSI* surgical site infections, *CRBSI* catheter related blood stream infection.

one; and coincidence of early onset SSI and pneumonia, one). Four of 61 patients with an early decrease in CRP (6.6%) had late onset SSIs (Table 1).

When a positive test was defined as a postoperative abnormal response of CRP, including a delayed decrease and second rise, examination of CRP for predicting postoperative infectious complications showed true positive results in 17 and false positive results in 22 patients. True negative results were recorded in 57 patients and four false negative results were observed. Except for cases of late onset SSI, CRP monitoring for early infectious complications showed true positive results in 14 patients and false positive results in 25 patients. True negative results were recorded in 61 patients, and no false negative result was observed. Sensitivity, specificity, PPV, and NPV for all postoperative infectious complications, as well as those, except for late onset SSI, are shown in Table 2.

Discussion

The postoperative course of primary reconstruction for large defects following oral cancer resection has complex and diverse complications. SSI often requires long-term wound treatment and prolonged hospital stays, which are a heavy burden for patients and medical staff. Although the incidence of postoperative wound infections after head and neck cancer surgery without administration of perioperative antibiotics ranges from 24–87% [13], some prospective studies recently reported that the wound infection rate has decreased in the range of 14–40% through prophylactic antibiotics [4,14]. The occurrence rate of SSI, particularly after oral cancer surgery, was reported as 19.8% by Liu et al. [2] and 21% by Cloke et al. [3] Postoperative pulmonary complications are also common (10–47%) in head and neck reconstructive surgery, and lead to longer hospital stays and increase mortality [15-20]. In our study, the occurrence rate of postoperative infectious complications was 21% (SSI, 13%; non-wound infection, 9%) under the administration of prophylaxis antibiotics.

Comprehension of the postoperative course in eventful cases and reliable screening tests for prediction of postoperative infections would contribute to appropriate treatment of postoperative infectious complications and improve postsurgical outcome. In some reports, postoperative CRP monitoring with a focus on abnormal CRP response (i.e., a steady or second rise in CRP from postoperative days 5 to

7) was considered to be a reliable predictor of SSI [7,11]. Kang et al. reported that the sensitivity, specificity, PPV, and NPV for an abnormal CRP response were 100%, 96.8%, 31.3%, and 100%, respectively, as a predictor for early onset SSI after spinal surgery [7]. Based on the time to clinical presentation, SSI can be categorized as early, delayed, or late onset. CRP monitoring in the early period after surgery might have a limitation in detecting late onset SSI, which might have a hematogenous origin or result from the intraoperative seeding of microbes, with infections remaining subclinical for an extended period [7]. All four false negative cases in this study were late onset SSI due to an infected old hematoma. This finding indicates that late onset SSI is difficult to predict only by perioperative CRP monitoring, as previously shown. Fujii et al. [11] reported that persistent elevation of CRP was predictive of incisional SSI (sensitivity, 71.4%; specificity, 83.1%) in colorectal surgery if pneumonia or anastomotic leakage was unlikely or excluded. Another report showed that a second rise or failure to achieve a decrease in postoperative CRP values had good sensitivity and a good predictive value for postoperative infections [21]. We defined a deviation from normal CRP kinetics after surgery as a second rise or delayed decrease. In the second rise group, all infectious complications were non-wound infection, while a delayed decrease in CRP was observed in early onset SSI cases. The sensitivity, specificity, PPV, and NPV for early infectious complications in our study were similar to those previously reported [7]. However, there are differences between oral oncologic surgery and spinal or colorectal surgery as follows. (1) Oral oncologic surgery has traditionally been considered clean-contaminated surgery. (2) Postoperative pulmonary complications are common among patients undergoing oral oncologic surgery with primary reconstruction requiring tracheostomy and planned postoperative mechanical ventilation in an intensive care unit. (3) There is a difference in surgical invasiveness between oral oncologic surgery and spinal or colorectal surgery.

Early identification of infections is still a challenge for clinicians. A previous meta-analysis reported that procalcitonin levels are more accurate markers for bacterial infections than CRP levels [22], while the usefulness of perioperative CRP monitoring in general surgery is generally accepted. Although Cole et al. [5] found no correlation between CRP levels and the occurrence of infection within the first 3 days after surgery, other studies have confirmed that CRP is not a good indicator of the presence of early postoperative infection [23]. We consider that a rise in CRP level after postoperative day 3 may indicate infection. Therefore, CRP has a clear role in monitoring response to treatment when infection is diagnosed [24]. Kang et al. mentioned that their management strategy for a postoperative abnormal CRP response, including a steady and second rise in CRP levels at postoperative

Table 2 Prediction of infectious complications

Infectious complications	Sensitivity	Specificity	PPV	NPV%
All	80.1	72.2	43.6	93.4
Except for late onset SSI	100	70.1	35.9	100

Abbreviations: SSI, surgical site infections; PPV, positive predictive value; NPV, negative predictive value.

day 5 or 7, was an immediate return to antibiotic therapy with a different regimen [7]. This strategy was decided upon because an abnormal CRP rise suggests that prophylactic antibiotics may be ineffective. When there is a postoperative abnormal CRP response with no clear evidence of intercurrent infection or other inflammatory processes, close observation for signs of SSI and serial monitoring of laboratory parameters are considered to be important [7].

In CRP "second rise" group in this study, all infectious complications were non-wound infections, treated with intravenous antibiotic therapies selected by the Division of Infectious Diseases Therapeutics in our hospital. CRP "delayed decrease" group in this study could be further classified into two patterns of kinetics as follows. (A) The maximum peak level of CRP on the 3rd day after surgery was so high with a subsequent steady decline, and CRP levels on postoperative day 7 could not recover within the normal range. (B) CRP levels within the first 3 days were not so high without a subsequent decrease between postoperative day 5 and 7. The former might not require prolonging or changing antibiotics in uncomplicated cases, irrespective of a high level of CRP. The latter should be kept under careful observation for signs of infection.

In conclusion, postoperative serial CRP screening is considered as one of the reliable indicators of postoperative infectious complications in oral oncologic surgery. A normal CRP response can rule out almost all postoperative infectious complications, except for late onset SSI, which is often caused by hematogenous origin. Therefore, late onset SSI can probably be prevented by intraoperative hemostasis and appropriate drainage.

Competing interests
The authors declare that they have no competing interests.

Authors' contributions
MA designed the study, performed the data analyses, and drafted the manuscript. SF and KH contributed to study concept and design. AS, TH, TS, and TM contributed to data collection and analysis. TK revised the article for important intellectual content. All authors read and approved the final manuscript.

Author details
[1]Department of Oral and Maxillofacial Surgery, Kobe University Graduate School of Medicine, Kusunoki-cho 7-5-1, Chuo-ku, Kobe 650-0017, Japan. [2]Department of Plastic Surgery, Kobe University Graduate School of Medicine, Kobe, Japan.

References
1. Robbins KT, Favrot S, Hanna D, Cole R. Risk of wound infection in patients with head and neck cancer. Head Neck. 1990;12:143–8.
2. Liu SA, Wong YK, Poon CK, Wang CC, Wang CP, Tung KC. Risk factors for wound infection after surgery in primary oral cavity cancer patients. Laryngoscope. 2007;117:166–71.
3. Cloke DJ, Green JE, Khan AL, Hodgkinson PD, McLean NR. Factors influencing the development of wound infection following free-flap reconstruction for intra-oral cancer. Br J Plast Surg. 2004;57:556–60.
4. Skitarelić N, Morović M, Manestar D. Antibiotic prophylaxis in clean-contaminated head and neck oncological surgery. J Craniomaxillofac Surg. 2007;35:15–20.
5. Cole DS, Watts A, Scott-Coombes D, Avades T. Clinical utility of perioperative C-reactive protein testing in general surgery. Ann R Coll Surg Engl. 2008;90:317–21.
6. Pepys MB. C-reactive protein fifty years on. Lancet. 1981;1:653–7.
7. Kang BU, Lee SH, Ahn Y, Choi WC, Choi YG. Surgical site infection in spinal surgery: detection and management based on serial C-reactive protein measurements. J Neurosurg Spine. 2010;13:158–64.
8. Pepys MB, Hirschfield GM. C-reactive protein: a critical update. J Clin Invest. 2003;111:1805–12.
9. Gabay C, Kushner I. Acute-phase proteins and other systemic responses to inflammation. N Engl J Med. 1999;340:448–54.
10. Mustard Jr RA, Bohnen JM, Haseeb S, Kasina R. C-reactive protein levels predict postoperative septic complications. Arch Surg. 1987;122:69–73.
11. Fujii T, Tabe Y, Yajima R, Tsutsumi S, Asao T, Kuwano H. Relationship between C-reactive protein levels and wound infections in elective colorectal surgery: C-reactive protein as a predictor for incisional SSI. Hepatogastroenterology. 2011;58:752–5.
12. Johnson JT, Myers EN, Thearle PB, Sigler BA, Schramm Jr VL. Antimicrobial prophylaxis for contaminated head and neck surgery. Laryngoscope. 1984;94:46–51.
13. Weber RS, Callender DL. Antibiotic prophylaxis in clean-contaminated head and neck oncologic surgery. Ann Otol Rhinol Laryngol Suppl. 1992;155:16–20.
14. Penel N, Fournier C, Roussel-Delvallez M, Lefebvre D, Kara A, Mallet Y, et al. Prognostic significance of wound infections following major head and neck cancer surgery: an open non-comparative prospective study. Support Care Cancer. 2004;12:634–49.
15. Rao MK, Reilley TE, Schuller DE, Young DC. Analysis of risk factors for postoperative pulmonary complications in head and neck surgery. Laryngoscope. 1992;102:45–7.
16. McCulloch TM, Jensen NF, Girod DA, Tsue TT, Weymuller Jr EA. Risk factors for pulmonary complications in the postoperative head and neck surgery patient. Head Neck. 1997;19:372–7.
17. Jones NF, Jarrahy R, Song JI, Kaufman MR, Markowitz B. Postoperative medical complications—not microsurgical complications—negatively influence the morbidity, mortality, and true costs after microsurgical reconstruction for head and neck cancer. Plast Reconstr Surg. 2007;119:2053–60.
18. Petrar S, Bartlett C, Hart RD, MacDougall P. Pulmonary complications after major head and neck surgery: A retrospective cohort study. Laryngoscope. 2012;122:1057–61.
19. Yeung JK, Harrop R, McCreary O, Leung LT, Hirani N, McKenzie D, et al. Delayed mobilization after microsurgical reconstruction: an independent risk factor for pneumonia. Laryngoscope. 2013;123:2996–3000.
20. BuSaba NY, Schaumberg DA. Predictors of prolonged length of stay after major elective head and neck surgery. Laryngoscope. 2007;117:1756–63.
21. Mok JM, Pekmezci M, Piper SL, Boyd E, Berven SH, Burch S, et al. Use of C-reactive protein after spinal surgery: comparison with erythrocyte sedimentation rate as predictor of early postoperative infectious complications. Spine. 2008;33:415–21.
22. Simon L, Gauvin F, Amre DK, Saint-Louis P, Lacroix J. Serum procalcitonin and C-reactive protein levels as markers of bacterial infection: a systematic review and meta-analysis. Clin Infect Dis. 2004;39:206–17.
23. Giannoudis PV, Smith MR, Evans RT, Bellamy MC, Guillou PJ. Serum CRP and IL-6 levels after trauma. Not predictive of septic complications in 31 patients. Acta Orthop Scand. 1998;69:184–8.
24. Khan MH, Smith PN, Rao N, Donaldson WF. Serum C-reactive protein levels correlate with clinical response in patients treated with antibiotics for wound infections after spinal surgery. Spine J. 2006;6:311–5.

11

Face and content validity of a novel, web-based otoscopy simulator for medical education

Brandon Wickens[1], Jordan Lewis[2], David P Morris[4], Murad Husein[1], Hanif M Ladak[1,2,3†] and Sumit K Agrawal[1,2,3,5*†]

Abstract

Background: Despite the fact that otoscopy is a widely used and taught diagnostic tool during medical training, errors in diagnosis are common. Physical otoscopy simulators have high fidelity, but they can be expensive and only a limited number of students can use them at a given time.

Objectives: 1) To develop a purely web-based otoscopy simulator that can easily be distributed to students over the internet. 2) To assess face and content validity of the simulator by surveying experts in otoscopy.

Methods: An otoscopy simulator, OtoTrain™, was developed at Western University using web-based programming and Unity 3D. Eleven experts from academic institutions in North America were recruited to test the simulator and respond to an online questionnaire. A 7-point Likert scale was used to answer questions related to face validity (realism of the simulator), content validity (expert evaluation of subject matter and test items), and applicability to medical training.

Results: The mean responses for the face validity, content validity, and applicability to medical training portions of the questionnaire were all ≤3, falling between the "Agree", "Mostly Agree", and "Strongly Agree" categories. The responses suggest good face and content validity of the simulator. Open-ended questions revealed that the primary drawbacks of the simulator were the lack of a haptic arm for force feedback, a need for increased focus on pneumatic otoscopy, and few rare disorders shown on otoscopy.

Conclusion: OtoTrain™ is a novel, web-based otoscopy simulator that can be easily distributed and used by students on a variety of platforms. Initial face and content validity was encouraging, and a skills transference study is planned following further modifications and improvements to the simulator.

Keywords: Otology, Otoscopy, Medical education, Simulation, Web-based, Simulator, Otitis media, Otitis media with effusion, Metrics, Evaluation

Introduction

Otologic diseases are highly prevalent, can significantly impair function, and are a costly burden to the healthcare system. Otitis media with effusion has affected 2.1% of the global population, and it can cause deficits in language acquisition and social interaction [1]. Acute otitis media is the most common reason antibiotics are prescribed for children in the United States [2]. Expertise in otoscopy is essential for assessing and diagnosing these illnesses, however studies have demonstrated the need for improved otoscopy education. In 1992, Fisher and Pfleiderer revealed that general practitioners possessed comparable otoscopy skills to medical students, thereby demonstrating room for improvement in otoscopy training [3]. Studies evaluating pediatric residents' assessment of ear disease determined a 41% accuracy rate and only a slight agreement between resident diagnosis and tympanometry [4,5]. Pichichero and Poole evaluated the ability of General Practitioners and Pediatricians to

* Correspondence: Sumit.Agrawal@lhsc.on.ca
†Equal contributors
[1]Department of Otolaryngology – Head and Neck Surgery, Western University, London, Ontario, Canada
[2]Department of Medical Biophysics, Western University, London, Ontario, Canada
Full list of author information is available at the end of the article

diagnose otitis media with effusion and acute otitis media, and their diagnostic accuracy rates were similar ranging from 36-51% [6,7].

Otoscopy simulators to date have primarily relied on physical models of the entire head, or of the ear in isolation [8-10]. These simulators have the advantage of high fidelity, as trainees use an actual otoscope to navigate through the synthetic ear and visualize the images of the tympanic membrane. However, physical simulators can be costly, they require dedicated space within the educational institution, they are 'single-user' making scheduling numerous trainees tedious, and distribution to developing nations may be difficult.

Recently, computer-based technology and web-based technology in medical education have been gaining in popularity [11-13]. Pure internet-based simulators are relatively low-cost in terms of servers and bandwidth, and they allow hundreds of students to use the platform simultaneously. Students can access the simulators on any internet-connected computer or mobile device, so they are not limited to their educational institution or particular scheduled times. Administrators and educators can also benefit with the ability to manage classes online, send reminder e-mails with links to the software, and track students' progress and results remotely. Achieving realism in computer simulators can be difficult, therefore the use of haptic devices for force feedback or hybrid-simulators may be necessary.

The primary objective of this study was to develop a novel web-based otoscopy simulator that could easily and inexpensively be deployed to any students with an internet connection. The secondary objective was to survey experts to establish face and content validity of the simulator.

Methods

Simulator development

The otoscopy simulator was designed and developed at Western University in the Auditory Biophysics Laboratory and is called OtoTrain. Models of the auricle and ear canal were created in Unity 3D (Unity Technologies, San Francisco, California), a gaming engine that works across desktop, mobile, web, and console-based platforms. The Unity plug-in allowed for real-time interaction with the 3D models of the ear over the internet.

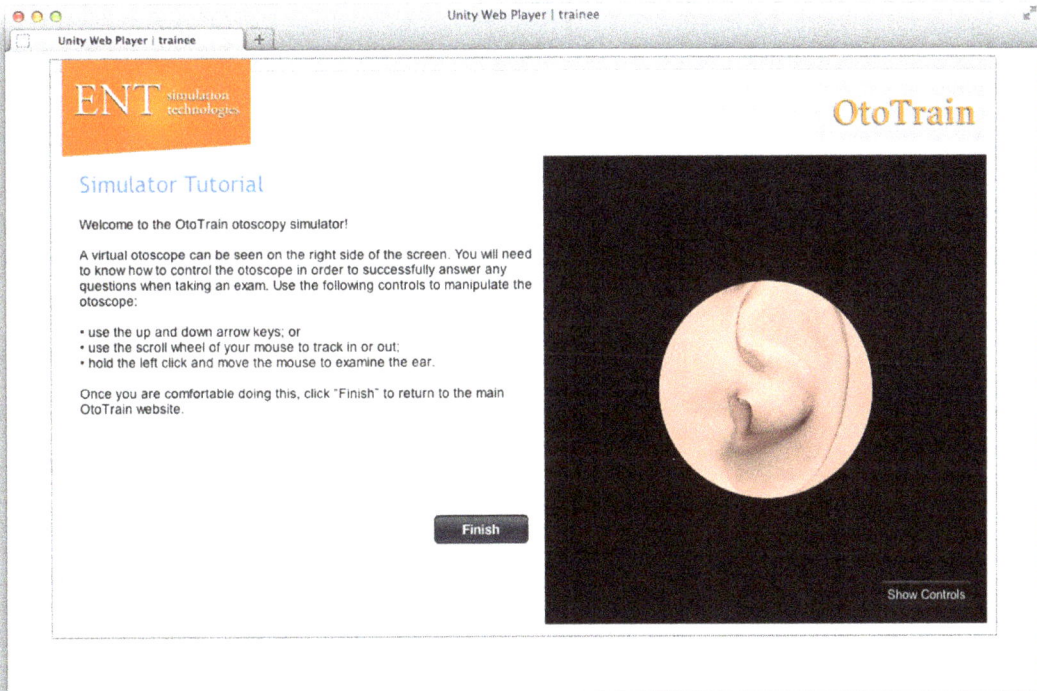

Figure 1 Otoscopy simulator tutorial module.

Users can log into the system as either an Administrator, Examiner, or Trainee. The Administrator module provides the ability to manage entire classes and e-mail addresses, create/delete accounts, and manage the program settings. The Examiner module allows the user to create custom exams with multiple-choice questions and a choice of pathologies. The latest version of the simulator allows examiners to upload tympanic membrane images from their personal collections, and these are dynamically attached to the 3D ear canal models within the simulator. Examiners can share their exams with other users, place them into 'study' mode (allows students to browse pathologies and receive the answers instantly), or place them into a formal 'exam' mode (students take an exam and the results are sent to the examiner). Examiners have the ability to send a link of their exam to an entire class, set time limits for completion, track which students have completed the exam, and automatically tabulate results.

Trainees can login to the simulator and learn otoscopic techniques, browse pathologies, or take a simulator tutorial (Figure 1). When browsing in 'study'

mode, the speculum is made translucent to ease the navigation down the ear canal and keep the students oriented (Figure 2). During the simulation, the virtual otoscopy is performed using a mouse/trackpad and keyboard. Feedback regarding the accuracy of the diagnosis and various metrics are immediately given when in 'study' mode (Figure 3). Current metrics include the percentage of tympanic membrane visualized, time to completion, and 'force' against the ear canal. The virtual 'force' is calculated in proportion to the displacement magnitude past the ear canal wall, and no actual haptic feedback is felt by the trainees. Trainees can then access further pathology descriptions and image examples to enhance their learning around each case (Figures 4 and 5).

OtoTrain validation
A comprehensive face and content validity questionnaire was developed by the authors as a validated tool assessing otoscopy simulation could not be found in the literature. The survey contained three assessment components. The first used a 7-point

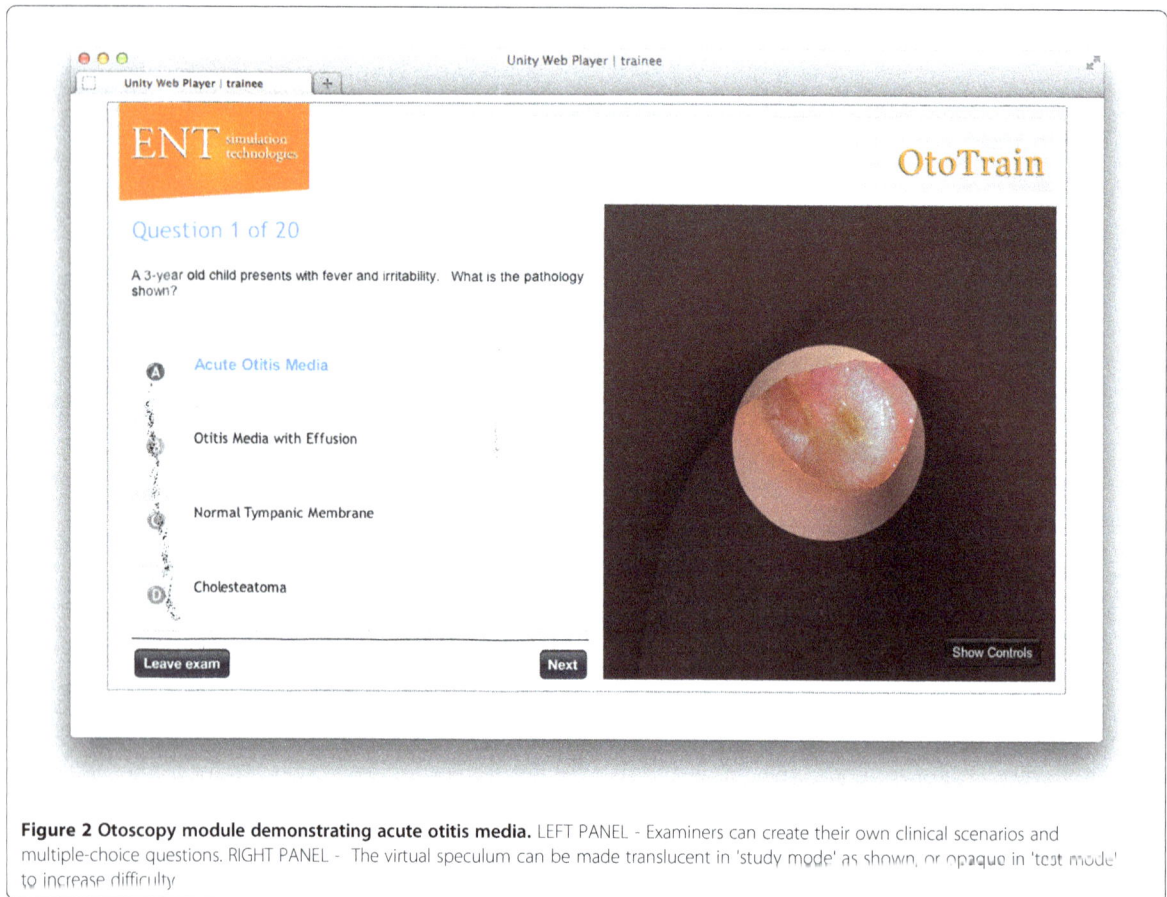

Figure 2 Otoscopy module demonstrating acute otitis media. LEFT PANEL - Examiners can create their own clinical scenarios and multiple-choice questions. RIGHT PANEL - The virtual speculum can be made translucent in 'study mode' as shown, or opaque in 'test mode' to increase difficulty.

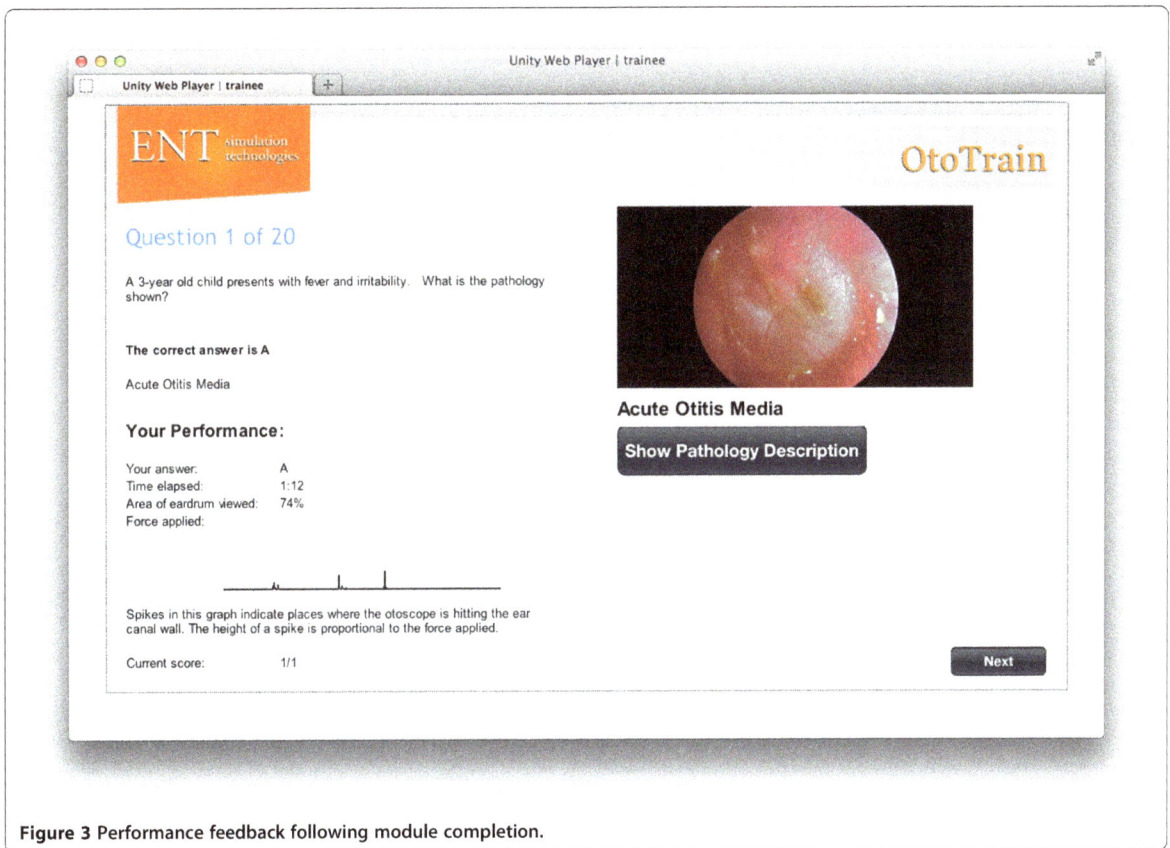

Figure 3 Performance feedback following module completion.

Likert scale (1 – strongly agree, 4 – neutral, 7 – strongly disagree) to assess the face and content validity of the simulator, applicability to training curriculum, and overall usability. The second component compared the otoscopy simulator to traditional lecture and atlas methods of otoscopy education, to assess whether experts felt this novel simulator would be beneficial. The third component solicited qualitative feedback using open-text questions regarding perceived advantages or limitations of the simulator, alternative applications and suggestions for improvement of the OtoTrain™ prototype. The survey was entered into an online survey tool, Survey Monkey (www.surveymonkey.com, Palo Alto, California).

Eleven experts actively involved in teaching otoscopy were contacted to evaluate the simulator and complete the assessments. The experts were based in the following academic institutions: Stanford University, Ohio State University, Dalhousie University, McGill University, University of Ottawa, University of Toronto, University of British Columbia, and the National Centre of Audiology.

An initial video oriented the experts to the simulator, and they were then given an unlimited time with access to the Administrator, Examiner, and Trainee modules. The results of the survey were then collected electronically.

Results

A total of eleven experts completed the survey. There were 7 males and 4 females, with a mean number of years in practice of 11.1 years (range, 1–18 years). By specialty, there were 5 Neurotologists, 5 Pediatric Otolaryngologists, and 1 Audiologist.

Face validity

The degree to which the simulator appears to be realistic was assessed using a 7-point Likert scale ranging from 1 (strongly agree) to 7 (strongly disagree). Two domains were assessed: (i) appearance of the normal/abnormal external auditory canal anatomy, and (ii) appearance of the normal/abnormal tympanic membrane (eardrum) anatomy. The results are tabulated in Table 1. The mean scores across both study domains measured at ≤ 3, falling between the "Agree", "Mostly Agree", and "Strongly Agree" categories. This was considered to be an acceptable realistic representation of the relevant anatomy.

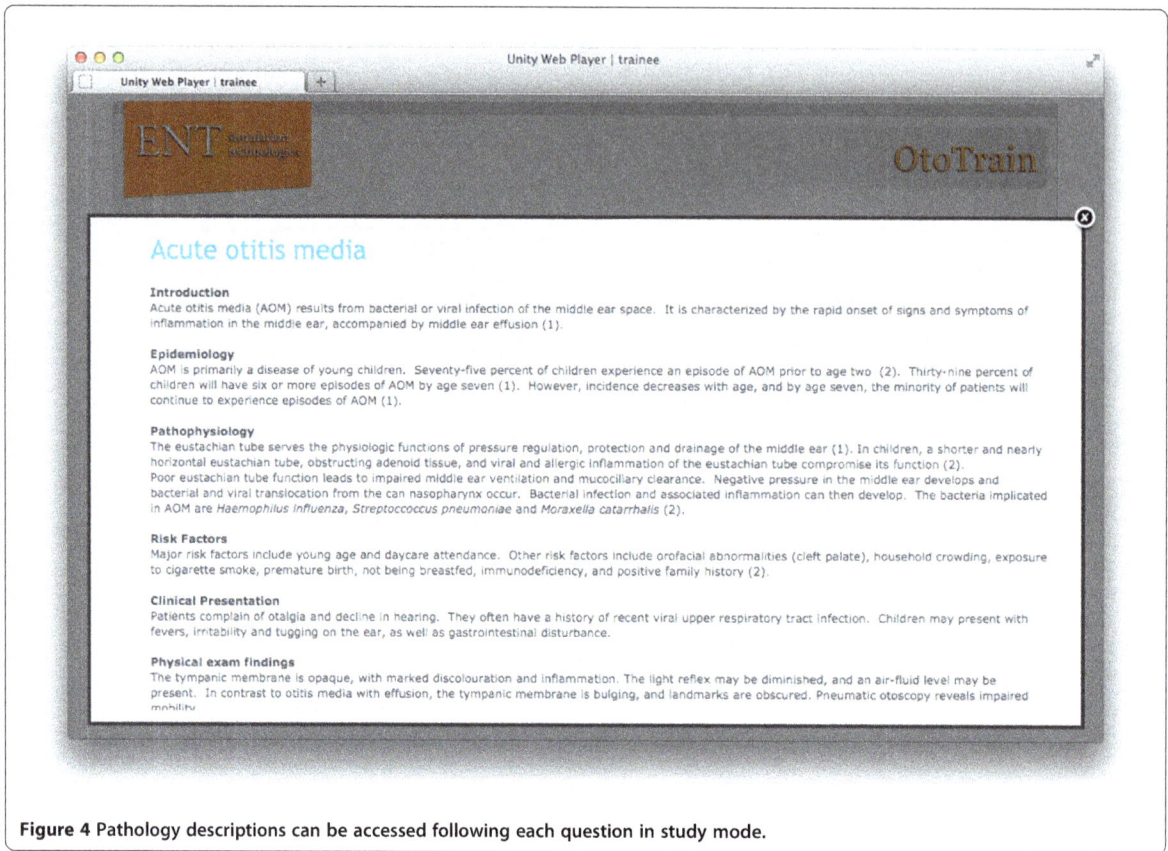

Figure 4 Pathology descriptions can be accessed following each question in study mode.

Content validity

The degree to which the simulator addresses all subject material and curriculum requirements was assessed using the same Likert scale across the following 3 domains: (i) assessment of the external auditory canal and tympanic membrane; (ii) exposure to adequate breadth of pathology; and (iii) utility as an introduction to otoscopy (Table 1). The mean scores across all three domains again measured ≤3, and were thus considered acceptable across all domains.

Applicability to the medical training curriculum

The global rating of the simulator characterized the success of the simulator overall (Table 1). This included the experts' opinions. individually and collectively, as to whether the simulator serves as a useful training tool for uptake by medical/audiology students, non-Otolaryngology residents, and Otolaryngology residents. The global rating also examined ease of use of the simulator, and whether the simulator should be recommended for use in medical education. The calculated means determined from the

statement parameters revealed consistently positive scores (≤3), and were considered acceptable across all domains.

Comparison of training methods

Experts ranked whether they felt that the OtoTrain™ simulator was superior, equivalent, or inferior to the traditional atlas- or lecture-based method of otoscopy education. Four domains were assessed: (i) learning tympanic membrane anatomy; (ii) learning external auditory canal anatomy; (iii) learning manual otoscopic technique; and (iv) ease of access/availability of the training method (Table 2). In each domain, the simulator tool was deemed superior to the atlas/lecture-based method, with the exception of learning tympanic membrane anatomy in which an equal percentage of experts considered it to be superior or equivalent.

Qualitative feedback

Although the means of all scores were ≤ 3, suggesting favourable responses to the otoscopy simulator overall,

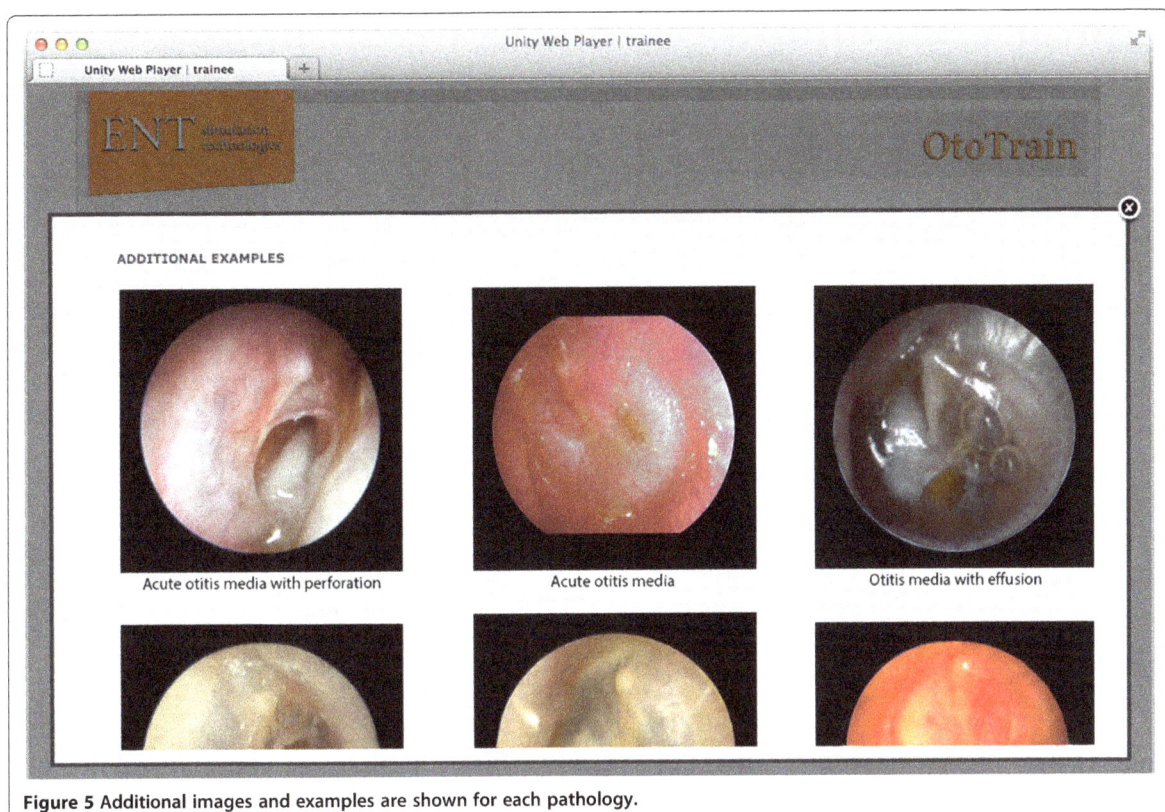

Figure 5 Additional images and examples are shown for each pathology.

several helpful suggestions were derived from the qualitative component of the survey. The most common suggested improvements included:

1. Need for haptic feedback (by using a device, such as a haptic arm, to simulate controlling and navigating the otoscope into the ear canal)
2. Need for greater emphasis on importance of pneumatic otoscopy (visualizing movement of eardrum due to various pressure changes)
3. Need for including more eardrum pathologies, such as eardrums with hearing aid complications, post-surgical scars, and different skin pathologies.

Other suggested refinements included simultaneously displaying both the left and right ear in the pathology pictures, including more pictures and less text when describing how to conduct otoscopy, and incorporating pictures of less obvious pathologies as student skill improves.

Discussion

The ability to perform accurate otoscopy is necessary for many medical and auditory professionals including Family Physicians, Pediatricians, Emergency Room Physicians, Nurses, and Audiologists. Despite its importance, diagnostic accuracy rates are low which necessitates improved teaching and experience in the early stages of training [4-7].

The results of the survey were encouraging with positive responses for face validity, content validity, and applicability to the medical training curriculum. Direct comparison against the traditional atlas/lecture method of teaching was also favourable for OtoTrain™.

The qualitative feedback section did highlight some limitations of a web-based solution for otoscopy simulation. The need for additional realism during the act of otoscopy was highlighted. This is a difficult problem to overcome when trainees are using inexpensive consumer hardware or mobile devices in order to access the simulator. One solution would be to incorporate an inexpensive haptic device to provide force feedback when navigating the otoscope, and this has already been programmed into the simulator. While this would be reasonable on a desktop or notebook computer, this would not work on portable/mobile devices. Another solution would be to develop an inexpensive hybrid model with a face 'mask' attached to a consumer

Table 1 Survey results

Domain	Mean Likert scale ranking[1] (SD) (n = 11)
Face validity	
Realistic representation of normal/abnormal external auditory canal anatomy	2.7 (1.5)
Realistic representation of normal/abnormal tympanic membrane anatomy	2.3 (1.3)
Content validity	
Teaches importance of assessing external auditory canal	2.4 (0.8)
Teaches importance of assessing entire tympanic membrane	2.2 (1.3)
Provides adequate breadth of pathologies	2.1 (1.4)
Is a useful introduction to otoscopy	1.5 (0.8)
Applicability to medical training	
Useful for training of medical students/ audiology students	1.5 (0.8)
Useful for training of non-Otolaryngology residents (Family Medicine, Paediatrics, Emergency Medicine, etc.)	1.7 (1.0)
Useful for training of Otolaryngology residents	2.5 (1.3)
Recommend for use in continuing medical education	1.8 (1.0)
User-friendly	1.7 (1.1)

[1]Likert scale ranking – 1- strongly agree, 4 – neutral, 7 – strongly disagree.

monitor. The advantage of a hybrid solution is that the trainee can hold and manipulate a real otoscope, feel the interaction between the speculum and the ear canal, and practice how to position their hands. This has been previously accomplished in ophthalmoscopy simulators, such as the Eyesi Direct Opthalmoscope Simulator (VRmagic GmbH, Mannheim, Germany), however its realism and efficacy would need further study.

The lack of tympanic membrane pathologies has also been addressed in the next version of the simulator. The examiner now has the ability to upload any photos in their personal collection to the simulator. These photos are then fit onto the end of the 3D ear canal so that they can be displayed interactively.

Pneumatic otoscopy is challenging to accurately simulate in a virtual-reality simulator. Physical simulators have recently incorporated pneumatic otoscopy [8,9], however in a virtual-reality system it would have to be displayed as an animation between a static and a pressurized tympanic membrane. The pressurization deformation could be estimated and applied to the image if actual pneumatic images are not available.

Advantages of internet-based learning have been established [11-13], with the primary advantages in this case being lower cost and wide accessibility around the world. Internet-based simulators can be used by hundreds of students simultaneously on mobile platforms anywhere. Examiners can also manage large classes of students remotely allowing for a great deal of flexibility. Also, in addition to being able to add unlimited tympanic membrane pathologies, virtual-reality simulators have the advantage of unlimited external auditory canal sizes, shapes/curvatures, and pathologies. The external auditory canal and meatus are typically static in most physical simulators.

Limitations of this study include the lack of direct comparisons against existing physical simulators. Experts were asked to compare OtoTrain™ against their existing teaching paradigm, which consisted of lectures/atlas-based teaching. However, high-fidelity, low-accessibility physical simulators may be used in conjunction with low-fidelity, high-accessibility virtual-reality simulators to maximize exposure and availability for trainees.

Finally, face and content validity only represent the initial stages of validation for any simulator. Modifications and updates to OtoTrain™ have already occurred based on the feedback from this study, and research ethics board approval has already been received for a skills transference study at Western University over the upcoming year. This will determine if the use of OtoTrain™ actually improves the diagnostic accuracy of medical students.

Conclusion

OtoTrain™ is a novel, web-based otoscopy simulator that can be easily distributed and used by students on a variety of platforms. Initial face and content validity was encouraging, and a skills transference study is planned following further modifications and improvements to the simulator.

Table 2 Comparison of training methods

Statement	Online simulator superior	Equivalent	Atlas or lecture superior	Unsure
Learning tympanic membrane anatomy	**45.5%**	**45.5%**	0.0%	9.1%
Learning external auditory canal anatomy	**63.6%**	36.4%	0.0%	0.0%
Learning otoscopy technique	**63.6%**	27.3%	0.0%	9.1%
Availability of training technique	**54.5%**	9.1%	27.3%	9.1%

Items in bold indicate the highest percentage in each domain.

Competing interests
The otoscopy simulator (OtoTrain™) described in this study was developed by researchers at Western University. This was done in collaboration with WORLDiscoveries, the business development arm of Western University and its affiliates. Agrawal and Ladak were both members of the development team.

Authors' contributions
BW designed the initial questionnaire, supervised distribution, performed data analysis, and wrote initial draft of manuscript. JL prepared the simulator, acquired the data, and aided with analysis. DM provided otoscopic images for the simulator, reviewed the questionnaire, and critically revised the manuscript. MH aided with simulator design, choice of tympanic membrane pathologies within simulator, and wrote pathologic descriptions. HL and SA designed the simulator, directed development and programming, conceived the study, supervised BW and JL, and wrote the final version of manuscript. All authors read and approved the final manuscript.

Author's information
Sumit K Agrawal and Hanif M Ladak were co-senior authors on this study.

Acknowledgements
Dr. Philip Doyle for reviewing and providing feedback on the questionnaire.

Reviewer exclusion
Please exclude reviewers who may have a potential conflict of interest with OtoTrain™.

Financial disclosure
Funding for this work was provided by the Ontario Centres of Excellence (OCE), Western Innovation Fund (WIF), and Natural Sciences and Engineering Research Council of Canada (NSERC).

Author details
[1]Department of Otolaryngology – Head and Neck Surgery, Western University, London, Ontario, Canada. [2]Department of Medical Biophysics, Western University, London, Ontario, Canada. [3]Department of Electrical & Computer Engineering, Western University, London, Ontario, Canada. [4]Division of Otolaryngology – Head and Neck Surgery, Department of Surgery, Dalhousie University, Halifax, Nova Scotia, Canada. [5]London Health Sciences Centre, Room B1-333, University Hospital, 339 Windermere Rd., London, Ontario N6A 5A5, Canada.

References
1. Vos T, Flaxman AD, Naghavi M, Lozano R, Michaud C, Ezzati M, et al. Years lived with disability (YLDs) for 1160 sequelae of 289 diseases and injuries 1990–2010: a systematic analysis for the Global Burden of Disease Study 2010. Lancet. 2012;380:2163–96.
2. Rovers MM, Schilder AG, Zielhuis GA, Rosenfeld RM. Otitis media. Lancet. 2004;363:465–73.
3. Fisher EW, Pfleiderer AG. Assessment of the otoscopic skills of general practitioners and medical students: is there room for improvement? Br J Gen Pract. 1992;42:65–7.
4. Pichichero ME. Diagnostic accuracy, tympanocentesis training performance, and antibiotic selection by pediatric residents in management of otitis media. Pediatrics. 2002;110:1064–70.
5. Steinbach WJ, Sectish TC, Benjamin Jr DK, Chang KW, Messner AH. Pediatric residents' clinical diagnostic accuracy of otitis media. Pediatrics. 2002;109:993–8.
6. Pichichero ME, Poole MD. Assessing diagnostic accuracy and tympanocentesis skills in the management of otitis media. Arch Pediatr Adolesc Med. 2001;155:1137–42.
7. Pichichero ME, Poole MD. Comparison of performance by otolaryngologists, pediatricians, and general practioners on an otoendoscopic diagnostic video examination. Int J Pediatr Otorhinolaryngol. 2005;69:361–6.
8. Davies J, Djelic L, Campisi P, Forte V, Chiodo A. Otoscopy simulation training in a classroom setting: A novel approach to teaching otoscopy to medical students. Laryngoscope. 2014;124(11):2594–7.
9. Morris E, Kesser BW, Peirce-Cottler S, Keeley M. Development and validation of a novel ear simulator to teach pneumatic otoscopy. Simul Healthc. 2012;7:22–6.
10. Volsky PG, Hughley BB, Peirce SM, Kesser BW. Construct validity of a simulator for myringotomy with ventilation tube insertion. Otolaryngol Head Neck Surg. 2009;141:603–8. e601.
11. Cook DA. Learning and cognitive styles in web-based learning: theory, evidence, and application. Acad Med. 2005;80:266–78.
12. Cook DA. The research we still are not doing: an agenda for the study of computer-based learning. Acad Med. 2005;80:541–8.
13. Cook DA, Levinson AJ, Garside S, Dupras DM, Erwin PJ, Montori VM. Internet-based learning in the health professions: a meta-analysis. JAMA. 2008;300:1181–96.

12

Does a mineral wristband affect balance? A randomized, controlled, double-blind study

Eva Ekvall Hansson[1*], Anders Beckman[2] and Liselott Persson[1]

Abstract

Background: Having good balance is a facilitating factor in the performance of everyday activities. Good balance is also essential in various sport activities in order to both get results and prevent injury. A common measure of balance is postural sway, which can be measured both antero-posteriorly and medio-laterally. There are several companies marketing wristbands whose intended function is to improve balance, strength and flexibility. Randomized controlled trials have shown that wristbands with holograms have no effect on balance but studies on wristbands with minerals seem to be lacking.

Objective: The aim of this study was to investigate if the mineral wristband had any effect on postural sway in a group of healthy individuals.

Study design: Randomized, controlled, double-blind study.

Material/Methods: The study group consisted of 40 healthy persons. Postural sway was measured antero-posteriorly and medio-laterally on a force plate, to compare: the mineral wristband, a placebo wristband, and without any wristband. The measurements were performed for 30 s, in four situations: with open eyes and closed eyes, standing on a firm surface and on foam. Analyses were made with multilevel technique.

Results: The use of wristband with or without minerals did not alter postural sway. Closed eyes and standing on foam both prolonged the dependent measurement, irrespective if it was medio-lateral or antero-posterior. Wearing any wristband (mineral or placebo) gave a small (0,22-0,36 mm/s) but not statistically significant reduction of postural sway compared to not wearing wristband.

Conclusion: This study showed no effect on postural sway by using the mineral wristband, compared with a placebo wristband or no wristband. Wearing any wristband at all (mineral or placebo) gave a small but not statistically significant reduction in postural sway, probably caused by sensory input.

Keywords: Postural control, Balance, Hologram, Force plate

Introduction

Having good balance is a facilitating factor in the performance of everyday activities [1]. Good balance is also essential in various sport activities in order to both get results and prevent injury [2]. Research about the effect of balance training on sports performance is however inconclusive [3]. Despite this, possibilities to improve balance and thereby possible enhancement of performance are attractive.

Balance has been defined as "Sensing the position of the body's centre of mass and moving the body to adjust the position of the centre of mass over the base of support provided by the feet", by Nashner *et al.* [4]. Several systems interact to maintain balance: vision, the somato-sensory system, and the vestibular organ. These systems interact and register inputs from the surroundings, which are integrated and processed in the central nervous system. The vestibulo-ocular reflex (VOR) coordinates eye and head movements, making it possible, for example, to walk and read signs at the same time [5]. Through the head-neck skeletomotor system, the cervico-ocular reflex interacts with the VOR, providing information about head movements in relation to the trunk [6]. Sensory receptors

* Correspondence: Eva.ekvall-hansson@med.lu.se
[1]Department of Health Sciences, Health Science Centre, Lund University, Baravägen 3, SE222 41 Lund, Sweden
Full list of author information is available at the end of the article

in the skin as well as mechanoreceptors in the muscles provide input as to how gravity affects the body [7, 8]. Input from these different parts of the balance system is constantly reconsidered and a response from the motor cortex is sent back. This means that even when standing still, the body is constantly in motion. This motion is called postural sway [1], and can be measured by using a force plate and measuring the movement of the center of pressure (COP) in the medio-lateral (ML) direction as well as in the antero-posterior (AP) direction [1, 9].

Wristbands and function
There are several companies that market wristbands aiming to improve functions such as balance, mobility/agility and strength [10–12]. The technology differs: holograms, ions, protons and minerals are claimed to influence function and well-being [10–12]. Therapists and coaches are often asked by patients and athletes about the efficacy of these wristbands and their impact on balance. Randomized controlled trials have shown that wristbands with holograms have no effect on balance [13, 14], but studies on wristbands with minerals seems to be lacking. Mineral wristbands are marketed to be able to dramatically improve balance by simply putting it on [12]. Therefore, it is important to perform studies on mineral wristbands as well, in order to provide therapists and coaches with adequate information about different wristbands, giving them possibilities to give correct advise to patients and athletes.

The aim of this study was therefore to investigate a mineral wristband's impact on postural sway in a group of healthy individuals, compared to a placebo wristband, and no wristband at all.

Methods
Subjects
The study group was 40 healthy volunteers, aged 20 to 69 years (mean 35 ± 17), of whom 25 (62 %) were women. They were 162 to 191 cm tall (mean 176 ± 8.5) with a body mass index 20.3 to 30.5 kg/m^2 (mean 23.7 ± 2.9). The inclusion criteria were no dizziness or balance problems, no neck pain, no newly acquired injury to the hip, knee, or foot for the last two months, and corrected visual impairment, if any. None of the participants had any hearing problems and none of them had used a wristband before. The subjects were selected among students and staff at Lund University.

Ethics
Participation in the study was strictly voluntary. All participants gave their informed consent before entering the study. The study was approved by the Regional Ethical Review Board in Lund no 2014/127.

Procedure
In this randomized double-blind study, the patricipants were tested on a force plate (Good Balance™, Metitur Ltd, Finland, http://www.papapostolou.gr/clientfiles/file/pdf/Good_Balance_Brochure.pdf) wearing the Bionic-sport wristband (The BIONICSPORT™, BionicFamily®, www.bionicband.com), a placebo wristband (without minerals but made of silicon and the same colour, weight and circumference as the mineral wristband), or no wristband. Tests were performed on the force plate with open and closed eyes and standing on 3 cm thick foam on the force plate with open and closed eyes.

All measurements were standardized and the tests were performed in the same room. Before the measurements, each participant received verbal and written information and signed a paper on the voluntary participation and filled in a report on personal data. Since the whole procedure took about 30 min, the participants was offered to drink a glass of water before the measure to reduce the risk of dehydration. The participants removed shoes, jewelry, watches, and electronic equipment such as mobile phones.

On the force plate, the participants were placed with the feet in a standardized position with 30° of external rotation, marked on the force plate. The neck was positioned in 20° of flexion, and the participants were asked to focus eyes on one spot on the wall, at a distance of 1.5 m, individually adjusted to height and neck position. This is to avoid proprioceptors from the neck to have an impact on the postural wobbling [15]. The participants could not see the force platform's computer screen during the measurements. The verbal instructions were standardized. The participants were instructed to keep the arms hanging freely and during the test not to speak. Each participant then performed a test measurement for 30 s with eyes open and on a firm surface, in order to familiarize themselves with the plate and the test approach.

The procedure was carried out without wristband, with the placebo wristband and with the mineral wristband. The order in which each of the three procedures was carried out, was randomly selected, using a random list.

The measurements were performed by two test-leaders. The same test-leader gave instructions to the participants, and applied the wristband to be used at each measurement. This test leader had no knowledge of which bracelet was used, or the randomized test scheme. Another test leader provided the first test leader with the wristbands according the random list, and documented the measurements into the computer system Good Balance TM, Metitur Ltd., Finland.

Equipment
The postural sway was measured by a computerized system, which consisted of a triangular plate with force

sensors at each corner. Force plate was connected to a PC where the program Good Balance TM, Metitur Ltd, Finland, was installed and synchronized with the plate. Based on signals from each corner of the force plate, the system analyzed the average speed of the movements based on the COP both ML and AP. These values are indicated in mm/s. The system corrects for any differences in the height and the COM of the various test subjects. The force plate was tested and calibrated prior to use and a basic calibration was implemented automatically every time the computer program was started. There were also automated checks every two hours. This model of force plates has been tested for validity and intrasession- and test-retest reliability [9, 16].

The mineral wristband was made of silicone and, according to the manufacturer, it contains mineralized surgical steel and has the "highest frequency" which therefore makes the greatest impact on balance [12]. The placebo wristband was also made of silicone and looked the same as the mineral wristband.

Statistical methods

Considering standard deviation for measures on the force plate [9] a power of 80 % and the significance level set at 0.05, a sample size of 30 subjects was required [17]. Since we also wanted to detect small differences between the groups, sample size was set to 40.

Due to the fact that the observations are repeated measures within the same subject, there is dependence between measurements. To correct for this deviation from the pre-requisites for a traditional regression model, we used a multilevel approach, where a correction for dependence is built into the model. [18, 19]. We regarded the repeated measures to be clustered within the subjects, thus giving a two level structure. The dependent variables used were ML and AP. The independent variables used were vision (eyes open or closed), surface (firm surface and foam) and wristband: without, placebo or mineral. Each dependent variable (ML, AP) was analyzed separately with all independent variables.

The multilevel analysis started with a so-called empty model, i.e. a model with only a fixed part and a random part. The fixed part models the effect of the mean that underlies all observations. The random part consists of a decomposition of the total variance into two levels: variance between subjects (second level) and between occasions within subjects.

The empty model was then extended by including the independent variables in the fixed part of the model (eyes, surface and wristband). Inclusion was made stepwise, but only the last model with all variables is presented.

Analysis was made with MlWin, v 2.30 [20] Residual (or restricted) maximum likelihood (REML) was used for all analysis. REML estimation takes into account the loss of degrees of freedom resulting from the estimation of the parameters of the fixed part. This has an indirect effect on the estimates of the fixed part.

The results are presented with 95 % confidence intervals [21].

A reduction in the total variance is an indicator of a better "fit" of the model, as is the reduction in the deviance.

Results

Standing with eyes open on a firm surface caused the smallest postural sway in all dimensions (ML 7,47 mm/s, AP 13,64 mm/s) and standing with eyes closed on foam prolonged the sway (ML +3,82 mm/s, AP +8,12 mm/s). The use of wristband with or without minerals did not alter the sway. The overall mean values and SD for each variable are displayed in Table 1 and each test is displayed in Table 2.

Multilevel analysis – fixed part

The sway in AP was almost 50 % higher than the sway in ML (Table 3). However, both measures show similar variations when the independent variables are introduced, i.e. a prolonging of sway when eyes are closed and the surface is non-firm (foam). However, the use of a wristband does not significantly alter the sway.

Multilevel analysis – random part

The empty model reveals for all outcomes a similar pattern, i.e. both random variance components (between subjects (second level) and between occasions within subjects) differ from zero. This justifies the use of a multilevel model. Similarly, the introduction of independent variables reveals an almost uniform pattern: Closed eyes and standing on foam both prolong the dependent measurement, irrespective if it is ML or AP. This also reduces the size of the random part, as an effect of a better model fit, also observed in the reduction in deviance shown in Table 3.

Table 1 Mean values and standard deviation (SD) for medio-lateral sway (ML) and anterior-posterior sway (AP)

		ML mm/s (SD)	AP mm/s (SD)
Overall mean		5.41 (2.59)	9.39 (4.49)
Eyes closed		6.58 (2.97)	11.70 (4.90)
Foam standing		6.15 (2.85)	11.20 (4.91)
Wristband	None	5.56 (2.59)	9.58 (4.49)
	Placebo	5.34 (2.68)	9.22 (4.51)
	Mineral	5.32 (2.50)	9.36 (4.50)

Table 2 Mean values and standard deviation (SD) for medio-lateral sway (ML), anterior-posterior sway (AP) in relation to proprioception, sight and wristband

Proprio	Eyes	Wristband	ML mm/s (SD)	AP mm/s (SD)
Firm	Open	Without	3.87 (1.16)	6.03 (2.07)
Firm	Shut	Without	5.66 (2.30)	9.35 (3.45)
Soft	Open	Without	4.91 (1.52)	8.78 (2.58)
Soft	Shut	Without	7.81 (3.14)	14.17 (4.90)
Firm	Open	Placebo	3.72 (1.03)	5.72 (1.76)
Firm	Shut	Placebo	5.60 (2.65)	9.18 (3.17)
Soft	Open	Placebo	4.53 (1.15)	8.00 (2.14)
Soft	Shut	Placebo	7.52 (3.41)	13.99 (5.27)
Firm	Open	Mineral	3.63 (1.25)	6.02 (1.64)
Firm	Shut	Mineral	5.53 (2.04)	9.40 (3.45)
Soft	Open	Mineral	4.75 (1.42)	8.03 (2.45)
Soft	Shut	Mineral	7.37 (3.18)	13.98 (5.18)

Discussion

In this study, the use of a mineral wristband did not affect postural sway, neither compared to wristband whitout minerals nor compared to no wristband at all. Standing with eyes open on a firm surface caused the smallest postural sway in all dimensions and standing with eyes closed on foam prolonged the sway, irrespective of which wristband was used or if no wristband was used. Closed eyes and standing on foam both prolong the dependent measurement, irrespective if it was ML or AP and also irrespective wristband or no wristband.

As shown in other randomized controlled trials, on other types of wristbands, there was no difference between placebo or mineral wristband [13, 14]. These studies were

similar to our in design, participants and one of them also used a force plate to measure balance [13].

Light touch of the skin has proven to affect postural sway among persons with balance deficits [22] and persons with poor ability to feel the direction of a tactile sensation can have reduced postural stability [23]. Thus, the small but statistically significant reduction in sway seen when using any of the wristbands in our study can be caused by the sensory information provided through the wristband's contact with the skin. Another explanation might be the expectation from the participants that without the wristband, balance would be worse. Studies about the placebo effect has shown that positive expectations increases the likelihood of reporting feeling better after surgery [24] and that dopamine receptors can be affected by treatment with placebo [25]. However, our study cannot answer whether the effect of the wristband is accentuated if the wearer believes that the wristband can improve performance.

The present study is a randomized controlled trial, where the same persons performed all the measures, the same protocol was used for all subjects and an independent person performed the randomization. The assessor was also blind to if the wristband used was placebo or mineral.

The subjects in our study only wore the wristband during the measurements. If wearing the wristband during a longer period of time or during sport activity or competition actually gives effect on results is not yet studied. We only measured static balance in this study, further studies is needed on dynamic balance, especially when performing a task. Further studies are also needed on the impact of mineral wristband on strength and flexibility. Also, the placebo effect has to be taken into

Table 3 Means and 95 % confidence intervals (CI) for fixed and random parts and deviance

		ML-speed mm/s (95 % CI) Empty model	mm/s (95 % CI) Full model	AP-speed mm/s (95 % CI) Empty model	mm/s (95 % CI) Full model
Fixed part					
Intercept		5,41 (5,18 - 5,64)	7,47 (6,90 - 8,04)	9,39 (8,60- 10,18)	13,64 (12,76 - 14,52)
Foam			1,48 (1,22 - 1,74)		3,54 (3,14 - 3,94)
Eyes closed			2,34 (2,08 - 2,60)		4,58 (4,18 - 4,98)
Wristband	None		0		0
	Placebo		−0,22 (−0,53 - 0,10)		−0,36 (−0,14 - 0,86)
	Mineral		−0,24 (−0,56 - 0,07)		−0,22 (−0,28 - 0,72)
Random Parts					
Variance					
Within subjects		4,25 (3,70 - 4,80)	2,14 (1,86 - 2,42)	14,6 (12,72 - 16,48)	5,43 (4,72 - 6,14)
Between subjects		2,43 (1,23 - 3,63)	2,61 (1,41 - 3,8)	5,54 (2,64 - 8,44)	6,31 (3,41 - 9,21)
Deviance		2139	1838	2718	2282

account when considering the effect of the wristband; a small increase in performance caused by the placebo effect when the athlete is convinced that the wristband will improve performance, is in fact a real improvement.

Conclusion

Wearing a mineral wristband did not affect postural sway in this group of healthy individuals, compared to a placebo wristband or no wristband at all. Wearing any wristband (mineral or placebo) gave a small but not statistically significant reduction of postural sway, probably caused by sensory input.

Competing interests
The authors declare that they have no competing interests.

Authors' contribution
EEH participated in the design of the study, carried out the randomization, participated in measuring postural sway and drafted the manuscript. AB carried out the statistical analysis and helped to draft the manuscript. LP participated in design of the study and in measuring postural sway and helped to draft the manuscript. All authors read and approved the final manuscript.

Acknowledgment
Thanks to Elin Berggren and Sanna Strandh Lorentzon for help with testing the first twenty subjects.

Author details
[1]Department of Health Sciences, Health Science Centre, Lund University, Baravägen 3, SE222 41 Lund, Sweden. [2]Department of Clinical Sciences in Malmö, Clinical Research Centre, Lund University, Jan Waldenströmsgata 25, SE205 02 Malmö, Sweden.

References
1. Rogind H, Lykkegaard JJ, Bliddal H, Danneskiold-Samsoe B. Postural sway in normal subjects aged 20–70 years. Clin Physiol Funct Imaging. 2003;23(3):171–6.
2. Ambegaonkar JP, Mettinger LM, Caswell SV, Burtt A, Cortes N. Relationships between core endurance, hip strength, and balance in collegiate female athletes. Int J Sports Phy Ther. 2014;9(5):604–16.
3. Zech A, Hubscher M, Vogt L, Banzer W, Hansel F, Pfeifer K. Balance training for neuromuscular control and performance enhancement: a systematic review. J Athl Train. 2010;45(4):392–403.
4. Nashner L, Shupert C, Horak F. Head-trunk movement coordination in the standing posture. Prog Brain Res. 1988;76:243–51.
5. Möller C. Dysfunction and Plasticity in Otoneurology with Emphasis on the Vestibular System. Linköping: Linköpings universitet; 1989.
6. Mergner T, Nasios G, Maurer C, Becker W. Visual object localisation in space. Interaction of retinal, eye position, vestibular and neck proprioceptive information. Exp Brain Res. 2001;141(1):33–51.
7. Magnusson M, Enbom H, Johansson R, Wiklund J. Significance of pressor input from the human feet in lateral postural control. The effect of hypothermia on galvanically induced body-sway. Acta Otolaryngol. 1990;110(5–6):321–7.
8. Stal F, Fransson PA, Magnusson M, Karlberg M. Effects of hypothermic anesthesia of the feet on vibration-induced body sway and adaptation. J Vestib Res. 2003;13(1):39–52.
9. Era P, Sainio P, Koskinen S, Haavisto P, Vaara M, Aromaa A. Postural balance in a random sample of 7,979 subjects aged 30 years and over. Gerontology. 2006;52(4):204–13.
10. Why wristbands for health? (In Swedish) 2014. Available from: www.goodbalance.se
11. Power Balance-Performance Technology 2014 [cited 2014]. Available from: www.powerbalance.se
12. BionicFamily. Bionic Sportsband 2011 [20130414]. Available from: www.bionicband.com.
13. Brice SR, Jarosz BS, Ames RA, Baglin J, Da Costa C. The effect of close proximity holographic wristbands on human balance and limits of stability: a randomised, placebo-controlled trial. J Bodyw Mov Ther. 2011;15(3):298–303.
14. Pothier DD, Thiel G, Khoo SG, Dillon WA, Sulway S, Rutka JA. Efficacy of the Power Balance Silicone Wristband: a single-blind, randomized, triple placebo-controlled study. J Otolaryngol Head Neck Surg. 2012;41(3):153–9.
15. Karlberg M. The Neck and Human Balance. Lund: Lund University, Sweden; 1995.
16. Bauer C, Groger I, Rupprecht R, Gassmann KG. Intrasession reliability of force platform parameters in community-dwelling older adults. Arch Phys Med Rehabil. 2008;89(10):1977–82.
17. Altman D. Practical Statistics for Medical Research. 9th ed. New York: Chapman&Hall/CRC; 1991. p. 611.
18. Maas C, Snijders T. The multilevel approach to repeated measures for complete and incomplete data. Qual Quant. 2003;37(1):71–89.
19. Quené H, van den Bergh H. On multi-level modeling of data from repeated measures designs: a tutorial. Speech Comm. 2004;43(1–2):103–21.
20. Rasbash J, Charlton C, Browne WJ, Healy M, Cameron B. MLwiN. 21st ed. University of Bristol: Centre for Multilevel Modelling; 2009.
21. Snijders T, Bosker R. Multilevel Analysis - An Introduction to Basic and Advanced Multilevel Modeling. Wiltshire: SAGE Publications; 1999.
22. Baldan AM, Alouche SR, Araujo IM, Freitas SM. Effect of light touch on postural sway in individuals with balance problems: a systematic review. Gait Posture. 2014;40(1):1–10.
23. Backlund Wasling H, Norrsell U, Göthner K, Olausson H. Tactile directional sensitivity and postural control. Exp Brain Res. 2005;166(2):147–56.
24. Flood AB, Lorence DP, Ding J, McPherson K, Black NA. The role of expectations in patients' reports of post-operative outcomes and improvement following therapy. Med Care. 1993;31(11):1043–56.
25. Lidstone SC. Great expectations: the placebo effect in Parkinson's disease. Handb Exp Pharmacol. 2014;225:139–47.

13

Prospective functional outcomes in sequential population based cohorts of stage III/ IV oropharyngeal carcinoma patients treated with 3D conformal vs. intensity modulated radiotherapy

Paul Kerr[1], Candace L Myers[2], James Butler[2,3], Mohamed Alessa[2], Pascal Lambert[2] and Andrew L Cooke[2,4*]

Abstract

Background and purpose: To compare early (3 and 6 month) and later (12 and 24 month) functional outcomes of stage III and IV (M0) oropharyngeal squamous cancer patients treated in sequential cohorts with 3D conformal (3DCRT) or intensity modulated radiotherapy (IMRT).

Patients and methods: 200 patients in sequential population based cohorts of 83 and 117 patients treated at a single institution with 3DCRT and then IMRT respectively were prospectively assessed at pre-treatment and 3, 6, 12 and 24 months post treatment. A standard functional outcomes protocol including performance status (KPS, ECOG), 3 Performance Status scales for Head and Neck (PSS-HN), the Royal Brisbane Hospital Outcome Measure for Swallowing (RBHOMS), Voice Handicap Index-10 (VHI-10) and self-rated xerostomia were applied.

Results: Mean age at diagnosis was 59 years. The primary site was base of tongue in 77 and tonsil or soft palate in 123 patients. Median follow up was 2.5 years for the second cohort. Concomitant therapy was used in 159 (79.5%). Overall survival at 3 years was 75.6% and 71.5% for IMRT and 3DCRT cohorts respectively (not significant). A multiple imputation technique was used to estimate missing values in order to avoid a healthy patient bias. KPS and ECOG reached nadirs at 3 to 6 months but approached baseline values at 12 to 24 months and did not differ by treatment. The 3 PSS-HN scales, Eating in Public ($p < 0.001$), Understandability of Speech ($p = 0.009$) and Oral Diet Texture ($p = 0.002$) and all showed significantly better outcomes in favor of IMRT. The RBHOMS showed a difference in favor of IMRT which appeared during 3 to 6 months ($p < 0.001$). The VHI-10 also showed a difference in favor of IMRT ($p = 0.015$). Self-rated xerostomia did not differ at 3 and 6 months but was significantly better in favor of IMRT after 12 months $p = 0.005$

Conclusions: A prospectively administered functional outcomes protocol showed meaningful differences in favor of IMRT over 3DCRT early (3–6 months) and later (12–24 months) in the treatment of oropharyngeal carcinoma with equivalent survival. These data support the adoption of IMRT as the standard radiation treatment method for patients with stage III and IV (M0) oropharyngeal squamous carcinoma. KPS and ECOG may not be sensitive to oropharyngeal cancer patients' functional outcomes by treatment.

Keywords: Oropharyngeal, Intensity modulated, Functional outcomes

* Correspondence: acooke1@cancercare.mb.ca
[2]Cancer Care Manitoba, Winnipeg, Manitoba, Canada
[4]Department of Radiation Oncology, CancerCare Manitoba, 675 McDermot Avenue, Winnipeg, Manitoba R3E 0 V9, Canada
Full list of author information is available at the end of the article

Background

Organ preservation protocols using chemo-radiotherapy for stage III and IV (M0) oropharyngeal squamous carcinoma have been developed to preserve anatomy and function. However acute and long term toxicities remain problems with the organ preservation approach. Long term toxicities related to radiation include chronic ulceration, xerostomia, pharyngeal constrictor dysfunction, esophageal stricture, impaired swallowing, PEG tube dependency, laryngeal edema and neck fibrosis [1,2]. However these specific narrow indicators of treatment related dysfunction may not necessarily correlate with broader quality of life and performance status which may be more meaningful for patients.

Intensity modulated radiation therapy [IMRT] offers an opportunity to generate dose distributions more conformal to the target volumes including tumor, involved nodes and areas at risk compared to its predecessor, 3D conformal radiotherapy (3DCRT) with relative sparing of surrounding normal tissues [3]. Reduction of the mean dose to the parotid gland by IMRT is feasible and correlates with a reduction in patient and observer-rated xerostomia [4]. Relative sparing of the pharyngeal, laryngeal and cervical esophageal swallowing structures outside the PTV is also possible with IMRT to avoid grade 3–4 late dysphagia and cervical esophageal stricture [5].

Two completed randomized phase III trials have compared the toxicity of IMRT with 3DCRT [6-8] in oropharyngeal cancer patients. The GORTEC 2004–01 is in progress [www.gortec.fr]. The trials are small, or had a heterogeneous population (i.e. included hypopharynx or larynx patients) or had endpoints that are limited to xerostomia and salivary function. One trial [8] used the EORTC QOL QLC-C30 with the Head and Neck Module (HN35) to assess 58 patients at least once. They concluded that IMRT when compared to 3DCRT resulted in clinically meaningful and statistically better QOL scores.

There are several non-randomized comparisons of IMRT vs. 2DRT or 3DCRT in head and neck patients (excluding NPC) [4,9-13] using a variety of instruments, heterogeneous populations and different time points for measurement which demonstrate patients treated with IMRT experience statistically meaningful improvements in several important QOL domains. IMRT has nevertheless been widely implemented with this limited information.

To address these issues we have prospectively collected standardized longitudinal clinical performance status and functional outcomes on 2 sequential population based cohorts of patients with stage III and IV(M0) oropharyngeal carcinoma treated at one institution.

Methods

The methodology has been described in a previous publication regarding oropharyngeal cancer patients treated with 3DCRT at this institution to 2008 [14]. All patients diagnosed with carcinomas of the head and neck and considered for curative intent between 2003 and 2011 were reviewed in a multi-disciplinary consensus conference to confirm site, histology and TNM stage and to determine treatment intent and modality(s). Patients were included in this study if they had American Joint Committee on Cancer (AJCC) stage III or IV (M0) squamous cell carcinoma of the oropharynx and were treated with 3DCRT or IMRT (after 2007), either with or without concomitant cisplatin or cetuximab and with curative intent (typically 66–70 Gy in 2 Gy fractions to gross disease). Neck irradiation was bilateral except in highly selected patients with cancers of the tonsil with N1 disease. Over the period of the two cohorts the selection and treatment polices for oropharyngeal stage III and IV cancers did not change except for the implementation of IMRT and the addition of cetuximab in some cases not eligible for cisplatin. Neck dissection for bulky neck nodes prior to or after radiation was allowed. Patients were excluded if they were treated with surgery alone, surgery to the primary tumor (with or without post-operative radiotherapy), or had a previous head and neck cancer within five years prior to diagnosis. Human papilloma virus [HPV] infection was not assessed in the early years of the study and is not included in the analysis.

The Manitoba Cancer Registry [MCR] is a comprehensive and accredited population-based registry for 1.2 million people. The MCR is a member of the North American Association of Central Cancer Registries which administers a program that reviews member registries for their ability to produce complete, accurate, and timely data. Fields include diagnosis coded using the International Classification of Diseases 10th revision for Canada (ICD-10-CA), age, and TNM stage. Medically necessary care is freely provided to all Manitobans without premiums or co-payments and non-participation in the plan is rare [www.gov.mb.ca/health/guide/2.html]. Therefore the registry and any derived cohort can be considered complete and population-based. All incident registry cases from 2003 to 2011 inclusive with oropharyngeal cancer were reviewed to ensure all cases were included.

Patients were assessed prospectively by one Speech Language specialist (CM) using a standardized clinical functional outcomes protocol at a pre-treatment visit and post-treatment at 3, 6, 12, 24 and 36 months. In the first year, assessments could vary by as much as +/− 1 month. At 24 and 36 months visits could vary within several months. Pre-treatment assessment was not a protocol standard until March of 2005. The following data were also collected: gender, age at diagnosis, weight at each visit, date of placement and removal of feeding tube if used, chemotherapeutic agents used, amifostine use, dose of radiotherapy, date of recurrence assessed clinically, radiographically or pathologically, site of recurrence, date of death, hospitalizations, tobacco use, and incidence of respiratory infections.

Functional outcomes protocol

The protocol was intended to capture functional outcomes beyond recurrence and survival consistent with the International Classification of Functioning, Disability and Health (ICF) 22–23. The protocol included 8 instruments which have proven inter-rater reliability and validity and are widely used in head and neck cancer patient assessments. The protocol was applied prospectively, in face to face interviews with patients by a single speech language pathologist (CM).

The Karnofsky Performance Status (KPS) scale [15] and the Eastern Cooperative Oncology Group (ECOG) toxicity and response criteria scale [16] are clinician-rated standard tools used to assess performance in activities of daily living.

The Performance Status Scale for Head and Neck Cancer Patients (PSS-HN) [17] is a clinician rated interview assessment tool that describes performance on three subscales: Eating in Public, Understandability of Speech and maximum Oral Diet Texture. Each PSS-HN scale has a 5 or 10 point ordinal scale (nominally from 0 to 100) with higher scores indicating better performance. The PSS-HN has good inter-rater reliability and ability to discriminate levels of functioning [18]. For graphic purposes but not for analysis the PSS-HN ordinal scales are here represented as 4 ranges for Eating in Public PSS-HN and Oral Diet Texture PSS-HN and 3 ranges for Understandability of Speech PSS-HN.

The Royal Brisbane Hospital Outcome Measure for Swallowing (RBHOMS) [19] is a clinician-rated 10-point scale which measures oral intake, swallowing function and relative dependence on enteral tube feeding. For graphic purposes the scale was collapsed into 4 ranges. The ranges were 1–3, (total tube dependence, NPO), 4–5, (reduced oral intake requiring partial or total tube feed supplementation), 6–7, (modified diet with no tube supplementation), and >8, (oral intake at optimum level).

The Voice Handicap Index-10 (VHI-10) [20] is a patient-rated scale with 10 questions with answers ranging from 0 (never) to 4 (always) for a total of 40 possible points with a higher score indicating worse self-perceived voice handicap. The VHI-10 has been collapsed into 3 ranges, 0–9 (never to almost never severe), 10–19 (sometimes severe), and > 20 (more than sometimes severe).

Finally self-rated xerostomia on a 0–10 scale from the Edmonton Self-Assessment Scale (ESAS) [21] was collected.

Statistical analysis

Overall survival (OS) and disease-free survival (DFS), for which events are recurrence without death and death from any cause, were measured from the time of diagnosis and compared by the logrank test. Patients with recurrence were followed and assessed until death or end of study follow-up. Patients were censored at the time of death, with or without recurrence.

Times for functional outcome assessments were measured from the date of the last radiation treatment. Compliance with the functional outcome protocol was measured as the percentage of patients administered a questionnaire out of all patients alive at that time. Missing assessments while patients were alive were considered to be missing at random (MAR) if they were the result of a conflict in schedule or because assessments were not systematically scheduled for pretreatment, 3 and 6 months at the beginning of data collection. Missing values were estimated using a multiple imputation bootstrap method [22]. Because the outcomes were skewed, the ICE procedure in *Stata 11.2* (StataCorp LP, College Station Tx) [23] was used for multiple imputations, which uses a conditional density approach. Pre-treatment outcomes were imputed first, using gender, stage, subsite, and age as predictors. Based on Graham [24] 20 imputations were used.

Post-treatment outcomes were then merged to the new pre-treatment dataset and imputed once, using gender, stage, subsite, age, month of assessment, and pre-treatment assessment as predictors. Results by treatment were compared with mixed logistic or ordinal models using GLLAMM in *Stata*. Adjustments to comparisons by treatment were made for variations in pre-treatment function.

Xerostomia was analyzed by mixed quantile regression using lqmm in **R** 2.15.2.

This study was approved by the University of Manitoba Health Research Ethics Board.

Results

From 2003 to 2011, 200 patients with stages III and IV (M0) squamous cell carcinoma of the oropharynx were treated with curative intent using 3DCRT (83) or IMRT (117) with or without concomitant therapy. Patient and treatment characteristics are shown in Table 1. One patient had a suspected tonsil primary but had only CIS on biopsy but had grossly involved regional nodes and has been included. Two significant differences were noted between the cohorts. Cetuximab was introduced for some IMRT patients not eligible for cisplatin (typically older or with renal impairment) and the lower number of 3 and 6 month assessments done in the 3DCRT group.

Median follow up is approximately 2.5 and 3.5 years for IMRT and 3DCRT patients respectively. Overall survival

Table 1 Sequential cohort patient characteristics

		IMRT (N = 117)	3DCRT (N = 83)	p
Age	mean (SD)	59.9 (9.0)	58.8 (9.5)	0.41
Gender	F (%)	18 (15.4)	19 (22.9)	0.20
	M	99 (84.6)	64 (77.1)	
T stage	1 or 0* (%)	28 (23.9)	14 (16.9)	0.52
	2	42 (35.9)	30 (36.1)	
	3	28 (23.9)	20 (24.1)	
	4	19 (16.2)	19 (22.9)	
N Stage	0 (%)	15 (12.8)	12 (14.5)	0.28
	1	16 (13.6)	18 (21.7)	
	2	83 (70.9)	51 (61.4)	
	3	3 (2.6)	2 (2.4)	
Stage	III (%)	20 (17.1)	19 (22.9)	0.37
	IV	97 (82.9)	64 (77.1)	
Primary site	Tongue Base (%)	41 (35.0)	36 (43.4)	0.24
	Tonsil, soft palate	76 (65.0)	47 (56.6)	
Concomitant	Cisplatin (%)	85 (72.6)	62 (74.7)	0.01
	Cetuximab	12 (10.3)	0 (0)	
	No	20 (17.1)	21 (25.3)	
Assessments	3 months (%)	95.7	72	<0.0001
	6	98.2	90.2	0.02
	12	92.2	90.8	0.96
	24	91.2	95.3	0.49

*1 patient had grossly involved tonsil but bx showed only CIS with gross nodes.

(OS) and disease-free survival (DFS) by treatment are shown in Figures 1 and 2. There was no significant difference between IMRT and 3DCRT for either OS (76 vs. 71% $p = 0.71$) or DFS (72 vs. 71% $p = 0.88$). Cause specific mortality (not shown) at 3 years was also not significantly different (17 vs 21%). Recurrence of any sort carried a poor prognosis. Only 1 patient with a local recurrence and 1 patient with a regional recurrence had successful surgical salvage and were alive without disease at the last follow up.

Functional outcomes

Functional outcomes are shown to 2 years of follow up. KPS is shown in Figure 3A. There is a nadir at the 3 month assessment with recovery to approximately pre-treatment values by 24 months but there is no difference by treatment ($p = 0.234$). ECOG is shown in Figure 3B. Similarly there is a nadir with recovery but there is only a non-significant trend by treatment in favor if IMRT ($p = 0.078$). On the other hand (data not shown) both KPS and ECOG were significantly predictive of death from any cause within 1 year irrespective of treatment.

All the following comparisons have been adjusted for baseline differences and death. PSS-HN results are shown in Figures 3C,D and E. Eating in Public PSS-HN (Figure 3C) shows a significant difference in favor of IMRT predicting no restriction vs. any restriction (100 vs. 75 and lower) OR 0.164 (95 %CI, 0.07-0.39 $p = <0.001$). For Eating in Public PSS-HN, at 12 and 24 months 83% and 82% of IMRT survivors had no restrictions compared to 49% and 64% of 3DCRT survivors respectively. The Understandability of Speech PSS-HN (Figure 3D) shows only <4% of patients with speech that was difficult to understand pretreatment and in the first 6 months. Thereafter no survivor was difficult to understand. Nevertheless a significant benefit in favor of IMRT (100 vs. 75 and lower) was noted, OR 0.294 (95% CI, 0.12-0.73 $p = 0.009$). Oral Diet Texture PSS-HN (Figure 3E) shows marked deterioration in both groups that did not recover to baseline even at 24 months with large subgroups preferring soft chewable food regardless of treatment. While little difference by treatment is seen at 3 and 6 months, there is a difference in favor of IMRT appearing at 12 and 24 months with an overall significant difference in favor of IMRT, OR 0.346 (95% CI, 0.18-0.67 $p = 0.002$). At 12 and 24 months 22% and 25% in the IMRT group had no Oral Diet Texture restrictions compared to 7% and 5% for 3DCRT survivors respectively.

The RBHOMS (Figure 3F) shows that pretreatment, fewer than 3% of patients in either group had partial or complete tube dependency. At 3 months, 46% in the 3DCRT group and 21 % in the IMRT group were partially or completely tube dependent. By 24 months partial tube dependency had declined to 3% in the 3DCRT group and 5% in the IMRT group and no survivor was totally tube dependent. Overall there was a significant benefit in favor of IMRT (8 vs. 7 or lower) OR 0.138 (95% CI, 0.06-0.33 $p < 0.001$).

The VHI-10 (Figure 3G) shows a significant benefit in favor of IMRT (0, 1–9 and 10+) OR 0.492 (95% CI, 0.28-0.87 $p = 0.015$) but function did not return to pretreatment levels.

Self-reported xerostomia (Figure 3H) shows little no difference by treatment at the 3 and 6 month assessments but there is a significant time-treatment interaction with improvements in favor of IMRT appearing at 12 months onward with a difference in median score of −1.232 (95% CI, −2.09—0.37 $p = 0.005$)

Discussion

The widespread implementation of IMRT in place of 3DCRT for head and neck cancer has been justified by surrogate end points such as dose volume histograms and uncontrolled series with various endpoints. Limited randomized controlled information comparing 3DCRT

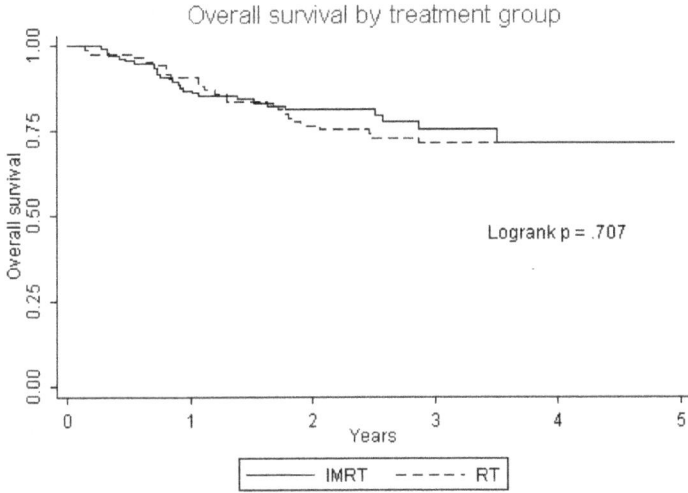

Figure 1 Overall survival.

to IMRT is available and only some of that data pertains to oropharyngeal carcinoma. Because narrow measures of salivary function or swallowing may not necessarily reflect patients' perceptions or overall functional outcome acutely or longer term, we have applied a functional outcomes protocol in order to more broadly assess outcomes. The population-based nature of our data implies that case selection beyond the actual indications for treatment has not occurred and that these results may be reliable and generalizable. Further, the prospective interview and self-rating based data are additional features that suggest our data are reliable indicators of patient function at various times after treatment.

One weakness of the study is that compliance was not 100% for all assessments and lower at 3 and 6 months for 3DCRT (Table 1). We have attempted to address this possible shortcoming by a multiple imputation technique that takes into account individual patient's scores to estimate missing values. At 12 and 24 months, where long term toxicities become important, assessment compliance was equivalent. Another weakness of the study is that for graphic purposes (but not for the statistical model analysis) we have censored patients who have died between assessments. Because death also censors functional assessments, some of the functional "improvement" seen over the months of follow up is due not only to recovery from the effects of treatment

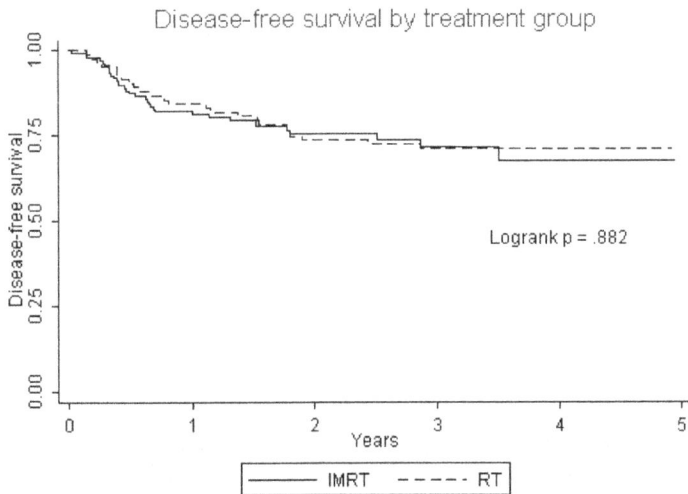

Figure 2 Disease free survival.

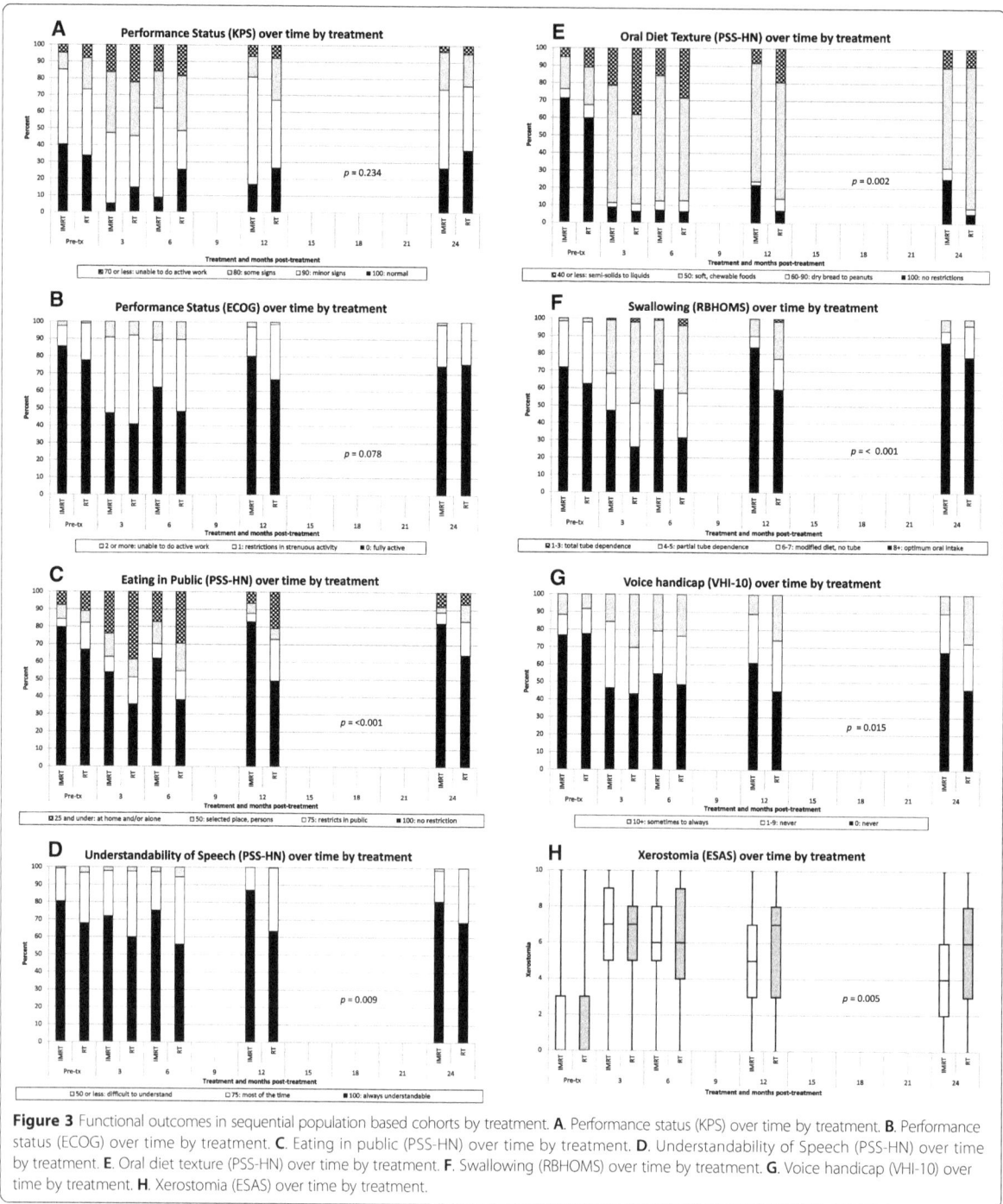

Figure 3 Functional outcomes in sequential population based cohorts by treatment. **A**. Performance status (KPS) over time by treatment. **B**. Performance status (ECOG) over time by treatment. **C**. Eating in public (PSS-HN) over time by treatment. **D**. Understandability of Speech (PSS-HN) over time by treatment. **E**. Oral diet texture (PSS-HN) over time by treatment. **F**. Swallowing (RBHOMS) over time by treatment. **G**. Voice handicap (VHI-10) over time by treatment. **H**. Xerostomia (ESAS) over time by treatment.

in survivors, but will instead be due to the deaths of those who are likely to have poor function. Thus the changes in functions graphically represented over time after treatment cannot be looked at as simply recovery of the cohort, but only a statement of the function of

the survivors at certain specific times after treatment. Also, the two cohorts differed somewhat in their baseline pre-treatment scores. As much as possible, we have adjusted the comparisons for the differences in the pre-treatment scores and the OR and p values we report are adjusted. We did not report on HPV because in the early years of the study this was not routinely measured. The similar demographics and survival of the two cohorts (Table 1, Figures 1 and 2) suggest that HPV status which can profoundly affect outcome [25] did not differ greatly between the two groups. Finally cetuximab was introduced during the IMRT cohort, primarily for those who would not be able to take cisplatin, such that percentage receiving cisplatin remained much the same in both cohorts, 74.7 vs 72.6%. If cetuximab added toxicity this would bias the results against IMRT.

We have documented both early post-treatment functional impairments (3 and 6 months) and those that occur later (12 and 24 months). The RBHOMS shows significant differences that appear soon after treatment at 3 to 6 months and the Eating in Public PSS-HN, Oral Diet Texture PSS-HN and self-rated xerostomia scale show differences that mostly appear at 12 to 24 months. IMRT in our study is therefore broadly superior to 3DCRT by different measures at different times and provides a persistent meaningful benefit to patients.

The effect of treatment on these functional outcomes is likely due to the effect of (chemo) radiation on multiple end points in composite including oropharyngeal mucous membranes, pharyngeal constrictors, taste and salivary gland function [7,26] but we cannot ascertain the degree to which any of these or any other component of eating contributes to these functional endpoints. Presumably the additional conformality afforded by IMRT in comparison to 3DCRT is responsible for the differences seen in our study.

Conclusions
In sequential population-based cohorts of 200 stages III and IV (M0) oropharyngeal cancer patients treated with 3DCRT and IMRT, with or without concomitant therapy OS and DFS did not significantly differ by treatment. While both treatments resulted in functional impairment at 3–6 months after treatment, significant differences were seen at 3 and 6 months in favor of IMRT as measured by RBHOMS, and later at 12 and 24 months as measured by the PSS-HN scales for Eating in Public, Oral Diet Texture, Understandability of Speech, the Voice Handicap Index (VHI) and xerostomia as assessed by the Edmonton Self-Assessment Score (ESAS). KPS and ECOG however did not show any differences by treatment. However, KPS and ECOG may not be sensitive to oropharyngeal cancer patients' functional outcomes by treatment.

IMRT maintained efficacy of treatment with improved functional outcomes indicating an improved therapeutic ratio compared to 3DCRT in patients with oropharyngeal squamous carcinoma stage III and IV(M0). These data support IMRT as the standard of care for curative (chemo) radiation for such patients.

It is unlikely given the established place IMRT has in the treatment of head and neck cancer that much additional data will be available from randomized controlled trials of IMRT vs. 3DCRT apart from the pending GORTEC 2004–01 trial.

Competing interests
The authors declare that they have no competing interests.

Authors' contributions
CM and JB provided collection and assembly of data. PK provided the concept and design of the manuscript. PL provided statistical data analysis and interpretation support. MA and ALC created/wrote and provided manuscript analysis. All authors have read and approved the final manuscript.

Author details
[1]Department of Otolaryngology, Winnipeg, Manitoba, Canada. [2]Cancer Care Manitoba, Winnipeg, Manitoba, Canada. [3]Department of Radiology, Winnipeg, Manitoba, Canada. [4]Department of Radiation Oncology, CancerCare Manitoba, 675 McDermot Avenue, Winnipeg, Manitoba R3E 0 V9, Canada.

References
1. Starmer HM, Tippett D, Webster K, Quon H, Jones B, Hardy S, et al. Swallowing outcomes in patients with oropharyngeal cancer undergoing organ preservation treatment. Head Neck. 2014;36(10):1392–7.
2. Saba NF, Edelman S, Tighiouart M, Gaultney J, Davis LW, Khuri FR, et al. Concurrent chemotherapy with intensity-modulated radiation therapy for locally advanced squamous cell carcinoma of the larynx and oropharynx: a retrospective single-institution analysis. Head Neck. 2009;31(11):1447–55.
3. Mendenhall WM, Amdur RJ, Palta JR. Intensity-modulated radiotherapy in the standard management of head and neck cancer: promises and pitfalls. J Clin Oncol. 2006;24(17):2618–23.
4. Vergeer MR, Doornaert PA, Rietveld D, Leemans CR, Slotman B, Langendijk J, et al. Intensity-modulated radiotherapy reduces radiation-induced morbidity and improves health-related quality of life: results of a nonrandomized prospective study using a standardized follow-up program. Int J Radiat Oncol Biol Phys. 2009;74(1):1–8.
5. Peponi E, Glanzmann C, Willi B, Huber G, Studer G. Dysphagia in head and neck cancer patients following intensity modulated radiotherapy (IMRT). Radiat Oncol. 2011;6:1.
6. Gupta T, Agarwal J, Jain S, Phurailatpam R, Kannan S, Ghosh-Laskar S, et al. Three-dimensional conformal radiotherapy (3D-CRT) versus intensity modulated radiation therapy (IMRT) in squamous cell carcinoma of the head and neck: a randomized controlled trial. Radiother Oncol. 2012;104(3):343–8.
7. Nutting CM, Morden JP, Harrington KJ, Urbano TG, Bhide SA, Clark C, et al. Parotid-sparing intensity modulated versus conventional radiotherapy in head and neck cancer (PARSPORT): a phase 3 multicentre randomised controlled trial. Lancet Oncol. 2011;12(2):127–36.
8. Rathod S, Gupta T, Ghosh-Laskar S, Murthy V, Budrukkar A, Agarwal J. Quality-of-life (QOL) outcomes in patients with head and neck squamous cell carcinoma (HNSCC) treated with intensity-modulated radiation therapy (IMRT) compared to three-dimensional conformal radiotherapy (3D-CRT): evidence from a prospective randomized study. Oral Oncol. 2013;49(6):634–42.
9. Lohia S, Rajapurkar M, Nguyen SA, Sharma AK, Gillespie MB, Day TA, et al. A comparison of outcomes using intensity-modulated radiation therapy and 3-dimensional conformal radiation therapy in treatment of oropharyngeal cancer. JAMA Otolaryngol Head Neck Surg. 2014;140(4):331–7.
10. Graff P, Lapeyre M, Desandes E, Ortholan C, Bensadoun RJ, Alfonsi M, et al. Impact of intensity-modulated radiotherapy on health-related quality of life for head and neck cancer patients: matched-pair comparison with conventional radiotherapy. Int J Radiat Oncol Biol Phys. 2007;67(5):1309–17.
11. Huang TL, Tsai WL, Chien CY, Lee TF, Fang FM. Quality of life for head and neck cancer patients treated by combined modality therapy: the

therapeutic benefit of technological advances in radiotherapy. Qual Life Res. 2010;19(9):1243–54.

12. Tribius S, Bergelt C. Intensity-modulated radiotherapy versus conventional and 3D conformal radiotherapy in patients with head and neck cancer: is there a worthwhile quality of life gain? Cancer Treat Rev. 2011;37(7):511–9.

13. McBride SM, Parambi RJ, Jang JW, Goldsmith T, Busse PM, Chan AW, et al. Intensity-modulated versus conventional radiation therapy for oropharyngeal carcinoma: long-term dysphagia and tumor control outcomes. Head Neck. 2014;36(4):492–8.

14. Myers C, Kerr P, Cooke AW, Bammeke F, Butler J, Lambert P. Functional outcomes after treatment of advanced oropharyngeal carcinoma with radiation or chemoradiation. J Otolaryngol Head Neck Surg. 2012;41(2):108–18.

15. Mor V, Laliberte L, Morris JN, Wiemann M. The Karnofsky Performance Status Scale, An examination of its reliability and validity in a research setting. Cancer. 1984;53(9):2002–7.

16. Oken MM, Creech RH, Tormey DC, Horton J, Davis TE, McFadden ET. Toxicity and response criteria of the Eastern Cooperative Oncology Group. Am J Clin Oncol. 1982;5(6):649–55.

17. List MA, Ritter-Sterr C, Lansky SB. A performance status scale for head and neck cancer patients. Cancer. 1990;66(3):564–9.

18. List MA, D'Antonio LL, Cella DF, Siston A, Mumby P, Haraf D, et al. The Performance Status Scale for Head and Neck Cancer Patients and the Functional Assessment of Cancer Therapy-Head and Neck Scale. A study of utility and validity. Cancer. 1996;77(11):2294–301.

19. Ward EC, Conroy A-L. Validity, Reliability and Responsivity of the Royal Brisbane Hospital Outcomes Measure for Swallowing. Asia Pacific J Speech Language Hearing. 1999;4:109–29.

20. Rosen CA, Lee AS, Osborne J, Zullo T, Murry T. Development and validation of the voice handicap index-10. Laryngoscope. 2004;114(9):1549–56.

21. Richardson LA, Jones GW. A review of the reliability and validity of the Edmonton Symptom Assessment System. Curr Oncol. 2009;16(1):55.

22. Curran D, Bacchi M, Schmitz SF, Molenberghs G, Sylvester RJ. Identifying the types of missingness in quality of life data from clinical trials. Stat Med. 1998;17(5–7):739–56.

23. Royston P. Multiple imputations of missing values; further update with ICE, with an emphasis on interval censoring. Stat J. 2007;4:445–64.

24. Graham JW, Olchowski AE, Gilreath TD. How many imputations are really needed? Some practical clarifications of multiple imputation theory. Prev Sci. 2007;8(3):206–13.

25. Lassen P, Eriksen JG, Hamilton-Dutoit S, Tramm T, Alsner J, Overgaard J, et al. Effect of HPV-associated p16INK4A expression on response to radiotherapy and survival in squamous cell carcinoma of the head and neck. J Clin Oncol. 2009;27(12):1992–8.

26. Eisbruch A, Schwartz C, Vineberg K, Damen E, Van As CJ, Marsh R, et al. Dysphagia and aspiration after chemoradiotherapy for head-and-neck cancer: which anatomic structures are affected and can they be spared by IMRT? Int J Radiat Oncol Biol Phys. 2004;60(5):1425–39.

Oncolytic activity of reovirus in HPV positive and negative head and neck squamous cell carcinoma

Timothy Cooper[1], Vincent L Biron[1], David Fast[2], Raymond Tam[3], Thomas Carey[4], Maya Shmulevitz[5*] and Hadi Seikaly[1*]

Abstract

Background: The management of patients with advanced stages of head and neck cancer requires a multidisciplinary and multimodality treatment approach which includes a combination of surgery, radiation, and chemotherapy. These toxic treatment protocols have significantly improved survival outcomes in a distinct population of human papillomavirus (HPV) associated oropharyngeal cancer. HPV negative head and neck squamous cell carcinoma (HNSCC) remains a challenge to treat because there is only a modest improvement in survival with the present treatment regimens, requiring innovative and new treatment approaches. Oncolytic viruses used as low toxicity adjunct cancer therapies are novel, potentially effective treatments for HNSCC. One such oncolytic virus is Respiratory Orphan Enteric virus or reovirus. Susceptibility of HNSCC cells towards reovirus infection and reovirus-induced cell death has been previously demonstrated but has not been compared in HPV positive and negative HNSCC cell lines.

Objectives: To compare the infectivity and oncolytic activity of reovirus in HPV positive and negative HNSCC cell lines.

Methods: Seven HNSCC cell lines were infected with serial dilutions of reovirus. Two cell lines (UM-SCC-47 and UM-SCC-104) were positive for type 16 HPV. Infectivity was measured using a cell-based ELISA assay 18 h after infection. Oncolytic activity was determined using an alamar blue viability assay 96 h after infection. Non-linear regression models were used to calculate the amounts of virus required to infect and to cause cell death in 50% of a given cell line (EC_{50}). EC_{50} values were compared.

Results: HPV negative cells were more susceptible to viral infection and oncolysis compared to HPV positive cell lines. EC_{50} for infectivity at 18 h ranged from multiplicity of infection (MOI) values (PFU/cell) of 18.6 (SCC-9) to 3133 (UM-SCC 104). EC_{50} for cell death at 96 h ranged from a MOI (PFU/cell) of 1.02×10^2 (UM-SCC-14A) to 3.19×10^8 (UM-SCC-47). There was a 3×10^6 fold difference between the least susceptible cell line (UM-SCC-47) and the most susceptible line (UM-SCC 14A) EC_{50} for cell death at 96 h.

Conclusions: HPV negative HNSCC cell lines appear to demonstrate greater reovirus infectivity and virus-mediated oncolysis compared to HPV positive HNSCC. Reovirus shows promise as a novel therapy in HNSCC, and may be of particular benefit in HPV negative patients.

Keywords: Reovirus, Head and neck cancer, Squamous cell carcinoma, HPV

* Correspondence: shmulevi@ualberta.ca; hadi.seikaly@albertahealthservices.ca
[5]Department of Medical Microbiology and Immunology, University of Alberta, 6-142 J Katz Group Centre for Pharmacy & Health Research, Edmonton, AB T6G 2E1, Canada
[1]Division of Otolaryngology - Head and Neck Surgery, Department of Surgery, University of Alberta, 1E4 University of Alberta Hospital, 1E4 Walter Mackenzie Center, 8440 112 St., Edmonton, AB T6G 2B7, Canada
Full list of author information is available at the end of the article

Background

Head and neck squamous cell carcinoma (HNSCC) is a devastating disease that affects all aspects of the patient's life, even in survivorship [1]. The management of patients with advanced stages of this disease requires a multidisciplinary and multimodality treatment approach which includes a combination of surgery, radiation, and chemotherapy. These toxic treatment protocols have significantly improved survival outcomes, especially in a distinct population of human papillomavirus (HPV) associated oropharyngeal cancer [2-7]. HPV is an important risk factor for a subset of HNSCC [8-10] and types 16 and 18 are particularly high risk for oncogenic transformation [11]. Patients with HPV associated head and neck cancer tend to be younger and less likely to have a significant history of smoking and alcohol consumption in comparison to those affected by non-HPV related head and neck cancer [8,12]. Advanced stage HPV negative HNSCC remains a challenge to treat because there is only a modest improvement in survival outcomes despite advances in therapy and the increasing toxicity of the different protocols [2,4-6]. This subset of patients, therefore, requires innovative and new treatment approaches.

The use of oncolytic viruses as a low toxicity adjunct cancer therapy is a novel and potentially effective treatment for HNSCC. One such oncolytic virus is Respiratory Orphan Enteric virus or reovirus [13-18]. Reovirus, from the family *Reoviridae*, is a non-enveloped, double stranded RNA virus that infects the upper respiratory and gastrointestinal tracts of humans with minimal symptoms [19]. Reovirus shows potent anti-tumor activity in a variety of tumor models, including models of HNSCC [20-27]. Multiple mechanisms mediate the strong specificity of reovirus towards cancer cells and especially towards cells with activated Ras signalling [16,28-33]. A proprietary formulation of the type 3 Dearing reovirus strain, called Reolysin®, is undergoing numerous phase I and phase II clinical trials and is currently in a phase III trial [19,34,35].

Susceptibility of HNSCC cells towards reovirus infection and reovirus-induced cell death has been previously demonstrated in both *in vitro* and mouse models [22,26,36,37], but the effectiveness and infectivity of reovirus in HPV positive and negative head and neck cancer cell lines has not been examined. The objectives of this study were to compare the infectivity and oncolysis of reovirus in HPV positive and negative HNSCC cell lines.

Methods
Cell lines
SCC-9, SCC-25, FaDU and L929 were purchased from ATC and maintained according to instructions. UM-SCC-14A, UM SCC 30, UM-SCC-47, and UM-SCC-104

were obtained from Dr. Thomas Carey at the University of Michigan and maintained according to instructions. UM-SCC-47 and UM-SCC-104 are both positive for high risk HPV 16 and express viral proteins E6 and E7 [38-40].

Virus
Reovirus serotype 3 Dearing was propagated in L929 cells and purified by ultracentrifugation on cesium chloride (CsCl) gradients as previously described [41]. Virus-infected cells were freeze-thawed and twice extracted with Vertrel XF (Dymar Chemicals) as previously described [41] and then layered onto 1.25- to 1.45-g/ml CsCl gradients. Virus was banded at 23,000 rpm for 5 h and dialyzed extensively against virus dilution buffer (150 mM NaCl, 15 mM $MgCl_2$, 10 mMTris, pH 7.4). Titers of purified reovirus preparations were obtained using standard plaque titration on L929 cells, and expressed as plaque forming units (PFU) per millilitre [32].

Seeding and infection of cells
Cells were counted using a TC20 automated cell counter (BioRad). 125 μL of cells at a concentration of 2.5×10^5 cells/mL were seeded into each well of a 96 well plate to achieve 100% confluence at time of infection. Serial dilutions of reovirus serotype 3 Dearing ranging from 4.8×10^8 to 1.43×10^1 PFU/mL (relative to L929 cells) were prepared in minimal essential media (MEM). Cells were incubated with 50 μl of virus at 37°C for 1 hour, then returned to virus-free complete medium for the remaining incubation period under standard tissue culture conditions.

Cell-based ELISA assay for infectivity
Eighteen hours after infection, cells were washed with PBS, fixed with methanol, and stored in blocking solution (Bovine serum albumin, PBS, Triton X-100). Cells were incubated with rabbit anti-reovirus primary antibody (1:5000, blocking solution), washed with PBS-T (PBS, Triton X-100) solution, then incubated with goat anti-rabbit alkaline phosphatase antibody (1:4000, blocking solution). Following extensive washes with PBS-T, 200 μL of P-nitrophenyl phosphate in diethanolamine buffer (1 mg/mL) was added to each well. Plates were incubated at room temperature for 80 minutes, and absorbance was measured at 405 nm using a spectrophotometer (EnVision Multilabel Reader, Perkin Elmer).

Alamar blue viability assay
Alamar blue is a commonly used indicator in cell viability assays [42]. At 96 hours after infection, 20 μL of 440 μM alamar blue in sterile PBS diluted 1:10 with ddH2O was added to each well of a 96-well plate. Following incubation for 2 hours at 37°C, fluorescence was measured at excitation/emission wavelengths of 544/590 nm respectively (Fluostar OPTIMA plate reader, BMG Labtech).

Calculation of 96 hour viability

Using the measured fluorescence from the alamar blue assay, viability at 96 h was calculated in the well infected with reovirus at a concentration of 2.40×10^8 PFU/mL. Fluorescence was averaged from two or more duplicates within each experiment. Viability was expressed as a percentage with 100% viability determined by the fluorescence of the uninfected cells and 0% viability calculated as an average of the fluorescence of wells containing media but not seeded with cells. Mean viability was calculated for each cell line from three or more independent experiments. Statistically significant outliers and experiments with technical issues related to uneven seeding of cells were excluded from analysis.

Calculation of EC_{50} values

Effective concentration 50 or EC_{50} is a term used in pharmacodynamics indicating the concentration required to have a 50% maximal effect. In the context of infection with a virus, we have defined EC_{50} to indicate the amount of virus needed to infect 50% of cells at 18 hours postinfection, as measured by a cell-based ELISA assay. To quantify reovirus-induced cell death, we have defined EC_{50} to indicate the amount of virus required to reduce cell viability to 50% (relative to untreated cells) at 96 hours postinfection, as measured by an alamar blue viability assay. Absorbance (infectivity) or fluorescence (cell viability) values were plotted against multiplicity of infection (MOI, PFU/cell). Baseline and maximum response were established from uninfected cells (maximum viability, minimum infectivity), media alone (minimum viability), or maximally-infected L929 cells (maximum infectivity). Mean absorbance or fluorescence at a given viral concentration was calculated as the mean of two or more duplicates within the same experiment. Three or more independent experiments were used to generate a dose–response curve for each cell line (Prism; Graph-Pad Software Inc., San Diego, CA). From this, EC_{50} values were calculated by fitting a standard equation for a sigmoidal dose–response curve.

Statistical analysis

Student's *t*-test was used to compare EC_{50} values for infectivity and oncolysis between cell lines. Student's *t*-test was also used to compare cell viability at 96 h. $P < 0.05$ was accepted as statistically significant.

Ethics

Institutional ethics review board approval was obtained from the University of Alberta Health Research Ethics Board prior to the commencement of the study.

Results

Infectivity

EC_{50} MOI for infectivity at 18 h indicates the number of reovirus particles per cell that were sufficient to achieve infection and active replication in 50% of cells at this time point. The HNSCC cell lines demonstrated variable susceptibility to infection by reovirus at 18 h. The cell lines listed from most to least susceptible to reovirus infection at 18 h and their corresponding EC_{50} MOI values (PFU/cell) were SCC-9 (18.6 ± 0.7), FaDU (28.4 ± 0.7), SCC-25 (51.2 ± 1.6), UM-SCC-14A (77.3 ± 3.1), UM-SCC-38 (651 ± 11), UM-SCC-47 (1425 ± 23), and UM-SCC-104 (3133 ± 86) (Figure 1). The most susceptible HNSCC cell lines were SCC-9 and FaDU. These cell lines required a mean of 18.6 and 28.4 virus particles per cell to achieve 50% infectivity at 18 h respectively. The least susceptible cell lines, UM-SCC-47 and UM-SCC-104, were both HPV positive. They required a mean of 1425 and 3133 virus particles per cell to achieve 50% infection, respectively. In comparing the two HPV positive cell lines individually to each of the 5 HPV negative cell lines, the HPV positive HNSCC cell lines were less susceptible to infection by reovirus with statistical significance ($p < 0.01$).

96 h viability

Differences in percent viability were also found between cell lines 96 h after infection with reovirus at a concentration of 2.40×10^8 PFU/mL. This equates to an MOI of 7.68×10^3 viral particles per cell. The mean percent viabilities for each cell line from least to greatest were UM-SCC-14A ($6.7 \pm 5.0\%$), FaDU ($10.9 \pm 3.7\%$), SCC-9 ($33.2 \pm 9.9\%$),

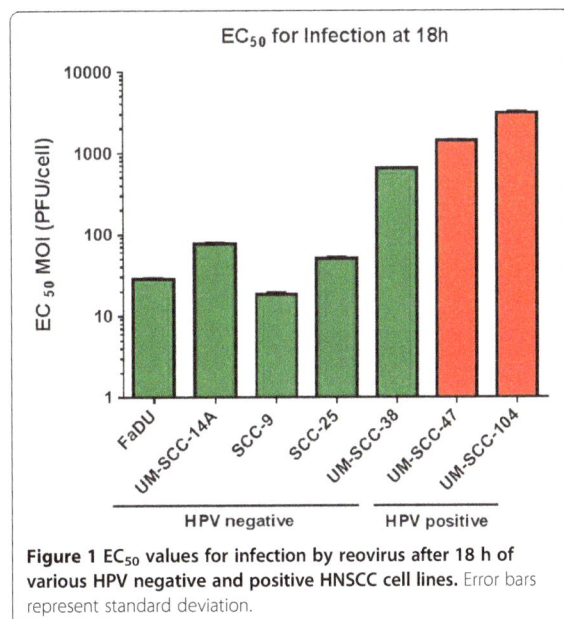

Figure 1 EC_{50} values for infection by reovirus after 18 h of various HPV negative and positive HNSCC cell lines. Error bars represent standard deviation.

SCC-25 (54.6 ± 21.5%), UM-SCC-104 (82.3 ± 6.5%), UM-SCC-38 (83.9 ± 16.3%), and UM-SCC-47 (97.2 ± 4.7%) (Figure 2). The two most susceptible cell lines to virally-induced cytotoxicity were UM-SCC-14A and FaDU which were both HPV negative. Of the three cell lines with the greatest viability at this time point, two were HPV positive (UM-SCC-104 and UM-SCC-47). UM-SCC-47 had more viable cells with statistical significance than all of the HPV negative cell lines except for UM-SCC-38 (p = 0.17). UM-SCC-104 had more viable cells with statistical significance than UM-SCC-14A, FaDU, and SCC-9 (all with p < 0.01). The HPV positive cell lines were highly resistant to onco-lysis by reovirus and showed only minimal viral-induced cytotoxicity at 96 h, even with high concentrations of reo-virus used for infection. Images taken from brightfield mi-croscopy at 96 hours after infection of the UM-SCC-14A, UM-SCC-47, and UM-SCC-104 cell lines demonstrate this difference (Figure 3).

Oncolysis

The head and neck cancer cell lines had variable EC_{50} values for cell death at 96 h. The HNSCC cell line most susceptible to reovirus was UM-SCC-14A (HPV nega-tive) with a mean EC_{50} MOI (PFU/cell) value of 102 (95%CI [93–112]). This means that 102 reovirus parti-cles per cell were sufficient to cause 50% cell death in this cell line. The remaining cell lines from most to least susceptible to reovirus-mediated oncolysis and their cor-responding EC_{50} MOI (PFU/cell) values were FaDU (388, CI[378–397]), SCC-9 (4.24×10^3, CI[4.00×10^3–4.49×10^3]), SCC-25 (1.07×10^4, CI[1.03×10^4–1.10×10^4]),

UM-SCC-38 (2.99×10^4, CI[2.80×10^4–3.18×10^4]), UM-SCC-104 (4.04×10^5, CI[2.62×10^5–6.23×10^5]), and UM-SCC-47 (3.19×10^8, CI[1.31×10^8–7.76×10^8) (Figure 4). The two HPV positive cell lines were more resistant to reovirus-mediated oncolysis in comparison to the HPV negative cell lines (p < 0.01 in all cases).

Discussion

The use of viruses in cancer therapy is a rapidly expand-ing area of research [13,16,23,27,34]. However, the use of viral oncolytic therapy has yet to make the transition from bench to bedside in standard practice. Reovirus was first shown to have an oncolytic effect in head and neck cancer cells by Ikeda et al. [22] using in vitro and in vivo models. This effect has been demonstrated in nu-merous head and neck cell lines [24,25,36,37]. The onco-lytic effect is believed to be independent of epidermal growth factor receptor (EGFR) activation and molecular predictors of response have yet to be identified [25]. Pre-clinical studies have shown the effectiveness of a com-bination of reovirus, paclitaxel and cisplatin in head and neck cancer lines [24]. Also, animal models have sug-gested a role for reovirus as an adjunct in surgically resected disease with positive margins [37]. Intravenously administered reovirus in combination with carboplatin and paclitaxel has been shown to have activity in advanced stage and recurrent head and neck cancer in a recently published phase I/II clinical trial [35]. An ongoing phase III trial is investigating intravenous reovirus in combin-ation with paclitaxel and carboplatin (Reo 018).

Reovirus has variable infectivity and oncolytic activity in head and neck cancer cell lines and the mechanism behind this variable susceptibility has yet to be eluci-dated but is likely multifactorial. Our findings suggest an important difference in the susceptibility of head and neck cancer cells to reovirus based on HPV status. The HPV negative cell lines used were much more suscep-tible than the HPV positive cells to both infection by reovirus and virus-mediated oncolysis. There was a >150 fold difference in the amount of virus required to infect 50% of cells in the most susceptible cell line (SCC-9) and the least susceptible cell line (UM-SCC-104). Simi-larly, there was a dramatic difference between oncolysis based on HPV status. There was a 3×10^6 fold difference in the EC_{50} values of the most susceptible cell line UM-SCC-14A (HPV negative) and the most resistant cell line UM-SCC-47 (HPV positive). For both infectivity at 18 h and oncolysis at 96 h, the HPV negative cells were more susceptible than the HPV positive cells by highly signifi-cant values. Our study is the first to compare the onco-lytic activity of reovirus in HPV positive and negative head and neck cancer cell lines. Also, it is the first to compare reovirus infectivity among head and neck can-cer cell lines.

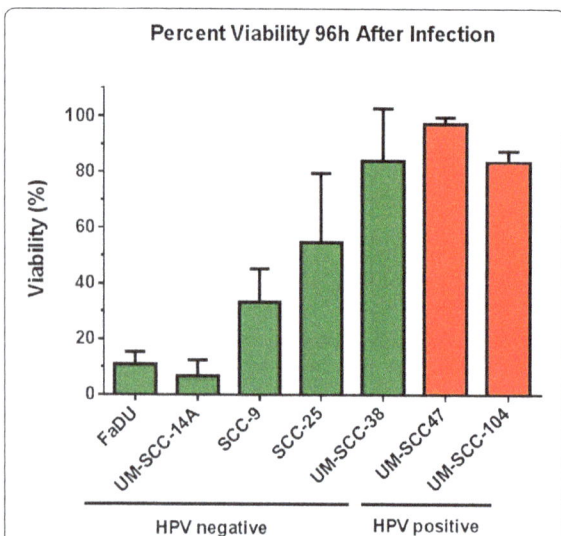

Figure 2 Percentage of viable cells of various HNSCC cell lines 96 h after addition of 2.40×10^8 PFU/mL dilution of reovirus. Mean values were taken from three or more independent experiments. Error bars represent standard deviation.

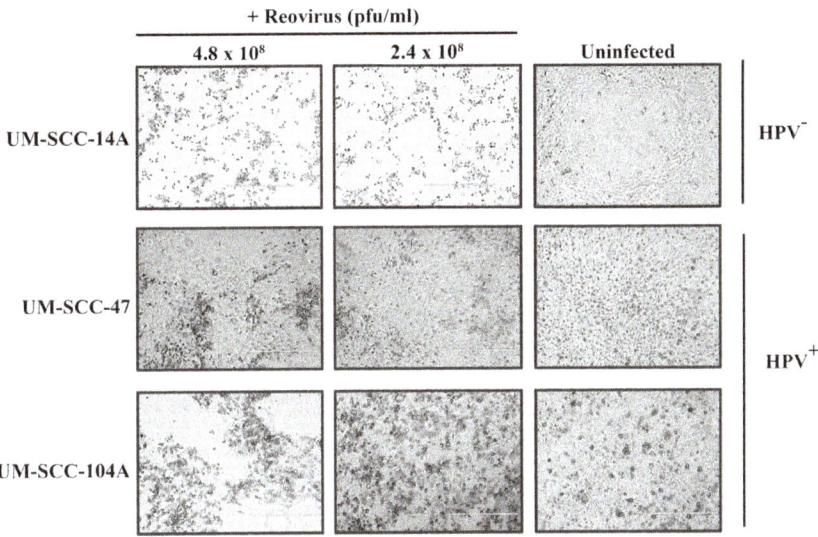

Figure 3 Brightfield microscopy of UM-SCC-14A, UM-SCC-47, and UM-SCC-104 cells 96 h after the addition of 4.8×10^8 and 2.4×10^8 PFU/mL reovirus dilutions according to experiment protocol compared to uninfected controls

HPV positive (vs negative) oropharyngeal squamous cell carcinoma (OPSCC) has been shown to have a more favourable response to treatment with surgical and non-surgical treatments [6,7]. However, when considering treatment with cetuximab, a monoclonal antibody that targets EGFR, a number of studies suggest HPV positive OPSCC tumors may be less responsive to this chemotherapeutic drug [43,44]. This is consistent with several studies showing an inverse relationship with HPV positivity [44]. It is important to note that both reovirus and

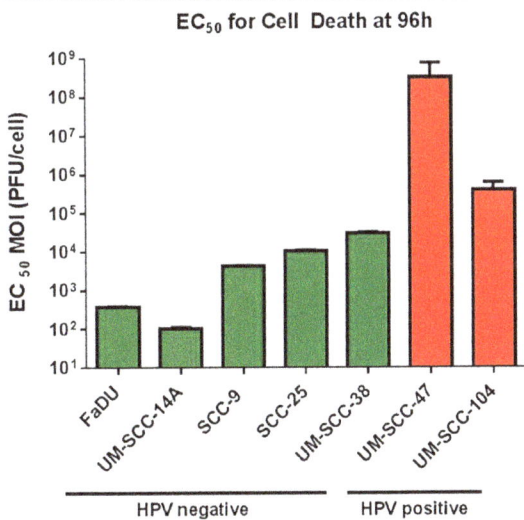

Figure 4 EC_{50} values for oncolysis 96 h after reovirus infection of various HPV negative and positive HNSCC cell lines. Error bars represent standard deviation.

cetuximab act on Ras-dependent pathways [44]. Taken together, our results showing resistance to reovirus in HPV-positive HNSCC cell lines could therefore be due to a lack of EGFR expression and its downstream Ras-dependent treatment response.

Novel therapies are needed in head and neck cancer, especially in patients with HPV negative malignancies. Conventional therapy is associated with substantial morbidity and long-term complications [1], and progress has been limited in the use of adjuvant therapy in patients with advanced stage HPV negative cancers [45]. Reovirus shows promise as a potential novel therapy in HPV negative head and neck cancer.

Further research is required to identify additional molecular markers for susceptibility to reovirus to identify patients most likely to benefit from adjunctive reovirus therapy. HPV negative patients, a group with a poor prognosis relative to those with HPV-related head and neck cancer, are identified as a group to target in future reovirus trials. Ongoing and future trials investigating reovirus in head and neck cancer may need to perform subgroup analysis based on HPV status.

Commonly described features of HNSCC cell lines include tumor subsite, staging, and treatment modalities utilized. Although clinically relevant, the smoking history of the patients from which these cell lines have been derived is not well described in the literature. The smoking status of the patients from which FaDU and SCC-9 were derived is not documented. The source of SCC-25 had an extensive history of smoking [46]. Of the cell lines obtained from Dr. Carey and the University of Michigan, UM-SCC-14A, UM-SCC-38, and UM-SCC-

104 were derived from smokers [47]. However, there is no laboratory documentation regarding the smoking status of the patient from which the HPV positive UM-SCC-47 cell line was derived. Despite this limitation in clinical history, numerous papers have delineated genotypic differences between these and other HNSCC cell lines [48].

There are several limitations to this study. The behavior of cell lines in *in vitro* experiments is variable. Confounding factors between the cell lines used beyond HPV status may have an impact on results. Head and neck cancer is a molecularly and genetically heterogeneous entity [48,49]. Therefore, caution must be used in generalizing the effect of reovirus on a selection of cell lines to all HPV positive or negative head and neck cancers. However, this study design allowed for a time and cost efficient way to test a hypothesis regarding the activity of reovirus and HPV positive and negative head and neck cancers. Further investigation into the effect of reovirus on additional HPV positive and negative cell lines as well as in HPV positive and negative animal models is warranted.

Conclusions

HPV negative cell lines appear to be more susceptible to reovirus infection and oncolysis than their HPV positive counterparts. Reovirus shows promise as a potential novel therapy in HPV negative head and neck cancer.

Ethics approval

Prior to commencement, health research ethics board approval was obtained from the University of Alberta Health Research Ethics Board.

Abbreviations

CsCl: Cesium chloride; EC_{50}: Effective concentration 50%; EGFR: Epidermal growth factor receptor; HNSCC: Head and neck squamous cell carcinoma; HPV: Human papillomavirus; $MgCl_2$: Magnesium chloride; MOI: Multiplicity of infection; OPSCC: Oropharyngeal squamous cell carcinoma; PBS: Phosphate buffered saline; PFU: Plaque forming units; RPM: Rotations per minute.

Competing interests

The authors declare that they have no competing interests.

Authors' contributions

TC contributed with conception and design, conduction of experiments, data collection, data analysis, writing and revision of the manuscript. VB contributed with conception and design, data analysis, and writing and revision of the manuscript. DF contributed with conduction of experiments, data collection, and critical revision of the manuscript. RT contributed with conduction of experiments, data collection, and critical revision of the manuscript. TEC contributed with conception and design and critical revision of the manuscript. MS contributed with conception and design, data analysis, and writing of the manuscript. HS contributed with conception and design, data analysis, and writing and revision of the manuscript. All authors have given final approval of the version to be published.

Authors' information

Hadi Seikaly and Maya Shmulevitz are co-senior authors.

Acknowledgements

We would like to acknowledge Heather Eaton, Adil Mohamed, Wong Kong Yip, Kevin James, Alicia Guenette, and Georgi Trifonov from Dr. Shmulevitz's laboratory for assistance with cell culture and reagents. We would also like to thank Dr. Carey's laboratory from the University of Michigan for collaborative contribution of cell lines and advice on cell line maintenance.

Financial Support/Disclosures

Funding from the Division of Otolaryngology Head – Neck Surgery, University of Alberta.

Author details

[1]Division of Otolaryngology - Head and Neck Surgery, Department of Surgery, University of Alberta, 1E4 University of Alberta Hospital, 1E4 Walter Mackenzie Center, 8440 112 St., Edmonton, AB T6G 2B7, Canada. [2]Faculty of Science 1-001 CCIS, University of Alberta, Edmonton, AB T6G 2E9, Canada. [3]Faculty of Medicine and Dentistry, University of Alberta, 2J2 WC Mackenzie Health Sciences Centre, Edmonton, AB T6G 2R7, Canada. [4]Department of Head and Neck Surgery, University of Michigan, 5311B Med Sci I, Ann Arbor, MI 48109-5616, USA. [5]Department of Medical Microbiology and Immunology, University of Alberta, 6–142 J Katz Group Centre for Pharmacy & Health Research, Edmonton, AB T6G 2E1, Canada.

References

1. Rutten H, Pop LA, Janssens GO, Takes RP, Knuijt S, Rooijakkers AF, et al. Long-term outcome and morbidity after treatment with accelerated radiotherapy and weekly cisplatin for locally advanced head-and-neck cancer: Results of a multidisciplinary late morbidity clinic. Int J Radiat Oncol, Biol, Phys. 2011;81(4):923–9.
2. Lau HY, Brar S, Klimowicz AC, Petrillo SK, Hao D, Brockton NT, et al. Prognostic significance of p16 in locally advanced squamous cell carcinoma of the head and neck treated with concurrent cisplatin and radiotherapy. Head Neck. 2011;33(2):251–6.
3. Laco J, Nekvindova J, Novakova V, Celakovsky P, Dolezalova H, Tucek L, et al. Biologic importance and prognostic significance of selected clinicopathological parameters in patients with oral and oropharyngeal squamous cell carcinoma, with emphasis on smoking, protein p16(INK4a) expression, and HPV status. Neoplasma. 2012;59(4):398–408.
4. Fakhry C, Westra WH, Li S, Cmelak A, Ridge JA, Pinto H, et al. Improved survival of patients with human papillomavirus-positive head and neck squamous cell carcinoma in a prospective clinical trial. J Natl Cancer Inst. 2008;100(4):261–9.
5. Cooper T, Biron V, Adam B, Klimowicz AC, Puttagunta L, Seikaly H. Prognostic utility of basaloid differentiation in oropharyngeal cancer. J Otolaryngol Head Neck Surg. 2013;42:57. 0216–42–57.
6. Ang KK, Harris J, Wheeler R, Weber R, Rosenthal DI, Nguyen-Tan PF, et al. Human papillomavirus and survival of patients with oropharyngeal cancer. N Engl J Med. 2010;363(1):24–35.
7. Bossi P, Orlandi E, Miceli R, Perrone F, Guzzo M, Mariani L, et al. Treatment-related outcome of oropharyngeal cancer patients differentiated by HPV dictated risk profile: A tertiary cancer centre series analysis. Ann Oncol. 2014;25(3):694–9.
8. Cardesa A, Nadal A. Carcinoma of the head and neck in the HPV era. Acta Dermatovenerol Alp Panonica Adriat. 2011;20(3):161–73.
9. El-Mofty SK, Patil S. Human papillomavirus (HPV)-related oropharyngeal nonkeratinizing squamous cell carcinoma: Characterization of a distinct phenotype. Oral Surg Oral Med Oral Pathol Oral Radiol Endod. 2006;101(3):339–45.
10. Gillison ML, Koch WM, Capone RB, Spafford M, Westra WH, Wu L, et al. Evidence for a causal association between human papillomavirus and a subset of head and neck cancers. J Natl Cancer Inst. 2000;92(9):709–20.
11. Nichols AC, Faquin WC, Westra WH, Mroz EA, Begum S, Clark JR, et al. HPV-16 infection predicts treatment outcome in oropharyngeal squamous cell carcinoma. Otolaryngol Head Neck Surg. 2009;140(2):228–34.
12. El-Mofty SK, Lu DW. Prevalence of human papillomavirus type 16 DNA in squamous cell carcinoma of the palatine tonsil and not the oral cavity, in young patients: a distinct clinicopathologic and molecular disease entity. Am J Surg Pathol. 2003;27(11):1463–70.

13. Coffey MC, Strong JE, Forsyth PA, Lee PW. Reovirus therapy of tumors with activated ras pathway. Science. 1998;282(5392):1332–4.

14. Duncan MR, Stanish SM, Cox DC. Differential sensitivity of normal and transformed human cells to reovirus infection. J Virol. 1978;28(2):444–9.

15. Hashiro G, Loh PC, Yau JT. The preferential cytotoxicity of reovirus for certain transformed cell lines. Arch Virol. 1977;54(4):307–15.

16. Maitra R, Ghalib MH, Goel S. Reovirus: a targeted therapeutic–progress and potential. Mol Cancer Res. 2012;10(12):1514–25.

17. Strong JE, Lee PW. The v-erbB oncogene confers enhanced cellular susceptibility to reovirus infection. J Virol. 1996;70(1):612–6.

18. Strong JE, Tang D, Lee PW. Evidence that the epidermal growth factor receptor on host cells confers reovirus infection efficiency. Virology. 1993;197(1):405–11.

19. Kyula JN, Roulstone V, Karapanagiotou EM, Melcher AA, Harrington KJ. Oncolytic reovirus type 3 (dearing) as a novel therapy in head and neck cancer. Expert Opin Biol Ther. 2012;12(12):1669–78.

20. Errington F, White CL, Twigger KR, Rose A, Scott K, Steele L, et al. Inflammatory tumour cell killing by oncolytic reovirus for the treatment of melanoma. Gene Ther. 2008;15(18):1257–70.

21. Etoh T, Himeno Y, Matsumoto T, Aramaki M, Kawano K, Nishizono A, et al. Oncolytic viral therapy for human pancreatic cancer cells by reovirus. Clin Cancer Res. 2003;9(3):1218–23.

22. Ikeda Y, Nishimura G, Yanoma S, Kubota A, Furukawa M, Tsukuda M. Reovirus oncolysis in human head and neck squamous carcinoma cells. Auris Nasus Larynx. 2004;31(4):407–12.

23. Norman KL, Coffey MC, Hirasawa K, Demetrick DJ, Nishikawa SG, DiFrancesco LM, et al. Reovirus oncolysis of human breast cancer. Hum Gene Ther. 2002;13(5):641–52.

24. Roulstone V, Twigger K, Zaidi S, Pencavel T, Kyula JN, White C, et al. Synergistic cytotoxicity of oncolytic reovirus in combination with cisplatin-paclitaxel doublet chemotherapy. Gene Ther. 2013;20(5):521–8.

25. Twigger K, Roulstone V, Kyula J, Karapanagiotou EM, Syrigos KN, Morgan R, et al. Reovirus exerts potent oncolytic effects in head and neck cancer cell lines that are independent of signalling in the EGFR pathway. BMC Cancer. 2012;12:368. 2407–12–368.

26. Twigger K, Vidal L, White CL, De Bono JS, Bhide S, Coffey M, et al. Enhanced in vitro and in vivo cytotoxicity of combined reovirus and radiotherapy. Clin Cancer Res. 2008;14(3):912–23.

27. Shmulevitz M, Marcato P, Lee PW. Unshackling the links between reovirus oncolysis, ras signaling, translational control and cancer. Oncogene. 2005;24(52):7720–8.

28. Marcato P, Shmulevitz M, Pan D, Stoltz D, Lee PW. Ras transformation mediates reovirus oncolysis by enhancing virus uncoating, particle infectivity, and apoptosis-dependent release. Mol Ther. 2007;15(8):1522–30.

29. Pan D, Pan LZ, Hill R, Marcato P, Shmulevitz M, Vassilev LT, et al. Stabilisation of p53 enhances reovirus-induced apoptosis and virus spread through p53-dependent NF-kappaB activation. Br J Cancer. 2011;105(7):1012–22.

30. Shmulevitz M, Lee PW. Exploring host factors that impact reovirus replication, dissemination, and reovirus-induced cell death in cancer versus normal cells in culture. Methods Mol Biol. 2012;797:163–76.

31. Shmulevitz M, Marcato P, Lee PW. Activated ras signaling significantly enhances reovirus replication and spread. Cancer Gene Ther. 2010;17(1):69–70.

32. Shmulevitz M, Pan LZ, Garant K, Pan D, Lee PW. Oncogenic ras promotes reovirus spread by suppressing IFN-beta production through negative regulation of RIG-I signaling. Cancer Res. 2010;70(12):4912–21.

33. Pan D, Marcato P, Ahn DG, Gujar S, Pan LZ, Shmulevitz M, et al. Activation of p53 by chemotherapeutic agents enhances reovirus oncolysis. PLoS One. 2013;8(1):e54006.

34. Black AJ, Morris DG. Clinical trials involving the oncolytic virus, reovirus: ready for prime time? Expert Rev Clin Pharmacol. 2012;5(5):517–20.

35. Karapanagiotou EM, Roulstone V, Twigger K, Ball M, Tanay M, Nutting C, et al. Phase I/II trial of carboplatin and paclitaxel chemotherapy in combination with intravenous oncolytic reovirus in patients with advanced malignancies. Clin Cancer Res. 2012;18(7):2080–9.

36. Brookes JT, Seikaly H, Lim T, Wong KK, Harris JR, Moore RB. Reovirus salvage of squamous cell cancer-contaminated wounds. J Otolaryngol. 2005;34(1):32–7.

37. Mechor B, Seikaly H, Wong K, Chau J, Uwiera R, Harris JR. Reovirus salvage of positive resection margin: a novel treatment adjunct. J Otolaryngol. 2006;35(2):97–101.

38. Zhao M, Sano D, Pickering CR, Jasser SA, Henderson YC, Clayman GL, et al. Assembly and initial characterization of a panel of 85 genomically validated cell lines from diverse head and neck tumor sites. Clin Cancer Res. 2011;17(23):7248–64.

39. Tang AL, Hauff SJ, Owen JH, Graham MP, Czerwinski MJ, Park JJ, et al. UM-SCC-104: a new human papillomavirus-16-positive cancer stem cell-containing head and neck squamous cell carcinoma cell line. Head Neck. 2012;34(10):1480–91.

40. Brenner JC, Graham MP, Kumar B, Saunders LM, Kupfer R, Lyons RH, et al. Genotyping of 73 UM-SCC head and neck squamous cell carcinoma cell lines. Head Neck. 2010;32(4):417–26.

41. Mendez II, Hermann LL, Hazelton PR, Coombs KM. A comparative analysis of freon substitutes in the purification of reovirus and calicivirus. J Virol Methods. 2000;90(1):59–67.

42. Rampersad SN. Multiple applications of alamar blue as an indicator of metabolic function and cellular health in cell viability bioassays. Sensors (Basel). 2012;12(9):12347–60.

43. Koutcher L, Sherman E, Fury M, Wolden S, Zhang Z, Mo Q, et al. Concurrent cisplatin and radiation versus cetuximab and radiation for locally advanced head-and-neck cancer. Int J Radiat Oncol, Biol, Phys. 2011;81(4):915–22.

44. Mirghani H, Amen F, Moreau F, Guigay J, Hartl DM, Lacau St Guily J. Oropharyngeal cancers: Relationship between epidermal growth factor receptor alterations and human papillomavirus status. Eur J Cancer. 2014;50(6):1100–11.

45. Burtness B, Bauman JE, Galloway T. Novel targets in HPV-negative head and neck cancer: overcoming resistance to EGFR inhibition. Lancet Oncol. 2013;14(8):e302–9.

46. Somers KD, Merrick MA, Lopez ME, Incognito LS, Schechter GL, Casey G. Frequent p53 mutations in head and neck cancer. Cancer Res. 1992;52(21):5997–6000.

47. Tang AL, Hauff SJ, Owen JH. UM-SCC-104: a new human papillomavirus-16-positive cancer stem cell-containing head and neck squamous cell carcinoman cell line. Head Neck. 2012;34(10):1480–91.

48. Biron VL, Mohamed A, Hendzel MJ, Alan Underhill D, Seikaly H. Epigenetic differences between human papillomavirus-positive and -negative oropharyngeal squamous cell carcinomas. J Otolaryngol Head Neck Surg. 2012;41 Suppl 1:S65–70.

49. Barber BR, Biron VL, Klimowicz AC, Puttagunta L, Cote DW, Seikaly H. Molecular predictors of locoregional and distant metastases in oropharyngeal squamous cell carcinoma. J Otolaryngol Head Neck Surg. 2013;42:53. 0216–42–53.

15

Predictors of round window accessibility for adult cochlear implantation based on pre-operative CT scan: a prospective observational study

Edward Park*, Hosam Amoodi, Jafri Kuthubutheen, Joseph M. Chen, Julian M. Nedzelski and Vincent Y. W. Lin

Abstract

Background: Cochlear implantation has become a mainstream treatment option for patients with severe to profound sensorineural hearing loss. During cochlear implant, there are key surgical steps which are influenced by anatomical variations between each patient. The aim of this study is to determine if there are potential predictors of difficulties that may be encountered during the cortical mastoidectomy, facial recess approach and round window access in cochlear implant surgery based upon pre-operative temporal bone CT scan.

Methods: Fifty seven patients undergoing unilateral cochlear implantation were analyzed. Difficulty with 1) cortical mastoidectomy, 2) facial recess approach, and 3) round window access were scored intra-operatively by the surgeon in a blinded fashion (1 = "easy", 2 = "moderate", 3 = "difficult"). Pre-operative temporal bone CT scans were analyzed for 1) degree of mastoid aeration; 2) location of the sigmoid sinus; 3) height of the tegmen; 4) the presence of air cells in the facial recess, and 5) degree of round window bony overhang.

Results: Poor mastoid aeration and lower tegmen position, but not the location of sigmoid sinus, are associated with greater difficulty with the cortical mastoidectomy. Presence of an air cell around the facial nerve was predictive of easier facial recess access. However, the degree of round window bony overhang was not predictive of difficulty associated with round window access.

Conclusion: Certain parameters on the pre-operative temporal bone CT scan may be useful in predicting potential difficulties encountered during the key steps involved in cochlear implant surgery.

Keywords: Round window, Cochlear implant, CT scan

Background

Cochlear implantation has become a widely accepted treatment option for patients with severe to profound sensorineural hearing loss. The benefits to the patient are well published in both pediatric and adult populations. Historically, the cochlear implant electrode was inserted through a cochleostomy, typically anterior-inferior to the presumed location of the round window. Currently, many large cochlear implant centres, including our own, have chosen the round window approach for the majority of electrode insertions. This was made possible mainly by the development of slimmer, atraumatic electrodes and through the popularization of the concept of "soft" hearing preservation surgical techniques [1].

There are several key surgical steps for a cochlear implant with the intention of a round window insertion. They include 1) cortical mastoidectomy; 2) opening the facial recess; and 3) round window membrane identification and opening. A cortical mastoidectomy is defined as a canal-wall-up mastoidectomy in which its main purpose is to establish the location of the mastoid antrum and allow access to the facial recess. The facial recess, also known as a posterior tympanotomy, is a well-established otologic surgical pathway that gains access to the middle ear without

* Correspondence: edward.park@utoronto.ca
Department of Otolaryngology – Head and Neck Surgery, Sunnybrook Health Sciences Centre, 2075 Bayview Avenue, Toronto, ON M4N 3M5, Canada

violating the tympanic membrane. Its borders are defined as the vertical segment of the facial nerve medially, the chorda tympanic nerve/tympanic annulus laterally and the incus buttress superiorly. This narrow, bony 3-dimensional space which comprises the facial recess can often be challenging to identify and expose in order to gain access to the round window located more posteriorly. Finally, the round window is usually partially hidden by the bony round window niche and this familiar landmark must be identified before the bony niche can be drilled away to fully expose the round window membrane. Once the round window membrane is fully exposed, then it can be opened to enter the perilymphatic space of the scala tympani before the electrode can be carefully and slowly inserted.

These well-established steps of cochlear implantation may be influenced by anatomical variations among patients, which can pose unanticipated technical challenges with respect to obtaining adequate surgical exposure. A pre-operative temporal bone CT scan, done routinely in many centres including ours, serves as a guide to the anatomical layout of the ear to be implanted. Our hypothesis is that by analyzing the pre-operative temporal bone CT scan, it may be possible to determine certain radiological features that can predict the level of difficulty with the aforementioned surgical steps. In turn, such information can help surgical trainees anticipate and prepare for technical challenges that may be encountered during the operation.

There are several previous studies that have assessed the relationship between the findings from pre-operative temporal bone CT scan and intraoperative findings of structural abnormalities during cochlear implant [2–4]. However, most of these studies have focused on cochlear patency/ossification and did not attempt to correlate intraoperative difficulties with pre-operative CT parameters. In the study by Woolley et al. [4], pre-operative CT findings were compared to intraoperative findings during pediatric cochlear implantation in a retrospective fashion, but there was no intraoperative grading to 'quantify' the difficulties associated with pertinent steps; instead, they described the difficulties and any intraoperative complications that occurred. In comparison, our study is a prospective study, which assessed the correlations between specific and easy-to-measure parameters on the pre-operative temporal bone CT and intraoperative difficulties with key surgical steps that were graded by the surgeon during cochlear implantation.

Methods
Study design
This was a prospective, observational study of consecutive cochlear implant surgeries with the goal of a round window insertion performed at an adult tertiary implant centre. All surgeries were performed by three surgeons who routinely perform round window electrode insertions. Patients with previous mastoid surgery, re-implantations, revision surgeries, and patients who were implanted via alternative techniques (e.g. transcanal) were excluded from the study.

Ethics, consent, and permissions
The study was approved by the ethics board at the Sunnybrook Health Sciences Centre and the consent for participation in research study was taken as part of the consent for cochlear implant surgery.

Subjects
A total of 57 patients who underwent unilateral cochlear implant with round window electrode insertion and had pre-operative high-resolution temporal bone CT scan were included. All patients had moderate to profound bilateral sensorineural hearing loss, which was unaidable with hearing aids. All patients underwent routine audiometric testing and pre-operative electronystagmography, as well as temporal bone CT scans. They also received pre-operative counseling from a cochlear implant audiologist as part of our screening protocol.

Intra-operative scoring of surgical difficulties
Difficulties encountered with each of the three key intraoperative steps - cortical mastoidectomy, access to the facial recess, and round window access - were scored according to the following scale: 1 = "easy", 2 = "moderate", 3 = "difficult". Scoring was performed by the primary surgeon, who was a staff otologist, or by the fully credentialed otology fellow. They were blinded to the potential predictors of difficulties with the aforementioned surgical steps on the pre-operative CT scan.

Analysis of pre-operative CT scan
Pre-operative temporal bone CT scans were analyzed by the primary author, who was blinded to the intraoperative scoring of surgical difficulties. The CT scan contained high-resolution images that are 0.625 mm thick with reconstructed coronal and sagittal images. The images were viewed in the standard bone window setting. The CT scan was analyzed for 1) degree of aeration of the mastoid; 2) location of the sigmoid sinus; 3) height of the tegmen, which correspond to difficulties associated with a cortical mastoidectomy, as well as 4) the presence of air cells around the facial recess, which relates to difficulty associated with performing the facial recess, and 5) degree of round window bony overhang, which relates to difficulties associated with round window access.

With respect to mastoid aeration, the mastoid on the ipsilateral side of cochlear implant was examined on axial images. The degree of its aeration was categorized as being either "well aerated", "moderately aerated", or "poorly aerated" (Fig. 1a-c).

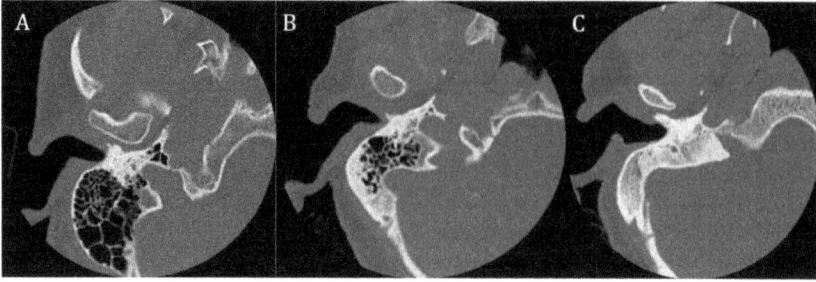

Fig. 1 Representative axial images of pre-operative high-resolution temporal bone CT scan showing mastoid that is (**a**) well aerated, (**b**) moderately aerated, and (**c**) poorly aerated

Location of the sigmoid sinus was measured on the same axial images as above. A straight line was first drawn through the mid-portion of the round window and the facial nerve, thus bisecting these landmarks. Subsequently, a perpendicular line from this axis to the most anterior aspect of the sigmoid sinus was drawn and measured (in mm) (Fig. 2).

To determine the height of the tegmen, a straight line was drawn through the axis of the horizontal semicircular canal on a coronal image. Subsequently, a perpendicular line from this axis to the lowest level of tegmen was drawn and measured (in mm) (Fig. 3). These three parameters were then compared to the intraoperative scoring of difficulty associated with the cortical mastoidectomy.

In addition, using the axial images, presence or absence of air cells around the facial recess was assessed (Fig. 4). This was correlated to the intraoperative scores of difficulties with access to facial recess.

Finally, the degree of round window bony overhang was measured by assessing four consecutive axial cuts, beginning with the most superior cut showing the round window membrane and proceeding inferiorly (Fig. 5). The number of cuts showing full thickness bony overhang around the round window was counted out of four. For instance, if there were two slices showing full thickness bony overhang, it was measured as 2/4 or 0.5. This variable was then compared to the intraoperative scoring of difficulty associated with round window access.

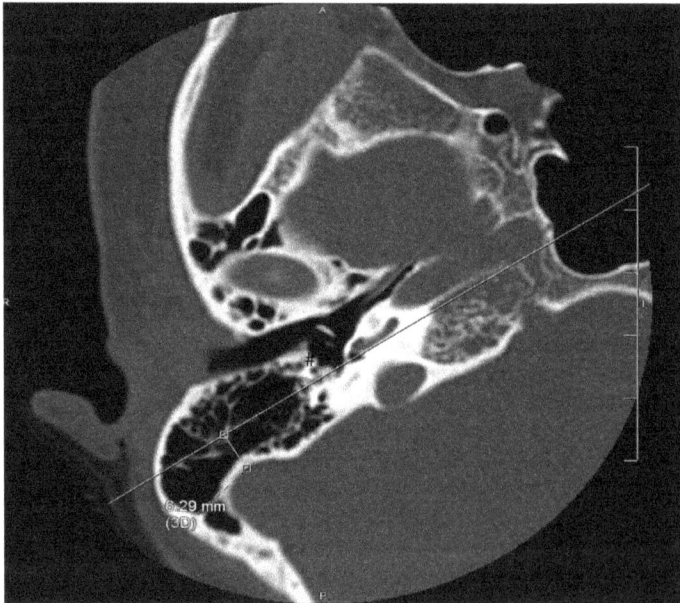

Fig. 2 Representative axial image of pre-operative high-resolution temporal bone CT scan illustrating the distance measured from the line drawn through round window (*) and facial nerve (#) to the anterior aspect of the sigmoid sinus

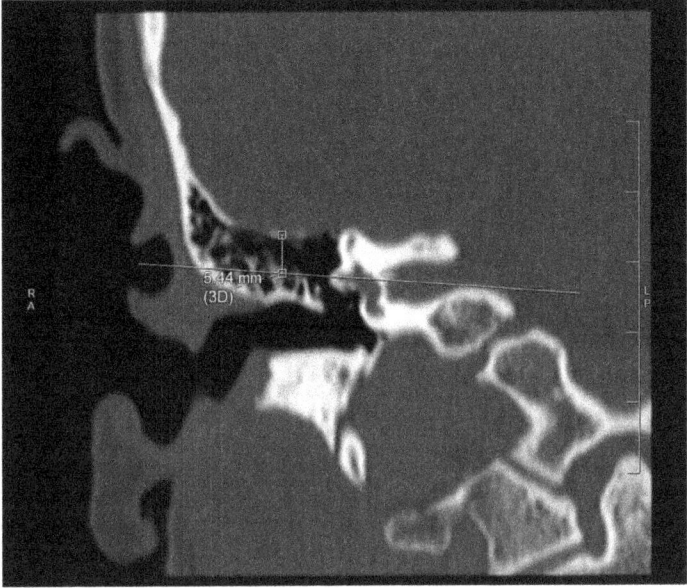

Fig. 3 Representative coronal image of pre-operative high-resolution temporal bone CT scan illustrating the distance measured from the line drawn through horizontal semicircular canal to the tegmen

Statistical analysis

A chi-square test of independence was used to find a potential relationship between difficulty with mastoidectomy and mastoid aeration, as well as a potential relationship between difficulty with accessing facial recess and presence/absence of facial recess air cell.

One-way analysis of variance (ANOVA) and student's t-test were used to compare the location of the sigmoid and the level of the tegmen between the three groups representing degrees of difficulties with mastoidectomy (i.e. "Easy", "Moderate", "Difficult"). In addition, one-way ANOVA and student's t-test were used to compare level

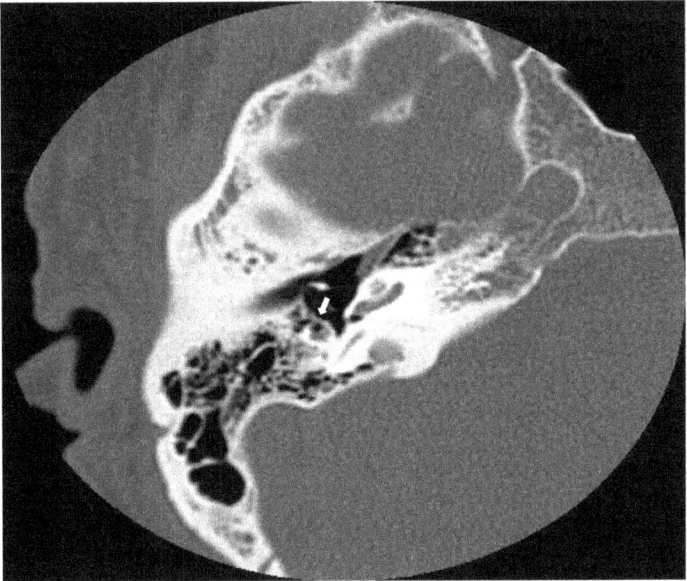

Fig. 4 Representative axial image of pre-operative high-resolution temporal bone CT scan illustrating an air cell (arrow) anterior to facial nerve

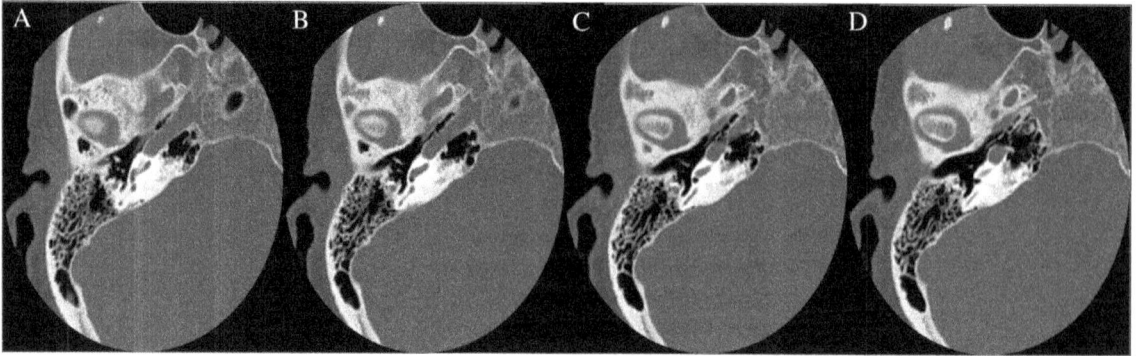

Fig. 5 Representative axial images of pre-operative high-resolution temporal bone CT scan illustrating bony overhang around round window in four consecutive slices from superior to inferior (**a** to **d**)

of round window bony overhang between the three groups of surgical difficulty.

Results
Demographics
The average age of subjects was 58 (range: from 21 to 84). There were 29 males and 28 females in the study. Twenty-eight patients underwent right cochlear implantation and 29 patients underwent left cochlear implantation.

Mastoidectomy
A chi-square test of independence was utilized to assess whether the difficulty encountered during the cortical mastoidectomy is related to the degree of mastoid aeration as assessed on the pre-operative temporal bone CT scan. The analysis revealed a chi-square value of 26.7 that is significant at the p-value of <0.001, demonstrating that lower degree of mastoid aeration is associated with higher level of difficulty during the cortical mastoidectomy.

The distance between the straight line drawn through the round window and the facial nerve, and the sigmoid sinus on the pre-operative CT scan provides an indication of how anterior the sigmoid sinus is. The mean distance was compared between the three groups, which corresponded to the levels of difficulty with the cortical mastoidectomy ("Easy" $=7.11 \pm 0.34$, "Moderate" $=6.39 \pm 1.74$, "Difficult" $=5.15 \pm 1.74$; mean SEM). One-way ANOVA revealed that the difference in mean distance of sigmoid sinus between the three groups is not statistically significant. When student's t-test was performed between the groups separately, none of the comparisons was statistically significant.

The height of the tegmen on pre-operative CT scan was analyzed in similar manner. The mean distance of tegmen from the axis of horizontal semicircular canal was significantly different between the three groups based on one-way ANOVA ("Easy" $= 5.50 \pm 0.22$, "Moderate" $= 4.36 \pm 0.46$, "Difficult" $= 3.11 \pm 0.35$, $p < 0.01$). The mean distance

for the "Moderate" group was significantly lower than the "Easy" group ($p = 0.05$), while the mean distance for the "Difficult" group tended to be lower than the "Moderate" group, although the difference was not statistically significant ($p = 0.06$) (Fig. 6).

Facial recess access
A chi-square test of independence was used to determine whether presence or absence of an air cell around the facial recess on pre-operative CT scan is a predictor for the degree of difficulty with accessing facial recess. The result shows that the presence or absence of an air cell around the facial nerve is significantly related to the degree of difficulty with accessing the facial recess ($p = 0.05$), with the presence of an air cell being associated with an 'easier' rating of facial recess.

Round window access
The degree of round window bony overhang was compared between the three groups corresponding to levels of difficulty associated with round window access using

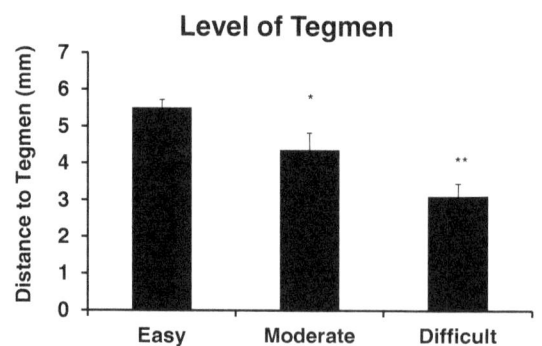

Fig. 6 Mean distance between the axis of the horizontal semicircular canal and the lowest level of the tegmen on coronal CT images among the three groups corresponding to the degree of difficulty associated with mastoidectomy. *: $p = 0.05$ vs "Easy", **: $p < 0.01$ vs "Easy"

one-way ANOVA. There was an overall statistical difference among the groups ($p = 0.02$). However, individual student's t-tests did not show statistically significant differences for all paired comparisons.

Discussion

The objective of this study was to determine if there are potential predictors of difficulties associated with the key surgical steps during cochlear implantation based on an analysis of the pre-operative temporal bone CT scan. These well-established steps include cortical mastoidectomy, facial recess, and round window exposure, which are not only important for successful insertion of the cochlear implantation electrode through the round window, but in fact are related since each subsequent step is dependent upon the previous steps being done properly and adequately. This study demonstrates that the difficulty associated with the cortical mastoidectomy is related to the degree of mastoid aeration and the height of the tegmen, and that the difficulty associated with facial recess is related to the presence/absence of an air cell around facial nerve.

Pre-operative CT scans are currently the standard of care for adult patients undergoing cochlear implantation. These images are routinely reviewed by the surgeon prior to surgery and a mental checklist is often performed to ensure that there are no anatomical obstructions to implant insertion. If there is any anatomical variation, the surgeon is not only better prepared intraoperatively, but a frank discussion can be undertaken with the patient preoperatively about alternative surgical steps, such as transcanal insertions or removal of the posterior canal wall.

However, there can be a high degree of variability in how the pre-operative CT scan is analyzed by the individual surgeon. Our goal was to formalize and standardize various radiological markers which can be used to prognosticate the potential challenges the surgeon may encounter during surgery. This planning is similar to obtaining a MRI to assess cochlear duct patency in post-meningitis patients who suffer profound sensorineural hearing loss and are requiring urgent cochlear implantation.

Our finding that decreased mastoid aeration and lower level of tegmen are associated with a greater level of perceived difficulty associated with cortical mastoidectomy is not surprising. In a sclerotic or small mastoid, identifying important landmarks required for subsequent steps, such as the identification of the lateral semicircular canal and incus body, is naturally more difficult. These are well established otologic landmarks that help the surgeon identify the location of the facial nerve and mastoid antrum. Without this identification, the risks of iatrogenic injury to the facial nerve and inner ear are significantly increased. Similarly, a low tegmen can also slow down the surgeon and make the exposure of the mastoid antrum

during cortical mastoidectomy more challenging. However, our findings do not rule out other anatomical or radiological markers that may contribute to technical challenges associated with mastoidectomy.

Interestingly, there was no significant association between the location of sigmoid sinus (in other words, how anterior its location is) and the degree of difficulty with mastoidectomy. It may be that even in patients whose mastoidectomy was "difficult", the sigmoid sinus was sufficiently away from the surgical field. This may also be related to the type of surgery. In cochlear implantation, most of the surgical dissection is located anterior to the sigmoid sinus within a limited mastoidectomy, as opposed to a wide, 'saucerized' cavity required for cholesteatoma or acoustic neuroma surgery.

Our results also show that the presence of an air cell around the facial recess on the preoperative CT scan is associated with lower degree of difficulty with facial recess access. Again, this is not surprising, as surgeons welcome the presence of an air cell in the facial recess, which is then used to confirm opening into the middle ear and guides rest of the facial recess enlargement.

During round window exposure, a thick bony overhang can pose problems for the surgeon. A thick bony overhang often precludes the true location and orientation of the round window. This overhang must be drilled away to expose the round window and to allow smooth insertion of the electrode into the perilymphatic space of the cochlea unhindered by bony obstructions. A thick bony overhang was assessed radiologically by assessing four consecutive axial cuts of the pre-operative CT scan. A thicker round window bony overhang was not associated with greater difficulty in accessing round window. It is likely that the orientation and size of the round window (i.e. how posterior it is), rather than thickness of the bony overhang, better predicts the difficulty with round window access, but this was not tested in our radiological markers. Most of the patients who received a cochlear implant also had little evidence of chronic mastoid disease, which made identification of the overhang easier.

There are several limitations with our study. The descriptors for difficulty associated with different steps of the cochlear implant are subjective and what is deemed as "difficult" vs "moderate", for instance, may vary widely between surgeons. Furthermore, only one investigator analyzed the CT images and therefore inter-observer reliability or variability is not known. This will be addressed in the future studies.

Conclusion

The results of our study show that 1) aeration of the mastoid and height of the tegmen may help predict the degree of difficulty with cortical mastoidectomy and 2) the presence of air cell around the facial recess may be a predictor of an easier facial recess.

These radiological parameters are relatively easy and quick to assess on readily available pre-operative temporal bone CT scan. They can form a pre-operative checklist that provides a formalized approach for the surgeons and, in particular surgical trainees, predict and, thus prepare for, potentially challenging cochlear implant cases.

Competing interests
The authors declare that they have no competing interests in this manuscript.

Authors' contributions
EP: carried out the retrieval of the data (pre-operative imaging), analysis of all data collected, including statistical analysis, and prepared the manuscript for submission. HA: helped with initial design of the study and initial data collection as one of the surgeons who performed the cochlear implant surgery and intraoperative scoring. JK: contributed to data collection as one of the surgeons who performed the cochlear implant surgery and intraoperative scoring. Also, he proof-read the manuscript. JMC: contributed to study design and data collection as one of the surgeons who performed the cochlear implant surgery and intraoperative scoring. JMN: contributed to study design and data collection as one of the surgeons who performed the cochlear implant surgery and intraoperative scoring. VYWL: as the principal investigator, he came up with the study idea/design and oversaw conduction of the study. He also contributed to data collection as one of the surgeons who performed the cochlear implant surgery and intraoperative scoring. He also proof-read the manuscript. All authors read and approved the final manuscript.

Acknowledgements
There was no source of funding for the authors or for the study itself.

References
1.   Arnoldner C, Lin VY. Expanded selection criteria in adult cochlear implantation. Cochlear Implants Int. 2013;14 Suppl 4:S10–3.
2.   Mueller DP. Temporal bone computed tomography in the preoperative evaluation for cochlear implantation. Ann Otol Rhinol Laryngol. 1989;98:346–9.
3.   Wiet RJ, Pyle GM, O'Connor CA, Russell E, Schramm DR. Computed tomography: how accurate a predictor for cochlear implantation? Laryngoscope. 1990;100(7):687–92.
4.   Wolley AL, Oser AB, Lusk RP, Bahadori RS. Preoperative temporal bone computed tomography scan and its use in evaluating the pediatric cochlear implant candidate. Laryngoscope. 1997;107:1100–6.

16

Thyroid Fine-needle aspiration biopsy: an evaluation of its utility in a community setting

Andre R Le[1]*, Gregory W Thompson[2] and Benjamin John A Hoyt[2]

Abstract

Background: Thyroid cancer rates are on the rise worldwide with over 5000 new cases estimated in Canada in 2012. The American Thyroid Association recommends the use of fine-needle aspiration biopsy (FNA) in the workup of thyroid nodules. Studies show that thyroid FNA accuracy may vary based on interpretation by cytopathologists in academic versus community centres. To date, there has been no literature published addressing the accuracy or utility of preoperative FNA in a Canadian community center. Our goals were to demonstrate the accuracy of thyroid FNA at our centre, and to compare our results to those published in the literature.

Methods: Medical records for patients who underwent thyroidectomy performed by two otolaryngologists in Fredericton, NB, between September 2008 and February 2013 were reviewed. 125 patients with 197 FNAs were analyzed. Fisher's Exact test was used to compare the malignancy rates in each FNA category, and Chi-Square test was used for FNA distribution comparison.

Results: The distribution of all FNA diagnoses at our centre was as follows: 38 (19%) benign, 100 (51%) inconclusive, 8 (4%) suspicious for malignancy, 2 (1%) malignant, and 49 (25%) unsatisfactory. FNA distribution was significantly different between our centre and comparison centres (Chi-Square p < 0.05). Our malignancy rates within each category using each FNA sample as a data point were 26.3%, 29.0%, 75%, 100% and 12.2% respectively. Comparison to other community studies revealed that we have significantly higher malignancy rates with benign FNAs (Fisher's exact p = <0.05). Analysis using our most malignant FNA data yielded similar results.

Conclusion: Thyroid FNA accuracy varies between institutions, and this may affect its utility in the workup of a thyroid nodule at some centres. Expert cytopathology opinions may be an asset in interpreting FNA samples in small community centres where volumes are relatively low, however our data do not support this assertion. It is essential that physicians continue to use clinical judgment first and foremost when evaluating thyroid nodules.

Keywords: Fine-needle aspiration, FNA, Thyroid, Nodule, Cytopathology, Thyroid cancer, Community

Background

It is estimated that the incidence of thyroid cancer has more than doubled in much of the developed world over the past few decades. In Canada, thyroid cancer annual incidence rates increased an average of 7% from 1998–2007. Over 5000 new cases were diagnosed in 2012 [1]. Theories have been postulated to explain this trend. It may be due to more frequent diagnostic imaging with an associated increase in radiation exposure. These tests may also be leading to the incidental discovery of earlier stage, asymptomatic thyroid cancers [1].

In the workup of thyroid nodules, one of the greatest challenges for physicians is to accurately identify which nodules have a high likelihood of harbouring malignant disease; thereby minimizing unnecessary surgical procedures and their associated risks in those with benign disease. The American Thyroid Association recommends fine needle aspiration biopsy (FNA) as a key step in the evaluation of thyroid nodules [2].

Thyroid FNA is an inexpensive, relatively safe test that may be performed in an outpatient setting. It is used to characterize thyroid nodules and to triage patients based on cytopathological results. It has been shown to demonstrate good specificity and sensitivity with respect to thyroid malignancy [3-5]. Before routinely using FNA in

* Correspondence: k55arl@mun.ca
[1]Memorial University Faculty of Medicine, S-1758B 300 Prince Phillip Drive, St John's, NL A1B 3 V6, Canada
Full list of author information is available at the end of the article

the workup of thyroid nodules, the malignancy rates of resected nodules were approximately fifteen percent; however, with current FNA practice these rates have reportedly increased to over fifty percent in some centres [6,7].

That said, there remain numerous limitations to FNA in the workup of thyroid nodules. For example, the skill of the aspirator and the expertise of the interpreting cytologist, both of which can vary from centre to centre, can dramatically affect accuracy of the test. Many papers have been published addressing this variability; however, the vast majority of them have been done in academic or tertiary care centres [8]. The number of studies done in a community setting is limited [8-10], and no data have been published from community centres in Canada. Given that most community centres have lower volumes than academic centres, and given that many community specialists have little sub-specialty or fellowship training, it is possible that the published accuracy of thyroid FNA may not truly reflect results seen in the community, thereby calling into question the utility of this test outside of tertiary centres.

As such, we decided to retrospectively review our experience at our Canadian community-based secondary hospital. We analyzed our thyroid FNA distribution and accuracy in the workup of thyroid nodules, and we compare these results to other international community centres [8-10] and to academic practices, including our closest major tertiary care referral centre [11].

Methods

The medical records for all patients who underwent thyroidectomy, performed by two otolaryngologists at the Dr. Everett Chalmers Hospital in Fredericton, NB, between September 2008 and February 2013 were retrospectively reviewed. The only patients excluded from our study were those who did not have a preoperative FNA. Examples of exclusions include cases of refractory hyperthyroidism and diffuse goiter with compressive symptoms in the absence of a dominant or suspicious nodule. A statistician was consulted throughout the study design and data review.

A total of 125 patients with 197 FNAs were included for analysis. The age and gender of each patient was recorded as well as the surgical procedure performed. Initially, each FNA was treated as a separate data point and our statistical analysis was carried out. Subsequently, the data were reorganized using only the most malignant FNA for those with more than one preoperative FNA, and the statistics were repeated. There lacked uniformity in reporting from one cytopathologist to the next, and the current Bethesda criteria were not always used. As such, the FNA results were classified into one of the following categories, in increasing order of suspicion: unsatisfactory; benign; inconclusive; suspicious for malignancy and malignant.

The distribution of the FNA results across the five categories was calculated. Using Chi-square test, the distribution at our centre was compared to data published from four other centres. Each preoperative FNA result was paired with the corresponding final pathological diagnosis from the surgical specimen. Fisher's exact test was used for comparison of malignancy rates per FNA category between centers. A p value of less than 0.05 was considered a statistically significant difference.

Ethics approval was provided by the Research Ethics Board for the Horizon Health Network.

Results

In total, 197 thyroid FNA samples from 125 patients, 102 females and 23 males, were reviewed. Their ages ranged from 15 to 78 years with a mean age of 50.10 +/− SD 13.25 years. They went on to have a diagnostic hemithyroidectomy (96), a total thyroidectomy (29).

The distribution of FNA diagnoses at our centre is demonstrated in Table 1. It shows the distribution when each FNA was considered a separate data point, as well as the distribution using only the most malignant FNA in those patients with more than one preoperative FNA.

The overall rate of thyroid cancer in our study was 28.8%. Table 2 demonstrates the rate of malignancy broken down by FNA category, once again including rates considering all FNA samples as distinct data points, as well as rates using only the most malignant FNA per patient.

Our results were then compared to three community-based centres [8-10] and one geographically close academic centre [11]. When using each FNA as a separate data point, our overall distribution across the categories was significantly different than all comparison centres (Table 3). When using only the most malignant FNA sample, the distribution at our centre remained significantly different than all but the geographically close academic centre (Table 4).

Table 5 shows the comparison of our malignancy rates to those of the four comparison centres using all FNA samples as distinct data points. Table 6 shows the same comparison using only our most malignant samples per thyroidectomy. Malignancies per FNA category yielded

Table 1 Distribution of preoperative thyroid FNA results as per diagnostic category

FNA Category	Percent of distribution	
Unsatisfactory	49/197: 24.9%	17/125: 13.6%*
Benign	38/197: 19.2%	22/125: 17.6%*
Inconclusive	100/197: 50.8%	76/125: 60.8%*
Suspicious for malignancy	8/197: 4.1%	8/125: 6.4%*
Malignant	2/197: 1.0%	2/125: 1.6%*

*using most malignant FNA for those patients with more than one preoperative FNA.
FNA: fine-needle aspiration biopsy.

Table 2 Malignancy rates per preoperative thyroid FNA diagnostic category

FNA Result	Malignancy rates	
Unsatisfactory	6/49: 12.2%	2/17: 11.8%*
Benign	10/38: 26.3%	4/22: 18.0%*
Inconclusive	29/100: 29%	22/76: 28.9%*
Suspicious for malignancy	6/8: 75%	6/8: 75%*
Malignant	2/2: 100%	2/2: 100%*
Overall	26.9%	28.8%*

*using most malignant FNA for those patients with more than one preoperative FNA.
FNA: fine-needle aspiration biopsy.

some interesting results. Using Fisher's Exact test, our malignancy rates in the setting of a benign FNA are significantly higher than those at the comparison community centres.

Discussion

Thyroid cancer rates continue to rise. Furthermore, the incidence of thyroid cancer in the setting of a thyroid nodule ranges from 20% to as low as 5%. FNA has been established as the gold-standard procedure in the workup of thyroid nodules to help clinicians determine whether or not a given nodule represents malignancy. Despite being ubiquitous in the workup of thyroid nodules in North America, the accuracy and utility of this apparently simple test can vary greatly from one centre to the next. In an effort to curb some of this variability, the American Thyroid Association (ATA) has created extensive guidelines addressing the indications for FNA, and the Bethesda system has been developed and widely accepted as the manner in which FNA samples should be cytopathologically interpreted and classified.

Cibas and Ali [12] claim that the routine use of FNA in the workup of a thyroid nodule has increased the malignancy rates in resected nodules from 14% to 50%. At our centre, we anecdotally observed a very high rate of benign nodules being resected despite the use of FNA in the preoperative workup. We also felt that we were seeing an unusually high number of inconclusive FNAs, and we began

to question the validity of FNA results at our institution. We hypothesized that the experience of the interpreting cytopathologists may be a contributing factor. Being a smaller secondary hospital, our volumes are relatively low compared to larger academic centres, and we do not have a dedicated head & neck pathologist reviewing all of our FNA specimens. We felt that it was possible that the relative inexperience of our pathologists when compared to the larger academic centres was leading to less accurate results from thyroid FNAs. If academic high-volume cytopathologists can produce more accurate and reliable results, then it may make sense for smaller volume centres to outsource their FNAs for interpretation by experts in centres of excellence. Our study was not powered to evaluate differences from one cytopathologist to the next.

In an effort to objectify our suspicions, we reviewed the literature and studied our data over a five-year period, comparing our results to those published. We felt it important to compare our results to those published from similar centres; however we were surprised to find no published studies addressing the accuracy and utility of FNA in a Canadian community centre. All Canadian data has been published at tertiary care hospitals. We chose our geographically closest academic centre as one of our comparison studies. We found three American studies done in community centres and we included all three in our analysis.

Our data show that only 28.8% of our resected nodules were malignant. The malignancy rates reported in the literature also seem to vary greatly, from as low as 12.0% to as high as 34.4% in the papers we chose as comparison studies. To our surprise, our overall malignancy rates were nearly identical to those published by our closest academic centre, and they were not significantly different than those published in the studies to which we compared. While it is reassuring that we aren't resecting more benign disease than others, it is very difficult to attribute these results to FNA accuracy as the FNA is but one of many tools used in the decision to proceed with surgery. Furthermore, we are still subjecting more than

Table 3 Comparison of preoperative FNA distributions between our center and other published centers shown as a percentage of all preoperative FNAs

FNA Result	Blansfield et al.*	Postma et al.*	Wu et al.*	Williams et al.*	Our center
Unsatisfactory	6.0%	0%	9.5%	14.2%	24.9%
Benign	24.0%	28.6%	28.5%	24.2%	19.2%
Inconclusive	46.4%	48.0%	52.0%	53.6%	50.8%
Suspicious for malignancy	7.7%	6.1%	8.1%	4.4%	4.1%
Malignant	15.8%	2.0%	8.6%	3.6%	1.0%
Total	34.4%	12.0%	21.7%	28.4%	26.9%

*Chi-square p < 0.05.
FNA: fine-needle aspiration.

Table 4 Comparison of preoperative FNA distributions between our center and other published studies shown as a percentage of all preoperative FNAs using the most malignant FNA per patient at our center

FNA Result	Blansfield et al.*	Postma et al.*	Wu et al.*	Williams et al.	Our center
Unsatisfactory	6.0%	0%	9.5%	14.2%	13.6%
Benign	24.0%	28.6%	28.5%	24.2%	17.6%
Inconclusive	46.4%	48.0%	52.0%	53.6%	60.8%
Suspicious for malignancy	7.7%	6.1%	8.1%	4.4%	6.4%
Malignant	15.8%	2.0%	8.6%	3.6%	1.6%
Total	34.4%	12.0%	21.7%	28.4%	28.8%

*Chi-square p < 0.05.
FNA: fine-needle aspiration.

70% of our thyroidectomy patients to surgery for benign disease.

We also found that our FNA results were inconsistent; we felt that an unusually high percentage of our samples were being reported as either unsatisfactory or inconclusive. Our data clearly support this suspicion, as our distribution was significantly different than that of the comparison centres. While there are many possible explanations for this discrepancy, including the skill of both the aspirator and the interpreter, it's difficult to clearly prove what factors are causative. But interestingly, when using only the most malignant FNA specimen in the analysis, our distribution was not significantly different than that of our closest teaching centre. This calls into question our assertion that the experience of our interpreting clinicians could be problematic.

Our most concerning finding is that 26.3% of our patients with FNAs that were reported as benign ultimately had well differentiated thyroid carcinoma. By limiting our analysis to only the most malignant specimens, that number decreases to 18.0%, still a very high false-negative rate. These results were significantly higher that those published at the other community centres, but interestingly not significantly higher than those of our closest academic centre. Wang et al., showed a statistically significant difference in false negative rates (10% vs 2%) between

community and academic centers [13]. Yeh et al., demonstrated a single false negative FNA delayed treatment by an average of more than two years resulting in patients experiencing higher rates of vascular and capsular invasion [14]. Subsequently, such patients were more likely to experience persistent disease at follow-up. The discrepancy between published results is difficult to conclusively explain, but selection bias may be playing a role. In our study and in Williams et al., only patients who went on to have thyroid surgery were included. There would have been many FNAs reported as benign in patients that did not go on to surgery during the study period, and thus not captured in our data set. Those that were included in our review likely had other concerning clinical features that resulted in them having surgery despite the results. A review of all FNAs performed would be more useful in comparing malignancy rates per FNA category to published norms. That said, our data once again refute our initial assertion that academic centre cytopathologists will yield more accurate data than those at our community centre.

A big limitation of our study is that our pathology department has not yet adopted the current Bethesda classification system, and the classification can even vary slightly from one interpreter to the next. This is not unique to our institution [9,10]. To compare our results to those published, we had to re-classify some FNAs to

Table 5 Comparison of malignancy rates per preoperative thyroid FNA diagnostic category between our center and other published studies

FNA Result	Blansfield et al.	Postma et al.	Wu et al.	Williams et al.	Our study
Unsatisfactory	0/11 = 0%	0/0 = 0%	3/21 = 14.2%	10/55 = 18.2%	6/49: 12.2%
Benign	3/44 = 6.8%*	0/28 = 0%*	2/63 = 3.1%*	15/94 = 16.0%	10/38: 26.3%
Inconclusive	25/85 = 29.4%	3/47 = 6%*	14/100 = 14.0%	55/208 = 26.4%	29/100: 29%
Suspicious for malignancy	8/14 = 57.1%	5/6 = 83%	10/18 = 55.6%	16/17: 94.1%	6/8: 75%
Malignant	27/29 = 93.1%	2/2 = 100%	19/19 = 100%	14/14 = 100%	2/2: 100%
Total	63/183 = 34.4%	10/83 = 12.0%	48/221 = 21.7%	110/388 = 28.4%	53/197 = 26.9%

*Fisher's exact p < 0.05.
FNA: fine-needle aspiration.

Table 6 Comparison of malignancy rates per preoperative thyroid FNA diagnostic category between our center and other published studies using the most malignant FNA per patient at our center

FNA Result	Blansfield et al.	Postma et al.	Wu et al.	Williams et al.	Our study
Unsatisfactory	0/11 = 0%	0/0 = 0%	3/21 = 14.2%	10/55 = 18.2%	2/17 = 11.8%
Benign	3/44 = 6.8%	0/28 = 0%*	2/63 = 3.1%*	15/94 = 16.0%	4/22 = 18.0%
Inconclusive	25/85 = 29.4%	3/47 = 6%*	14/100 = 14.0%	55/208 = 26.4%	22/76 = 28.9%
Suspicious for malignancy	8/14 = 57.1%	5/6 = 83%	10/18 = 55.6%	16/17 = 94.1%	6/8 = 75.0%
Malignant	27/29 = 93.1%	2/2 = 100%	19/19 = 100%	14/14 = 100%	2/2: 100%
Total	63/183 = 34.4%	10/83 = 12.0%	48/221 = 21.7%	110/388 = 28.4%	36/125 = 28.8%

*Fisher's exact p < 0.05.
FNA: fine-needle aspiration.

fit into one of the chosen categories. We also had to group two categories in at least one of the comparison studies. Until all published data use uniform and current classification, comparison will remain a challenge.

This study is retrospective and is therefore potentially subject to confirmation bias. However, we did not have the authority or the resources to randomize our FNAs into two groups and outsource the "academic centre" cohort to another centre. Ideally these retrospective data support our concerns and open the door to resources for future prospective randomized research.

Our FNAs are primarily done by our radiology department under ultrasound-guidance. However, there is not a department-wide standard for technique used and not all FNAs were done with guidance. This could also be seen as a limitation. A less skilled aspirator may see a higher percentage of unsatisfactory biopsies. Biopsies taken without ultrasound guidance may not even sample the target nodule and may only get surrounding thyroid tissue. Standardized guided aspiration should be the standard at all centres, particularly when publishing data and comparing to published norms.

Lastly, volume is obviously a limitation. Our study is not adequately powered to compare to larger academic studies. However, if assessing the accuracy of FNA done in a low-volume community centre, a well-powered study is virtually impossible if done at a single centre. A multi-centre randomized trial is needed to truly assess whether low-volume centres produce less accurate FNA data in the workup of thyroid nodules.

Conclusions

FNA remains a key tool in the investigation of thyroid nodules. Despite its use, surgeons continue to resect a very high percentage of benign disease because of uncertainty with respect to its malignant potential. Until a more accurate non-invasive diagnostic test is developed, it is important that we continue to refine our FNA technique to improve its accuracy. Regardless, clinical judgment remains of paramount importance in interpreting FNA results in the context of a given patient. Our review

is the first Canadian community-based study to analyze the utility of preoperative FNA in terms of final thyroidectomy pathology. Despite our suspicion, our data do not support our hypothesis that low-volume community centre FNAs will be less accurate than those done in academic centres. That being said, it is possible that our study's limitations prevented us from finding the real answer. Our study does show statistically significant variability in FNA distribution between our study and all three of the comparison community studies. It also shows significantly higher malignancy rates in benign FNA specimens between our centre and the three community centres. This variability may be the result of study design; of discrepancies, inconsistencies in technique or in interpretation of the FNA itself; or of difference in regional practice patterns as all three were international studies. Regardless, consistency is needed in both the aspiration and interpretation of FNAs in all centres. With consistent methodology, further prospective studies will be better able to address whether or not high-volume academic centres can produce more accurate and reliable FNA results in the workup of thyroid nodules.

Abbreviations
FNA: Fine-needle aspiration biopsy.

Competing interests
The authors declare that they have no competing interests.

Authors' contributions
AL: retrospectively reviewed data, collected and organized data, performed literature review, prepared manuscript. BH: developed research question, interpreted the results, gave conceptual direction, helped prepare manuscript. GT: developed research question, interpreted the results, gave conceptual direction. All authors read and approved the final manuscript.

Acknowledgements
We thank Dr. Yanqing Yi of Memorial University Faculty of Community Health and Humanities for assistance in the development and execution of our statistical analysis.

Author details
[1]Memorial University Faculty of Medicine, S-1758B 300 Prince Phillip Drive, St John's, NL A1B 3 V6, Canada. [2]Department of Otolaryngology – Head & Neck Surgery, Zone 3, Horizon Health Network, 700 Priestman St, Fredericton, NB E3B 5 N5, Canada.

References

1. Canadian Cancer Society's Advisory Committee on Cancer Statistics. Canadian Cancer Statistics 2013. Toronto, ON, Canada: Canadian Cancer Society; 2013.

2. American Thyroid Association (ATA) Guidelines Taskforce on Thyroid Nodules and Differentiated Thyroid Cancer, Cooper DS, Doherty GM, Haugen BR, Hauger BR, Kloos RT, et al. Revised American thyroid association management guidelines for patients with thyroid nodules and differentiated thyroid cancer. Thyroid Off J Am Thyroid Assoc. 2009;19:1167–214.

3. Kuru B, Gulcelik NE, Gulcelik MA, Dincer H. The false-negative rate of fine-needle aspiration cytology for diagnosing thyroid carcinoma in thyroid nodules. Langenbeck's Arch Surg. 2010;395:127–32.

4. Porterfield JR, Grant CS, Dean DS, Thompson GB, Farley DR, Richards ML, et al. Reliability of benign fine needle aspiration cytology of large thyroid nodules. Surgery. 2008;144:963–9.

5. Ogilvie JB, Piatigorsky EJ, Clark OH. Current status of fine needle aspiration for thyroid nodules. Adv Surg. 2006;40:223–38.

6. Hamberger B, Gharib H, Melton III LJ, Goellner JR, Zinsmeister AR. Fine-needle aspiration biopsy of thyroid nodules: impact on thyroid practice and cost of care. Am J Med. 1982;73:381–38.

7. Yassa L, Cibas ES, Benson CB, Frates MC, Doubilet PM, Gawande AA, et al. Long-term assessment of a multidisciplinary approach to thyroid nodule diagnostic evaluation. Cancer. 2007;111:508–16.

8. Wu HH-J, Rose C, Elsheikh TM. The Bethesda system for reporting thyroid cytopathology: an experience of 1,382 cases in a community practice setting with the implication for risk of neoplasm and risk of malignancy. Diagn Cytopathol. 2012;40:399–403.

9. Blansfield JA, Sack MJ, Kukora JS. Recent experience with preoperative fine-needle aspiration biopsy of thyroid nodules in a community hospital. Arch Surg. 2002;137:818–21.

10. Postma DS, Becker MO, Roberts A, Gilleon S, Soto J. Thyroidectomy in a community hospital: Findings of 100 consecutive cases. ENT Ear Nose Throat J. 2009;88:30.

11. Williams BA, Bullock MJ, Trites JR, Taylor SM, Hart RD. Rates of thyroid malignancy by FNA diagnostic category. J Otolaryngol-Head Neck Surg. 2013;42:61.

12. Cibas ES, Ali SZ. The Bethesda system for reporting thyroid cytopathology. Thyroid Off J Am Thyroid Assoc. 2009;19:1159–65.

13. Wang CC, Friedman L, Kennedy GC, Wang H, Kebebew E, Steward DL, et al. A large multicenter correlation study of thyroid nodule cytopathology and histopathology. Thyroid. 2011;21:243–51.

14. Yeh MW, Demircan O, Ituarte P, Clark OH. False-negative fine-needle aspiration cytology results delay treatment and adversely affect outcome in patients with thyroid carcinoma. Thyroid. 2004;14:207–15.

17

Bilateral vocal fold immobility: a 13 year review of etiologies, management and the utility of the empey index

Maria K. Brake[1] and Jennifer Anderson[2*]

Abstract

Background: Bilateral vocal fold immobility (BVFI) is a rare diagnosis causing dyspnea, dysphonia and dysphagia. Management depends on respiratory performance, airway patency, vocal ability, and quality-of-life priorities. The authors review the presentation, management and outcome in patients diagnosed with BVFI. The utility and efficacy of the Empey index (EI) and the Expiratory Disproportion Index (EDI) are evaluated as an objective monitoring tools for BVFI patients.

Methods: A 13-year retrospective review was performed of BVFI patients at St. Michael's Hospital, University of Toronto, a tertiary referral centre for laryngology.

Results: Forty-eight patients were included; 46 presented with airway obstruction symptoms. Tracheotomy was required for airway management in 40 % of patients throughout the course of their treatment, which was reduced to 19 % at the end of the study period. Twenty-one patients underwent endoscopic arytenoidectomy/cordotomy. Non-operative management included continuous positive airway pressure devices. Pulmonary function testing was carried out in 29 patients. Only a portion of the BVFI patients met the defined upper airway obstruction criteria (45 % EI and 52 % EDI). Seven patients had complete pre- and post-operative PFTs for comparison and all seven had ratios that significantly improved post-operatively which correlated clinically.

Conclusion: The EI and EDI have limited use in evaluating patients with who have variable upper airway obstruction, but may be helpful in monitoring within subject airway function changes.

Keywords: Bilateral vocal fold immobility, Bilateral vocal cord immobility, Glottis stenosis, Cordotomy, Arytenoidectomy, Empey, Expiratory disproportion index

Background

Bilateral vocal fold immobility (BVFI) is a rare diagnosis that can be due to paralysis or fixation of the vocal folds, and frequently associated with significant morbidity and disability. Depending on the underlying etiology, vocal fold position and compensatory behaviour, varying degrees of dyspnea, dysphonia and dysphagia occur [1–3].

Determining the need for surgery, as well as assessing outcomes can be difficult due to the variability in etiology, symptoms and limited BVFI patient population.

Investigations available to assess the airway function include imaging, physical examination with endoscopy, pulmonary function testing (PFT), sleep studies and validated quality of life questionnaires. Parameter ratios of individual PFT values have been proposed as a potential objective measure of upper airway function. One such measure is the Empey Index (EI), which was described in 1972 as a marker of upper airway obstruction by Duncan Empey [4–6]. The index is the ratio of forced expiratory volume in 1 s (FEV_1) in milliliters to the peak expiratory flow rate (PEFR) in litres per minute. The respiratory physiology is described elsewhere [4–6] but can be summarized as follows:

* Correspondence: andersonj@smh.ca
[2]St. Michael's Hospital, Department of Otolaryngology – Head and Neck Surgery, University of Toronto, 30 Bond St. 8C-129, ON M5B 1 W8 Toronto, Canada
Full list of author information is available at the end of the article

The ratio of FEV₁ is predominantly determined by the properties of the small intrathoracic airways and less affected by upper airway stenosis than PEFR. In the setting of upper airway stenosis, the ratio increases.

In normal subjects and in patients with lung diseases (asthma, chronic bronchitis and others) the EI ratio was found to be less than 10 (ml/l/min). In comparison, Empey discovered that patients with known upper airway obstruction, including those with bilateral vocal fold fixation, all had values greater than 10 and a mean of 14 [4].

When Nouraei *et al.* re-evaluated this ratio in 2013, they proposed a modified ratio calculation of $FEV_1/$ PEFR × 100, termed the expiratory disproportion index (EDI), using the SI units of FEV_1 (L) and PEFR (L/s) [6]. In studying the utility of the EDI, they found that benign upper airway stenosis subjects had a mean of 76 ± 17 s. Their study also found that the degree of stenosis correlated with a higher EDI value. For practicality, multiplying EI ratio by six will allow conversion to EDI units.

It is not clear whether these ratios can be useful in the BVFI population, which includes a large proportion of bilateral vocal fold paralysis patients. In this report, the authors review the presentation, management and outcome in patients diagnosed with BVFI at a laryngology clinic in a tertiary referral academic centre. Within this group, the utility and efficacy of the EI and EDI are evaluated as an objective monitoring tool for BVFI patients.

Material and methods

A retrospective cohort study was undertaken at an academic, tertiary-care laryngology clinic in Toronto, Canada. All patients diagnosed with BVFI between January 1, 2001 and Dec 31, 2013 were included. Collected data included demographics (age, gender), etiology of BVFI, past medical history, pulmonary function testing (flow volume loop, FEV1 and PEFR), relevant surgeries, history of tracheotomy, decannulation, and post-operative complications. The hospital electronic medical record system was used to review transcriptions, clinic notes, pathology reports, operative notes and pulmonary function results to collect the data.

The data was analyzed using GraphPad Prism® version 6.02. Descriptive statistics were calculated for demographics, EI, and EDIs ratios. The Wilcoxon Matched Pairs Signed Rank Test was used to compare the paired pre- and post- operative EIs and EDIs. Unpaired parametric t-tests were used to compare the EI/EDI ratios between mean ages patients that underwent airway surgery, specifically a cordotomy/artenoidectomy, versus the group that did not. Chi-squared testing was used to determine if the rates of cordotomies, tracheostomy or decannulation varied between number of cormorbities. In all cases $p < 0.05$ was considered statistically significant. Ethics approval was obtained from the St. Michael's Hospital Research Ethics in Toronto, Canada.

Results

A total of 48 patients with bilateral vocal fold immobility were identified from the institutional laryngology database. The mean age of presentation was 52 years, with ages ranging from 15 – 83 years. Thirty-five (73 %) of the patients were female. Thirty-three of the patients (69 %) were diagnosed with bilateral vocal fold paralysis, twelve (25 %) with joint fixation, and one was documented as a combination. Two patients were unable to be categorized given the information available. Seven patients (17 %) were documented as smokers. Demographics are outlined Table 1.

Presentation

The primary complaint for the majority of patients (75 %) presenting to the clinic was that of dyspnea such as stridor, exercise intolerance, and airway obstruction when supine. Vocal complaints were the presenting complaint in 6 patients (12.5 %), followed by two with dysphagia or aspiration (4 %). Two patients (4 %) were seen on the recommendation of the referring doctor but reported to be without symptomatic complaints otherwise.

Etiology

The etiology of BVFI in the study population, in decreasing order of incidence, included thyroid disease or associated surgery, intubation-related injury, congenital,

Table 1 Patient demographics bilateral vocal fold immobility (*n* = 48)

Demographics (*n* = 48)	n (%)
Gender	
Male	13 (27 %)
Female	35 (73 %)
Documented Smokers	7 (17 %)
Diagnosis	
Bilateral Vocal Fold Paralysis	33 (68 %)
Joint Fixation	12 (25 %)
Combination	1 (2 %)
Unknown	2 (4 %)
Presentation	
Airway Obstruction	36 (75 %)
Dysphonia	6 (13 %)
Dysphagia/Aspiration	2 (4 %)
Other	2 (4 %)
Unknown	2 (4 %)

central neurological disorders, autoimmune disease, and surgery or cancer of cardiothoracic origin (Fig. 1).

Of the sixteen patients who suffered from bilateral vocal fold paralysis secondary to thyroid surgery, it was noted that 44 % (7) had their surgery outside of Canada and the pathology could not be determined.

A head and neck cancer diagnosis was present in eleven (23 %) patients. Four of these patients (36 %) had BVFI secondary to direct malignant invasion of the nerve or larynx. The other seven (64 %) developed BVFI from cancer treatment interventions: three with post-radiation polyneuropathy and four from injury or intentional transection during surgery for their disease.

Tracheotomy

Nineteen BVFI patients (40 %) required a tracheotomy for airway management at some point in their management. Nine patients with tracheotomy opted to undergo further surgical treatment with the intent to decannulate. To date, eight of these have been decannulated at the time of manuscript preparation.

Three patients were decannulated without surgical intervention. Overall, 17 % (8) of the 48 BVFI patients continued to require a tracheotomy for airway control (see Fig. 2 for full details). There was no statistical significance between the tracheostomy-dependent groups, the groups who were decannulated or the groups that did not require tracheostomies in terms of ages or comorbidities.

Surgical intervention

Of the 46 patients who complained of airway obstruction, twenty one patients (44 %) underwent a unilateral cordotomy and arytenoidectomy in order to improve the upper airway. The remaining 25 patients either had mild symptoms or medical comorbidities that prohibited a cordotomy/arytenoidectomy.

Revisions were required in seven (33 %), including five patients with persistent airway symptoms and two due to granuloma formation. Of the patients requiring

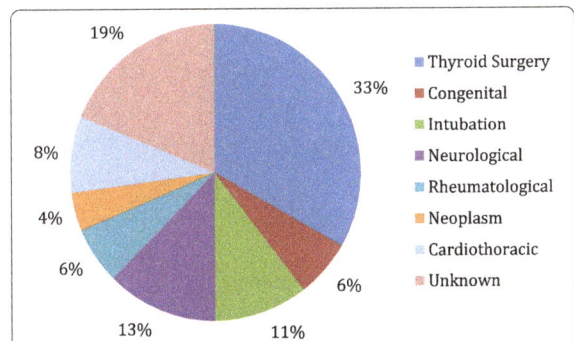

Fig. 1 Etiologies of BVFI in the study population

revisions, four (44 %) of the seven had BVFI secondary to fixation: two cases of post-glottic stenosis, one case of a Teflon granuloma, and a fourth case secondary to SLE-related joint fixation.

Two patients required multiple revisions (see the flow chart in Fig. 3 for full details). In one instance the patient had notable weight gain and recurrence of Reinke's edema in the setting of paralysis attributed to Charcot-Marie-Tooth disease. This individual required a contralateral cordotomy/arytenoidectomy, followed by an external approach vocal cord lateralization via laryngofissure. After the final procedure, the patient was able to achieve decannulation. The second patient had the aforementioned Teflon granuloma and associated sequelae.

There was no significance between cordotomy and non-cordtomy groups in terms of ages or comorbidities; there was also no significance for these same variables when comparing the revision cordotomy groups to the single-surgery patients.

Two patients underwent medialization thyroplasty for lateralized vocal folds in order to improve vocal function and reduce aspiration. In both of these cases, the etiology of their BVFI was congenital resulting in widely patent glottis and poor voice.

Empey ratio

A total of 81 PFTs had been completed on 60 % (29) of the patient population. The surgical group ($n = 21$) had 49 PFTs done in total, with this group referring specifically to patients having undergone a cordotomy/arytenoidectomy and/or revision. In the non-surgical group ($n = 25$), 32 PFT studies were done as part of their evaluation. Only twelve (41 %) of the 29 patients who underwent full PFT studies met the defined EI criteria for upper airway obstruction. Fifteen patients (52 %) had EDI values which fell within the mean range of 76 ± 17 as described by Nouraei *et al.* [4].

The EI and EDI were separated into surgical and non-surgical groups for comparision. Within the surgery group, comparision was also completed between subgroups: last pre-operative value, first post-operative value, all pre-operative values and all post-operative values. It should be noted that some patients only had pre-operative values while some others only had post-operative values. There was no significance found between the mean EI and EDI ratios in the non-surgical and surgical groups, nor between any of the subcategories.

Seven patients had complete PFT data allowing for comparison from pre to post cordotomy/arytenoidectomy. The Wilcoxon Matched-Pairs Signed Rank Test (WSRT) was completed on the Empey ratios and EDI for this subgroup which showed a significant increase post-surgery ($p = 0.0156$), which also correlated with clinical airway improvement. One patient was initially found to

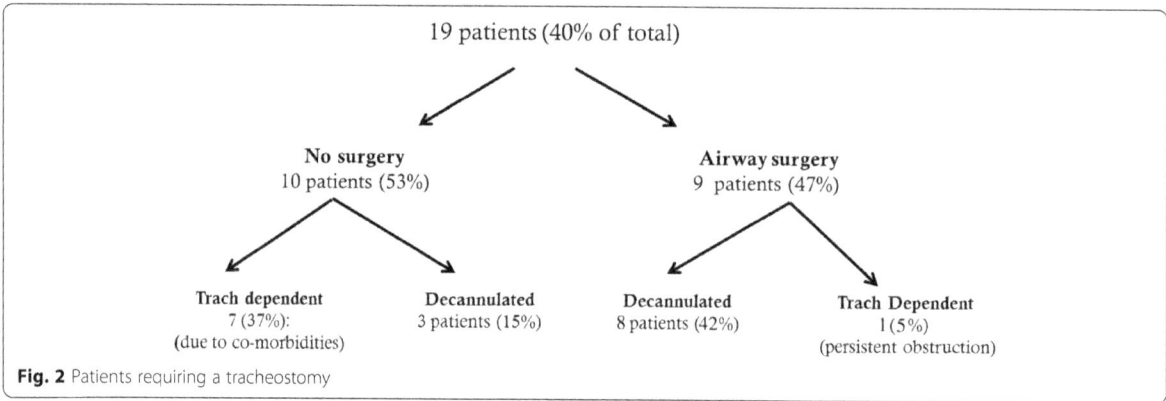

Fig. 2 Patients requiring a tracheostomy

have a post-operative granuloma, worsening dyspnea and an elevated EI (10.53) and EDI (63.17). A PFT was repeated following revision surgery and the final value was used as the post-operative value for comparision.

Nineteen patients did not have records of PFTs in their charts; two had medical reasons for not pursuing further surgical treatment (both had long term tracheotomy) and three others had mild symptoms that did not warrant intervention. Other patients could not complete the PFT tasks due to airway limitations (with a corked tracheotomy tube). It is unclear how many PFTs were performed at outside institutions and were not added to our institutional electronic medical record.

Other management

The majority of patients (56 %) underwent laryngeal computer tomography. Ten patients of 46 (21 %) were recommended to use home continuous positive airway pressure (CPAP) devices secondary to the diagnosis of obstructive sleep apnea on the basis of abnormal sleep studies attributable to their upper airway pathology. Of these patients, five patients were post-operative from a cordotomy/arytenoidectomy and the remaining five patients did not undergo any surgical airway intervention.

Discussion

Airway obstruction is the most disabling symptom in patients with BVFI. In both glottic stenosis and bilateral vocal fold paralysis, the primary goal is to provide a stable increase in glottic airway with minimal compromise in voice quality. Airway management depends on a variety of factors, including their degree of upper airway obstruction, underlying respiratory function, voice demands and quality of life priorities. Long-term tracheostomy, which was the only treatment available until 1922 [7–9], may be an appropriate option in some patients

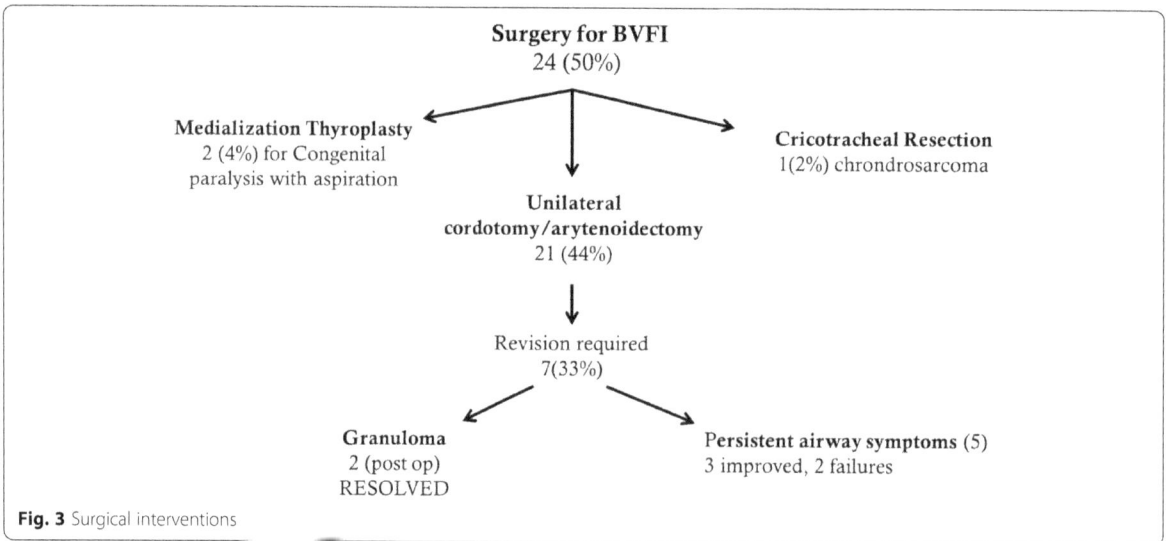

Fig. 3 Surgical interventions

for either quality of life preference (voice quality) or for medical reasons. Other patients may choose to undergo surgical procedures in order to improve glottic airway patency, potentially at the risk of increased dysphonia and aspiration, in order to have the tracheotomy tube removed.

Chevalier Jackson was the first to introduce surgical treatment in BVFI via an open approach cordectomy and ventriculocordectomy [10]. Poor voice and swallowing outcome prompted modifications: submusocal resection of the true vocal cord [11], extralaryngeal arytenoidectomy with arytenopexy to the ipsilateral strap muscles [12], 'arytenoidectomy via a thyroid alar window [13], and arytenoid abduction with lateral suture by Woodman [14]. Techniques were further improved with the introduction of the transoral arytenoidectomy in 1948 by Thornell [15]' and the application of endoscopic carbon dioxide laser [16–18].

Dennis and Kashima popularized the use of endoscopic posterior glottic cordotomy in 1989, which remains the most common surgical option, either as a unilateral [19] or bilateral intervention [20]. Other reports have been published with variations on these procedures including suture techniques [21–23], mucosal approaches [24] and equipment [10].

In our cohort, bilateral vocal fold immobility was most frequently caused by bilateral recurrent nerve paralysis after thyroid surgery, (Fig. 1). A twenty –year review of the etiology of bilateral vocal fold immobility was completed by at Cleveland Clinic in [25]. The percentages of BVFI attributed to thyroid surgery, intubation, cardiothoracic malignancy, neurological disease and radiation were within 3 % or less of the rates quoted in the 20-year review; our cohort also had a higher rates of idiopathic/unknown causes (19 % vs 11.4 %) as well as rheumatologic disease (6 % vs 2.7 %).

The majority of patients (75 %) presented with complaints of dyspnea secondary to paramedian positioned vocal folds and inadequate airway. Rarely, patients can present with bilaterally lateralized vocal folds; in our case two patients presented in this fashion and underwent Type I thyroplasty. Both of these patients were found to have congenital etiologies, suggesting a high vagal or central pathology other than the recurrent laryngeal nerve dysfunction.

Many patients in our series did not require surgery due to mild symptoms, and were monitored clinically via regular clinical examinations which included laryngoscopy and serial PFTs.

The decision to treat is based on the severity of symptoms, functionality and patient priorities. For some, optimal vocal quality is worth living with a tracheostomy, but for most, decannulation of their tracheotomy, or improvement of their airway obstruction symptoms is

the primary goal of treatment. Of the 21 patients who underwent a cordotomy, 2 (10 %) failed to improve and continued to required tracheotomy, in keeping with the literature in this population [2, 9]. No major complications occurred in the surgical treatment group.

CPAP has been shown to effectively manage sleep apnea without surgical intervention in patients with bilateral vocal cord paralysis and tracheal stenosis [26]. Our patients who are borderline in terms of symptoms or those who are unwilling or unfit to undergo a permanent airway modifying surgery may benefit from nocturnal CPAP. Sleep studies are often performed on these patients, as well as those undergoing corking trials, prior to decannulation [27].

Pulmonary function testing is currently proposed as the one of the most useful objective evaluation of the respiratory system, although application to upper airway obstruction has been problematic both as a diagnostic and quantitative measure. The ratio of FEV1 and PEFR expressed either as EI or as EDI, has been proposed as a useful tool in identifying upper airway obstruction [4, 6].

In our cohort, surprisingly, only half of the patients (41 % of EI/52 % of EDI) met the published criteria for upper airway obstruction, despite the diagnosis of BVFI and 96 % having presented with variable degrees of airway symptoms. The proposal by Nourai [4] to utilize EDI as a diagnostic tool for upper airway obstruction was based on PFT results in laryngotracheal stenosis patients ($n = 184$). However, the pathophysiology of glottis obstruction is unique in bilateral vocal fold paralysis wherein the inspiratory flow is more adversely affected than the expiratory flow based on the Bernoulli effect [28]. This rationale may explain why our BVFI cohort, consisting of predominantly bilateral vocal fold paralysis, were found to have a much lower mean ratio of EDI (52) than was reported by Nourai in fixed obstruction patients (76). Since bilateral vocal fold paralysis is predominantly an inspiratory obstruction, It may be more appropriate to quantified bilateral vocal fold paralysis using a ratio containing an inspiratory parameter, such as peak inspiratory flow rate (PIFR).

Regardless, the subgroup of seven patients who underwent a cordotomy/arytenoidectomy and who also had complete pre- and post- PFT data, did show a statistically significant increase in EDI/EI postoperatively, which also correlated with clinical airway improvement. Although it is difficult to draw a conclusion regarding the utility of this ration based the small sample size, these findings do suggest these proposed ratios still may have some utility in objectively monitoring patients' airway status.

In bilateral vocal fold paralysis, emerging research has shown that in a highly selected patients, re-innervation of the recurrent laryngeal nerve using a phrenic nerve rootlet maybe be effective in providing active abduction

[29]. There is also some evidence that transecting the RLN branch between the PCA and interarytenoid may prevent aberrant reinnervation and help avoid synkinesis; other have taken the approach of selectively reinnervating the adductors and the PCA muscles separately, with goals of isolated abduction during respiration while maintaining good adduction for voice production [28]. Reinnervation techniques of the RLN are still primarily in the research stage, but there are positive preliminary outcomes suggesting promise for bilateral vocal cord paralysis patients in the future, particularly in younger BVFI patients.

Conclusion

Bilateral vocal fold immobility is a challenging condition to manage due to the significant morbidity associated with the condition. Adequate airway management using endoscopic cordotomies/arytenoidectomy can achieve symptom improvement and decannulation for the majority of patients. CPAP ventilation can be a useful adjunct for those patients who continue to experience upper airway obstruction while sleeping.

Pulmonary function testing has much potential for the utility in the monitoring of these patients but ideal parameters in the setting of upper airway obstruction is still unclear. In our cohort of BVFI patients, EI/EDI ratios were not overly reliable in identifying bilateral vocal cord immobility, unlike in previously published reports. This different could be due to anatomic differences of BVFI versus the previous studies, which were based on subglottic stenosis – a fixed obstruction. Additional prospective data collection on this patient population, including evaluation of parameter ratios that include PFT inspiratory flow values may help us to further understand the utility of pulmonary function testing in objectively monitoring patients with obstructive symptoms secondary to bilateral vocal cord immobility.

Competing interests
The authors declare that they have no competing interests.

Authors' contributions
MB participated in the study design, reviewed the charts, collected the data, participated with the statistical analysis and drafted the manuscript. JA conceived of the study and helped to draft the manuscript. Both authors read, edited and approved the final manuscript.

Acknowledgements
The authors would like to acknowledge Carmen McKnight for her assistance in completing the ethics proposal, acquisition of data and data analysis. Thank you to Michelle Kwok for her help with the literature review.

Author details
[1]Department of Otolaryngology – Head and Neck Surgery, University of Toronto, Ontario, Canada. [2]St. Michael's Hospital, Department of Otolaryngology – Head and Neck Surgery, University of Toronto, 30 Bond St. 8C-129, ON M5B 1 W8 Toronto, Canada.

References

1. Olthoff A, Zeiss D, Laskawi R, Kruse E, Steiner W. Laser microsurgical bilateral posterior cordectomy for the treatment of bilateral vocal fold paralysis. Ann Otol Rhinol Laryngol. 2005;114:599–604.
2. Ozdemir S, Tuncer U, Tarkan O, Kara K, Surmelioglu O. Carbon dioxide laser endoscopic posterior cordotomy technique for bilateral abductor vocal cord paralysis: a 15-year experience. JAMA Otolaryngol Head Neck Surg. 2013;139:401–4.
3. Segas J, Stavroulakis P, Manolopoulos L, Yiotakis J, Adamopoulos G. Management of bilateral vocal fold paralysis: experience at the University of Athens. Otolaryngol Head Neck Surg. 2001;124:68–71.
4. Empey DW. Assessment of upper airways obstruction. Br Med J. 1972;3:503–5.
5. France JE, Thomas MJ. Clinical use of the empey index in the emergency department. Emerg Med J. 2004;21:642–3.
6. Nouraei SAR, Nouraei SM, Patel A, Murphy K, Giussani DA, Koury EF, et al. Diagnosis of laryngotracheal stenosis from routine pulmonary physiology using the expiratory disproportion index. Laryngoscope. 2013;123:3099–104.
7. Tucker HM. Laryngeal paralysis: aetiology and management. Otolaryngology. Philadelphia: Harper and Raw Publishers; 1980. p. 1–11.
8. Cheung EJ, McGinn JD. The surgical treatment of bilateral vocal fold impairment. Operative Techniques in Otolaryngology-Head and Neck Surgery. 2007;18:144–55.
9. Dursen G, Gokcan K. Aerodynamic, acoustic and functional results of posterior transverse laser cordotomy for bilateral abductor vocal cord paralysis. J Laryngol Otol. 2006;120:282–8.
10. Jackson C. Ventriculocordectomy: a new operation for the cure of goitrous glottic stenosis. Arch Surg. 1922;4:257–74.
11. Hoover W. Bilateral abductor paralysis: operative treatment of submucous resection of the vocal cord. Arch Otolaryngol. 1932;15:337–55.
12. King B. A new and function restoring operation for bilateral abductor cord paralysis. JAMA. 1939;112:814–23.
13. Kelly J. Surgical treatment of bilateral paralysis of the abductor muscles. Arch Otolaryngol. 1941;33:293–304.
14. Woodman D. A modification of the extralaryngeal approach to arytenoidectomy for bilateral abductor paralysis. Arch Otolaryngol. 1946;43:63–5.
15. Thornell W. Intralaryngeal approach for arytenoidectomy in bilateral abductor paralysis of the vocal cords. Arch Otolaryngol. 1948;47:505–8.
16. Manolopoulos L, Stavroulaki P, Yiotakis J, Segas J, Adamopoulos G. CO$_2$ and KTP-532 laser cordectomy for bilateral vocal fold paralysis. J Laryngol Otol. 1999;113:637–41.
17. Ossoff R, Sisson GA, Duncavage JA, Moselle H, Andrews PE, McMillan WG. Endoscopic laser arytenoidectomy for the treatment of bilateral vocal cord paralysis. Laryngoscope. 1984;94:1293–7.
18. Ossoff RH, Duncavage JA, Krespi YP, Shapshay SM, Sisson Sr GA. Endoscopic laser arytenoidectomy revisited. Ann Otol Rhinol Laryngol. 1990;99:764–71.
19. Dennis D, Kashima H. Carbon dioxide laser posterior cordectomy for treatment of bilateral vocal cord paralysis. Ann Otol Rhinol Laryngol. 1989;98:930–4.
20. Khalifa MC. Head neck surg. simultaneous bilateral posterior cordectomy in bilateral vocal fold paralysis. Otolaryngol Head Neck Surg. 2005;132(2):249–50.
21. Moustafa H, ElGuindy A, ElSherief S, Targam A. The role of endoscopic laterofixation of the vocal cord in the treatment of bilateral abductor paralysis. J Laryngol Otol. 1992;106(1):31–4.
22. Katilmiş H, Oztürkcan S, Başoğlu S, Aslan H, Ilknur AE, Erdoğan NK, et al. New technique for the treatment of bilateral vocal cord paralysis: vocal and ventricular fold lateralization using crossing sutures with thyroplasty technique. Acta Otolaryngol. 2011;131(3):303–9.
23. Hyodo M, Nishikubo K, Motoyoshi K. Laterofixation of the vocal fold using an endo-extralaryngeal needle carrier for bilateral vocal fold paralysis. Auris Nasus Larynx. 2009;36(2):181–6.
24. Benninger MS, Hseu A. Laser surgical management of bilateral vocal fold immobility. Operative Techniques in Otolaryngology-Head and Neck Surgery. 2011;22:116–21.
25. Rosenthal-Swibel L, Benninger MS, Deeb RH. Vocal fold immobility: a longitudinal analysis of etiology over 30 years. Laryngoscope. 2007;117:1864–70.

26. Wiest GH1, Ficker JH, Lehnert G, Hahn EG. Secondary obstructive sleep apnea syndrome in a patient with tracheal stenosis and bilateral recurrent paresis. Successful treatment with nasal continuous positive airway pressure therapy. Dtsch Med Wochenschr. 1998;123(17):522–6.

27. Wolter NE and Anderson J. Polysomnography: Assessment of decannulation readiness in chronic upper airway obstruction. Laryngoscope 2014;124(11):2574-8. doi:10.1002/lary.24836

28. Woodson G. Upper airway anatomy and function. In: Johnson J, Rosen C, Bailey B, editors. Bailey's head and neck surgery – otolaryngology. 5th ed. Philadelphia, Pa: Wolters Kluwer Health/Lippincott Williams & Wilkins; 2014. p. 865–77.

29. Marina MB1, Marie JP, Birchall MA. Laryngeal reinnervation for bilateral vocal fold paralysis. Curr Opin Otolaryngol Head Neck Surg. 2011;19(6):434–8.

18

Informed consent: do information pamphlets improve post-operative risk-recall in patients undergoing total thyroidectomy: prospective randomized control study

Hussain Alsaffar*, Lindsay Wilson, Dev P. Kamdar, Faizullo Sultanov, Danny Enepekides and Kevin M. Higgins

Abstract

Background: Informed consent consists of basic five elements: voluntarism, capacity, disclosure, understanding, and ultimate decision-making. Physician disclosure, patient understanding, and information retention are all essential in the doctor-patient relationship. This is inclusive of helping patients make and manage their decisions and expectations better and also to deal with any consequences and/or complications that arise. This study investigates whether giving patients procedure-specific handouts pre-operatively as part of the established informed consent process significantly improves overall risk-recall following surgery. These handouts outline the anticipated peri-operative risks and complications associated with total thyroidectomy, as well as the corrective measures to address complications. In addition, the influence of potential confounders affecting risk-recall, such as anxiety and pre-existing memory disturbance, are also examined.

Methods: Consecutive adult (≥18 years old) patients undergoing total thyroidectomy at a single academic tertiary care referral centre are included. Participants are randomly assigned into either the experimental group (with pamphlets) or the control group by a computerized randomization system (Clinstat). All participants filled out a Hospital Anxiety and Depression Scale (HADS) and they are tested by the physician for short-term memory loss using the Memory Impairment Screen (MIS) exam. All patients are evaluated at one week post-operatively. The written recall questionnaire test is also administered during this clinical encounter.

Results: Forty-nine patients are included - 25 of them receive verbal consent only, while another 24 patients received both verbal consent and patient education information pamphlets. The overall average of correct answers for each group was 83 % and 80 % in the control and intervention groups, respectively, with no statistically significant differences. There are also no statistically significant differences between the two groups, in both interview duration, in time between interviews, and in recall tests. No correlation is also apparent between the pre-op HADS score and the recall questionnaire overall score.

Conclusions: A pre-operative thyroid surgical information pamphlet alone might not be sufficient to enhance patient test scores and optimally educate the patient on their expected care pathway in thyroid surgery. Supplementation with alternative means of patient education perhaps using emerging technologies needs to be further investigated.

Keywords: Informed consent, Pamphlets, Post-operative risk-recall, Total thyroidectomy and patient education

* Correspondence: haskfu2@yahoo.com
Sunnybrook Health Sciences Centre, University of Toronto, Toronto, ON, Canada

Background

Informed consent consists of basic five elements: voluntarism, capacity, disclosure, understanding, and ultimate decision-making [1]. Physician disclosure, patient understanding, and information retention are essential in the doctor- patient relationship. This is inclusive of helping patients make and manage their decisions and expectations better and also dealing with any consequences and/or complications that arise.

There are many factors that can affect understanding and information retention. Some examples include, the language of communication, the psychological impact of diagnosis, the intellectual characteristics of an individual, the educational status, the level of general fund of knowledge, and the preexisting conditions affecting memory impairment and social support [2].

The understanding and retention of peri-operative expectations, possible complications, and appropriate corrective action plans can possibly avert catastrophic outcomes, unnecessary emergency visits, and decrease patient anxieties.

To enhance verbal communication, other means have been used such as pamphlets; multimedia and/or web based interactive media. Studies, especially in clinical trials [3], have demonstrated that the singular act of signing consent paperwork alone does not correlate with understanding the overall comprehensive picture of the consent, nor does it reflect on the overall quality of process. Total thyroidectomy, as it is one of the most common procedures in head and neck surgical practice with a widely understood risk profile, is chosen as the test procedure.

Objectives

It is important to investigate whether giving patients procedure-specific handouts pre-operatively as part of the established informed consent process significantly improves overall risk-recall following surgery. These handouts outline the anticipated peri-operative risks and complications associated with total thyroidectomy, as well as the corrective measures to address some of those complications. In addition, the influences of potential confounders affecting risk-recall, such as anxiety and pre-existing memory disturbance are also examined.

Methods

Consecutive adult (≥ 18 years old) patients undergoing total thyroidectomy at a single academic tertiary care referral centre are included. Patients included in the study who undergo total thyroidectomy are based on pre-operative cytopathology that is suggestive or is stratified as a high risk for thyroid cancer with Bethseda V or VI cytopathology. This also means that patients demonstrated no cognitive impairment, patients signed pre-operative consent paperwork, and patients are

English-speaking, or they are able to effectively utilize available translational services. Participants are randomly assigned into either the experimental group (with pamphlet), or the control group with a computerized randomization system.

All patients are given verbal informed consent by senior staff surgeons. This included a review of possible post-operative complications and the associated risks and the benefits for the procedure. Signs and symptoms of major complications are carefully explained to the patient and the best corrective action plans explicitly outlined. In order to ensure uniformity and consistency of the verbal consent process, the senior staff surgeons involved in the study followed a standardized script (see Additional file 1: A.1). Concurrently, patients are asked to complete the Hospital Anxiety and Depression Scale (HADS) and they are screened for short-term memory loss using the Memory Impairment Screen (MIS) by the study coordinator [4].

In the experimental group, additional pamphlets are provided at the beginning of the interview, which is discussed point-by-point after patients are instructed and give time to read the pamphlet in its entirety. The pamphlet is a pre-existing pamphlet that is used at our institution. Translational services are offered to both control and experimental interventions as necessary. (See Additional file 1: A.2)

All participants underwent total thyroidectomy. All patients are also screened for renal dysfunction and they are prepared and sent home with prophylactic calcium and Vitamin D3 oral supplements in accordance with well-established clinical practice norms. Patients are evaluated one-week post-operatively for wound inspections, biochemical follow-ups, suture removals, and voice assessments. The written recall test is administered during this clinical encounter.

The recall test is a 12 - point multiple-choice test with two principal domains. The first six questions test patients on information in relation to the described post-operative risks; the second six questions test information in relation to the management of those highlighted post-operative complications and appropriate corrective action steps. (See Additional file 1: A.3).

Patient demographics, ethnicity, native language, interview duration, time to surgery while on a waiting list, HADS score, cognitive status, post-operative complications, unplanned clinic or emergency room visits, post-operative PTH, Vitamin D and ionized calcium levels are all collected. Statistical analysis are conducted with SPSS with $p < 0.05$ considered significant for a two-tailed testing.

Results

Fifty consecutive patients are enrolled in the study by two senior head and neck surgeons. One patient withdrew

Table 1 Participants demographics, cognitive status and language

	Control group	Intervention group	P value
Total number	24	25	
Gender			N/A
Male	6 (25 %)	11 (44 %)	
Female	18 (75 %)	14 (56 %)	
Mean age (years)	48 (27–77)	50 (34–74)	0.697
Cognitive impairment	None	None	N/A
Require translator	None	2	N/A

from the study because he deferred his surgery. Of the forty-nine patients, 25 received verbal consent only, while 24 received both verbal consent and patient education information pamphlets. The mean age was 48 (27–77) years and 50 (34–74) years in the control and in the intervention groups, respectively. There are no statistically significant differences in age between the two groups with $P = 0.697$. None of the study population demonstrated cognitive impairments, while two patients in the intervention group required translational services. Patient demographic details are listed in Table 1.

Overall score
The overall average correct answer for each group was 83 % (25–100 %) and 80 % (35.3–94.2 %) in the control and intervention groups, respectively, with no statistically significant differences (Fig. 1). There is also no statistical significance between answers to the questions that are in the pamphlets in comparison to questions that are not in the pamphlets (Q4, Q5, Q6, Q11, and Q12).

Overall score, interview duration and waiting time
The mean interview durations are 16.9 (5–40) and 15.8 (5–30) minutes in control and in intervention groups, respectively. The duration of two patients at the interview

who required translators in the intervention group are 20 and 30 min, respectively. There are also no statistically significant differences between the two groups in regards to both interview duration and in time between interview and in recall tests ($p = 0.663$ and 0.629, respectively). This is in reference to Table 2. Further analysis between these two factors using a Pearson correlation coefficient test showed an inverse correlation between time duration with consents and with interviews in respect of an overall score correlation (−0.291) ($P = 0.093$). A notable trend towards statistical significance is also observed. For the interview duration, parametric Pearson correlation tests showed positive correlations between interview duration and overall score (0.243) with statistical significance ($P = 0.042$) (Figs. 2 and 3).

Relation of anxiety and depression score with overall score
All patients filled the HADS questionnaire. Pre-operative anxiety scores are borderline in 10 patients (41.6 %) and none in the control group. In the interventional group, six (24 %) are borderline and three (12 %) have abnormal scores. On the other hand, pre-operative depression scores are borderline in one patient for each group. There are no statistically significant differences between the two groups in both anxiety and in depression score with a P value of 0.842, 0.4163, respectively (See Table 3). There are also no correlations between the pre-op HADS score and the overall score of the recall test.

Post-operative complication
Immediate post-operative parathyroid hormone (PTH) was within normal range (1.6–6.9 pmol/L) with no symptomatic hypocalcaemia. There are no unplanned clinic or emergency room visits during the first week post-operatively. All calcium and Vitamin D3 supplementation, that were given preoperatively as prophylaxis

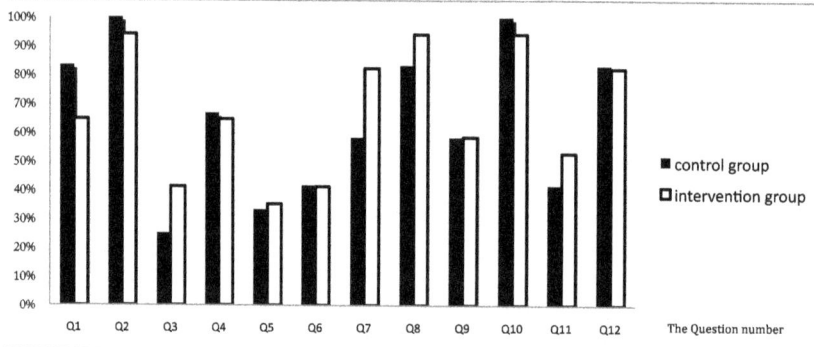

Fig. 1 Percentages of correct answers for each question in the two groups

Table 2 Duration of interview, time lapse to test recall and post-operative complication

	Control group	Intervention group	P value
Mean interview duration (mins)	16.9	15.8	0.633
Duration between consent – test recall (Days)	68 (14–181)	75 (9–266)	0.629

preoperatively, were stopped by the third post-operative based on previously established best practice protocols.

Discussion

Aside from legal and ethical requirements, informed consent serves as an important role in patient education in regards to post-operative expectations, consequences, and complications. It is apparent that patient satisfaction correlates strongly with the amount of information received [5, 6]. The process of informed consent often occurs in one or two encounters in the outpatient clinic before surgery. This is typically done verbally and occasionally through the use of information pamphlets or through the use of audiovisual aids. This can lead to possible information overload, resulting confusion and poor information retention [7]. Previous research indicates that, just five minutes after a consultation, patients already forget half of what the doctor told them. The percentage of retained information can be raised from approximately 20 to 50% by providing visual or written information as additional support [8, 9].

This paper investigates whether presenting patients with procedure-specific handouts pre-operatively significantly improves overall risk-recall following total thyroidectomy. In addition, it examines the influence of potential confounders affecting risk-recall such as anxiety and pre-existing memory disturbances. In our study, the addition of a pre-operative handout in thyroid surgery did not improve the overall test score on post-operative recall testing between the two groups. There are no statistically significant differences between the overall test scores and the waiting times for surgery and interview durations, however there is a noticeable trend toward the negative impact of the former and positive impact of the latter. There are no correlations between pre-operative anxiety and depression and between overall recall.

Pre-operative written information demonstrates improvements in recalls on admission [10–12].

Chan et al. [10] studied the effect of written leaflets with illustrations on the ability to list three complications in 93 patients undergoing thyroid surgery. The

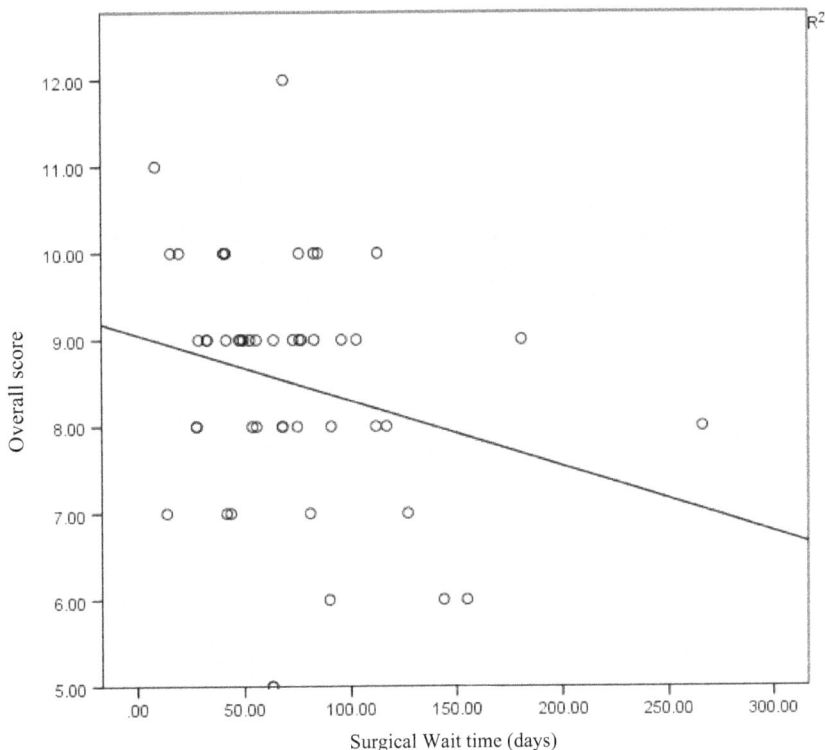

Fig. 2 Simple linear regressions plot between surgical wait time (days) and overall scores

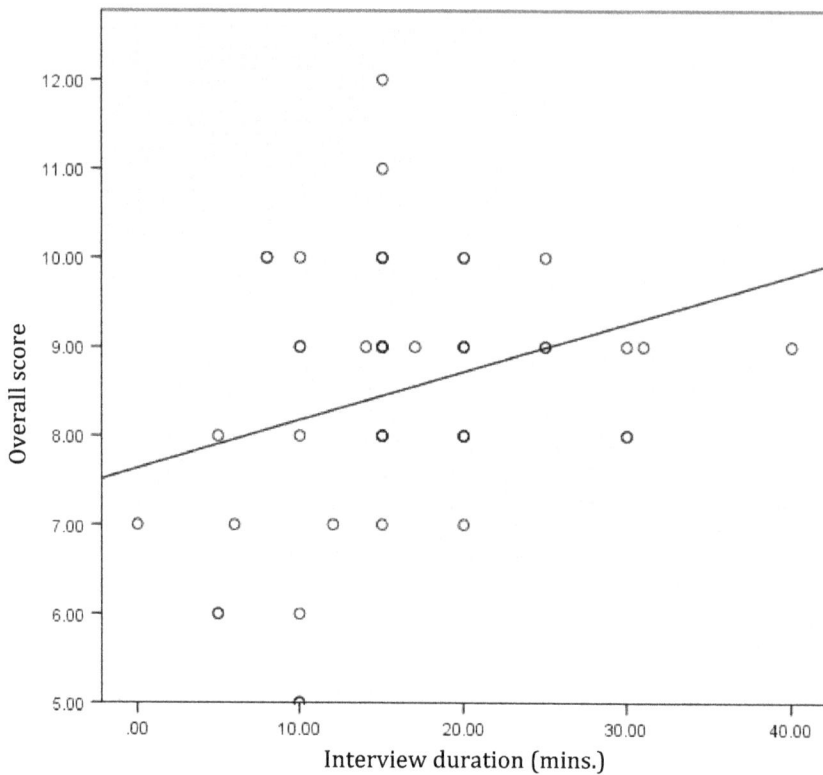

Fig. 3 Simple linear regressions plot between duration of interview and overall score

overall recall rates are 30.6 and 50.4 % between the control and intervention groups, respectively. Similarly, in our study waiting time is not a factor between groups (average wait time to surgery of 33 days). Siau et al. reported that patients prefer to receive information leaflets and reading them subsequently demonstrated improved recall of the nature of the procedures and risks in adult tonsillectomy [13]. With regards to patient satisfaction, a cohort of patients with no significant differences between control and intervention groups for the Hospital Anxiety and Depression Scale, Clode-Baker et al. found that patients were more satisfied with information they had received and they felt less confronted by information on arrival for the hospital stay [14]. Ihedioha et al. conducted a randomized control trial to assess additional benefits of

video education when combined with a written pamphlet in the psychological preparedness of patients undergoing elective colorectal surgery [15]. No differences in short-term outcomes in the hospital or in the complication rates are observed. Another important category of educational tools are web-based platforms. Advancements in social media and improved Internet access permit easy, accessible, interactive, and comprehensive tools for informed consent delivery. Farval et al. conducted a randomized control trial comparing the quality of informed consent provision in order to augment discussions with online education resources. The result is a statistically significant increase in patient knowledge with an average score of 69.25 % correct answers in the intervention group as compared to 47.38 % in the control arm with a higher patient

Table 3 Anxiety and depression scores in the two groups

	Anxiety score			Depression score		
	Control	Intervention	P value	Control	Intervention	P value
Mean score	6.54	6.36	0.842	3.5	2.92	0.416
Normal	14	16	n/a	23	24	n/a
Borderline	10	6	n/a	1	1	n/a
Abnormal	0	3	n/a	0	0	n/a

satisfaction (p = 0.043). There are no statistically significant differences in anxiety scores with P value of 0.195.

Unlike these studies, our study has an emphasis on testing not only the inherent complication risk-recalls for medico-legal purposes, but also testing a critical educational component in respect to the corrective action plans post-operatively. Our study reveals a higher overall average recall score than other studies in both groups (80 and 83 %). This fact may relate to the multiple choice question format and study power. A limitation is that that we used a recall test which is developed for the purposes of this study, however, it has not been validated as a method of assessment.

Despite the importance of pamphlets in patient satisfaction, risk conveyance, and addressing complications, pamphlets per se might not be sufficient to optimally educate the patient on their pre-operative care pathway in thyroid surgery. Future directions point to an expansion of web-based platforms coupled with embedded informational videos which are currently being rolled out.

Conclusion

A pre-operative thyroid surgical information pamphlet alone might not be sufficient to enhance patient test scores and optimally educate the patient on their expected care pathway in thyroid surgery. Supplementation with alternative means of patient education perhaps using emerging technologies needs to be further investigated.

Additional file

Additional file 1: The script read for risk listing (See A.1). The Pamphlet (See A.2). Risk-recall questionnaire test (See A.3). (DOCX 810 kb)

Abbreviations
HADS: Hospital anxiety and depression scale; MIS: Memory impairment screen; PTH: Parathyroid hormone.

Competing interests
The authors declare that they have no competing interests.

Authors' contributions
H. A., acquisition of data, or analysis and interpretation of data, drafting the manuscript. D. P. K. contributions to conception and design. L. W. contributions to conception and design and acquisition of data. F. S. acquisition of data. D. E. contributions to conception and design. K. M. H. contributions to conception and design, critically revised the manuscript. All authors read and approved the final manuscript.

Acknowledgements
None.

References
1. Lidz CW. The therapeutic misconception and our models of competency and informed consent. Behav Sci Law. 2006;24:535–46.
2. Falagas ME, Korbila IP, Giannopoulou KP, Kondilis BK, Peppas G. Informed consent: how much and what do patients understand? Am J Surg. 2009; 198:420–35.
3. Jefford M, Moore R. Improvement of informed consent and the quality of consent documents. Australia lancet oncology. 2008;9:485–93.
4. Buschke H, Kuslansky G, Katz M, Stewart WF, Sliwinski MJ, Eckholdt HM, et al. Screening for dementia with the memory impairment screen. Neurology. 1999;52:231.
5. Krishel S, Baraff LJ. Effect of emergency department information on patient satisfaction. Ann Emerg Med. 1993;22:568–72.
6. Robbins JA, Bertakis KD, Helms LJ, Azari R, Callahan EJ, Creten DA. The influence of physician practice behaviors on patient satisfaction. Fam Med. 1993;25:17–20.
7. Hutson MM, Blaha JD. Patients' recall of preoperative instruction for informed consent for an operation. J Bone Joint Surg Am. 1991;73:160–2.
8. Kitching JB. Patient information leaflets – the state of the art. J R Soc Med. 1990;83:298–300.
9. Gauld VA. Written advice: compliance and recall. J R Coll Gen Practice. 1981; 31:553–6.
10. Chan Y, Irish JC, Wood SJ, et al. Patient education and informed consent in head and neck surgery. Arch Otolaryngol Head Neck Surg. 2002;28:1269–74.
11. Winterton RIS, Alaani A, Loke D, et al. Role of infor-mation leaflets in improving the practice of informed consent for patients undergoing septoplasty. J Laryngol Otol. 2007;121:134–7.
12. Langdon IJ1, Hardin R, Learmonth ID. Informed consent for total hip arthroplasty: does a written information sheet improve recall by patients? Ann R Coll Surg Engl. 2002;84:404–8.
13. Siau D1, List RJ, Hussin N, Woolford TJ. Do printed information leaflets improve recall of the procedure and risks in adult tonsillectomy? How we do it. Clin Otolaryngol. 2010;35:503–6.
14. Clode-Baker E1, Draper E, Raymond N, Haslam C, Gregg P. Preparing patients for total hip replacement: a randomized controlled trial of a preoperative educational intervention. J Health Psychol. 1997;2:107–14.
15. Ihedioha U, Vaughan S, Mastermann J, Singh B, Chaudhri S. Patient education videos for elective colorectal surgery: results of a randomized controlled trial. Colorectal Dis. 2013;15:1436–41.

19

Brief electrical stimulation after facial nerve transection and neurorrhaphy: a randomized prospective animal study

Adrian Mendez[1*], Hadi Seikaly[1], Vincent L. Biron[1], Lin Fu Zhu[2] and David W. J. Côté[1,3]

Abstract

Background: Recent studies have examined the effects of brief electrical stimulation (BES) on nerve regeneration, with some suggesting that BES accelerates facial nerve recovery. However, the facial nerve outcome measurement in these studies has not been precise or accurate.

The objective of this study is to assess the effect of BES on accelerating facial nerve functional recovery from a transection injury in the rat model.

Methods: A prospective randomized animal study using a rat model was performed. Two groups of 9 rats underwent facial nerve surgery. Both group 1 and 2 underwent facial nerve transection and repair at the main trunk of the nerve, with group 2 additionally receiving BES on post-operative day 0 for 1 h using an implantable stimulation device. Primary outcome was measured using a laser curtain model, which measured amplitude of whisking at 2, 4, and 6 weeks post-operatively.

Results: At week 2, the average amplitude observed for group 1 was 4.4°. Showing a statistically significant improvement over group 1, the group 2 mean was 14.0° at 2 weeks post-operatively ($p = 0.0004$). At week 4, group 1 showed improvement having an average of 9.7°, while group 2 remained relatively unchanged with an average of 12.8°. Group 1 had an average amplitude of 13.63° at 6-weeks from surgery. Group 2 had a similar increase in amplitude with an average of 15.8°. There was no statistically significant difference between the two groups at 4 and 6 weeks after facial nerve surgery.

Conclusions: This is the first study to use an implantable stimulator for serial BES following neurorrhaphy in a validated animal model. Results suggest performing BES after facial nerve transection and neurorrhaphy at the main trunk of the facial nerve is associated with accelerated whisker movement in a rat model compared with a control group.

Background

Facial neuromuscular disorders and functional impairment resulting from facial nerve injury are common and can be severe [1]. Aesthetic impairments also impart an affliction leading to social isolation and further emotional distress. Together these can lead to depressive symptoms and mental health issues, which further exacerbate their functional disabilities [2]. There are

several clinical factors that have been identified that further impact peripheral nerve function recovery following nerve injury including time to repair, type of repair, and the age of the patient [3]. In an effort to optimize recovery, specific repair techniques are utilized that have been shown to improve outcome. The basic requirement is to appose the cut ends of the nerve in such a fashion as to minimize scar formation and preserve the optimal blood supply [4]. In cases of sharp nerve division with minimal gap, direct end-to-end nerve repair is indicated [5]. Tension-free suture repair remains the preferred treatment option as tension will result in scaring and poor regeneration [4, 5].

* Correspondence: amendez@ualberta.ca

This study will be presented at the Canadian Society of Otolaryngology-Head and Neck Surgery Annual Meeting (June 2015, Winnipeg MB).

[1]Department of Surgery, Division of Otolaryngology-Head and Neck Surgery, University of Alberta, Edmonton, AB, Canada

Full list of author information is available at the end of the article

Despite advances in microsurgical technique, functional recovery following facial nerve transection injury remains suboptimal [6]. Synkinesis, or axonal regeneration from the proximal stump into inappropriate distal pathways, has long been recognized as a significant contributing factor to poor functional recovery [7]. Previous studies have shown that electrical stimulation affects morphological and functional properties of neurons including nerve branching, rate and orientation of neurite growth, rapid sprouting, and guidance during axon regeneration [8, 9]. Specifically, Gordon et al. examined the effect of electrical stimulation on regeneration after nerve transection in a rat sciatic nerve model [6]. The authors were able to demonstrate that electrical stimulation dramatically accelerated both axonal regeneration as well as preferentially reinnervated motor nerves over sensory branches. The authors also found short-term, 1-h periods of stimulation were as effective as long-term stimulation lasting days to weeks [6].

Animal studies have begun to investigate the effects of electrical stimulation on the facial nerve. In 2008, Lal et al. demonstrated that electrical stimulation accelerates facial nerve recovery [1]. In 2012, Foecking et al. confirmed these findings and also demonstrated that single 30-min sessions of stimulation were as effective in improving facial nerve function as prolonged stimulation [10]. However, the outcome model employed by these studies relied on video observation, potentially introducing error.

In 2010, Hadlock et al. studied the effect of electrical stimulation on the facial nerve in a rat model using a precise functional outcomes model capable of detecting micrometer movements of rat whisking [2]. The authors were able to demonstrate improvement in facial nerve functional outcomes in the first 8 weeks. However, the study employed a facial nerve stimulation technique that introduced stimulation prior to nerve injury [2]. In a generalizable clinical setting, this would be less applicable to repair following an unplanned resection or injury.

A recently developed, validated animal model adapted from Heaton et al. was employed to precisely and accurately measure facial nerve function [11]. The objective of this study was to evaluate facial nerve outcomes using BES employed after nerve transection in our validated animal model.

Methods

Study design

This prospective randomized control animal trial was conducted at the Surgical Medical Research Institute (SMRI) at the University of Alberta. A previously validated rat facial nerve model was used [11]. Ethics approval was obtained from the Animal Care and Use Committee (ACUC) overseen by the University Animal Policy and Welfare Committee (UAPWC) at the University of Alberta in Edmonton, Alberta [AUP00000785].

Study subjects

Eighteen female Wistar rats (Charles River Laboratories, Canada) weighing 200–220 g were used for this study. Sample size was calculated based on the study by Heaton et al., which employed a similar outcome measure, powered to detect a difference of 10° in whisking [11]. All rats were housed in pairs at the Health Sciences Laboratory Animal Services (HSLAS) at the University of Alberta. Rats were weighed and handled daily 2 weeks prior to the commencement of the study to reduce animal stress during the study. The 18 rats were block randomized into two groups of 9. Each animal underwent unilateral facial nerve transection and repair at the main trunk of nerve. Group 2 additionally received brief electrical stimulation for 1 h following nerve repair. Facial nerve functional outcome assessment was collected at 2, 4, and 6 weeks post-operatively.

Facial nerve functional outcome assessment

The facial nerve functional outcome assessment model employed in this study was based on the model previously described and validated by Heaton et al. [11]. This model employs a head fixation device, body restraint, and bilateral photoelectric sensors to detect precise whisker movements as an objective measure for facial nerve function.

Head implant

In order to ensure proper head fixation during whisker movement measurement, an implantable head fixation device was required. An animal head implant was bioengineered for this purpose. The implant is composed of acrylic and long threaded screws.

Body restraint

Based on the design described by Heaton et al., a custom body restraint device for the rat subjects was bioengineered (Metalworks Engineering Shop, University of Alberta, Edmonton, AB) [11]. Our body restraint apparatus consisted of a half-pipe (ABS-DWV IPEX Drainway) measuring 7.6 cm in diameter and 30 cm in length. Three Velcro® straps were then fastened across the top of the half-pipe for added restraint. A steel bar spanning across the half pipe provided a fixation point for the head implant as well as functioned to support the laser micrometers. Along the anterior portion of the half-pipe we added a circular platform to support the weight of the rat's head while placed in the apparatus (Fig. 1).

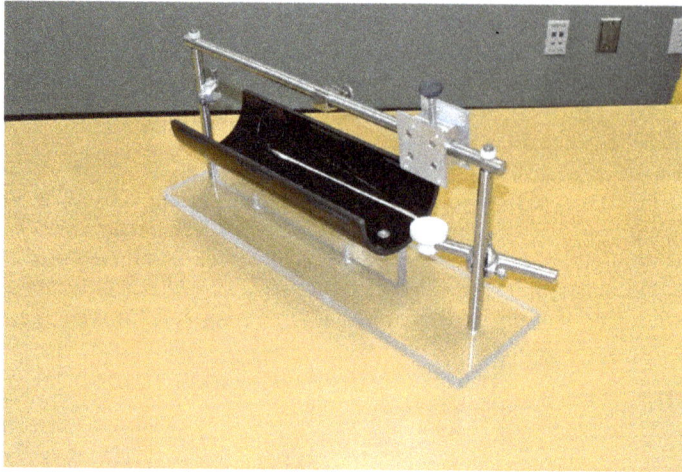

Fig. 1 Customized body restraint

Tracking whisker movement

Two pairs of photoelectric sensors (Rx-Laser Micrometer, Metralight Inc., San Mateo, Ca) were placed along each side of the subject's face in order to track whisker movement. Thin tubing 1.5 mm in diameter was placed over a midline whisker on either side of the subject's face to facilitate tracking by the laser micrometer. The laser micrometers were placed at 17° from the midline along each side of the face and this was considered parallel to the lateral surface of the face and positioned 10 mm from the origin of the tracked whisker on each side of the face.

The laser micrometer was comprised of an emitter, which produced a 780 nm wavelength light curtain, and a detector composed of a 28 mm linear array of 4000 charge-coupled devices (CCD scanline). A 5 cm vertical distance separated the emitter and detector, producing a laser curtain. Movement detected within the laser curtain sent a digital signal that could then be recorded. The laser micrometers were calibrated to avoid detection of objects less than 1 mm in size to prevent tracing of multiple whiskers. The calibrated laser curtain detected only the marked whisker.

Data acquisition

Whisker movement was elicited in each subject by providing a scented stimulus (chocolate milk). The laser micrometers themselves were connected to a 32-Channel Digital I/O Module (NI 9403, National Instruments, Dallas, Tx), which received digital output from the laser micrometers. The I/O module was connected to a PC through a CompactDAQ chassis (cDAQ-9174, National Instruments, Dallas, Tx). The I/O module acquired the laser micrometer signal at a sampling rate of 1 kHz. LabVIEW (LabVIEW Full

Development System, National Instruments, Dallas, Tx) software was used as the interface for data acquisition.

Surgical procedure

All subjects underwent both facial nerve surgery and head implantation surgery during the same anesthetic. Group 2 additionally received 1 h of BES following nerve repair while remaining anesthetized. All rats were first anesthetized with 3–4 % isoflurane. Subjects were then maintained under general anesthesia using 1.5 % isoflurane. Fur was then removed from the right side of the face and the top of the head using an electric shaver.

Facial nerve surgery

Facial nerve surgery was completed on the right side on all subjects. A small incision was made just inferior to the right ear bony prominence. Under microscopic visualization, the parotid gland was visualized, everted, and retracted out of the surgical field. Distal branches of the facial nerve were identified just inferior to the parotid bed. These were followed proximally until the main trunk of the facial nerve was identified. Once identified, the main trunk and upper and lower bifurcation of the facial nerve were carefully dissected. A single transection of the main trunk of the facial nerve was made using straight microscopic scissors; the cut nerve ends were then immediately repaired using a direct end-to-end technique. Using 9-0 sutures, four simple interrupted sutures were made within the proximal and distal epineural nerve endings. Care was taken to ensure proper nerve alignment.

Brief electrical stimulation

Along with facial nerve repair, animal subjects in group 2 received brief electrical stimulation. The stimulation

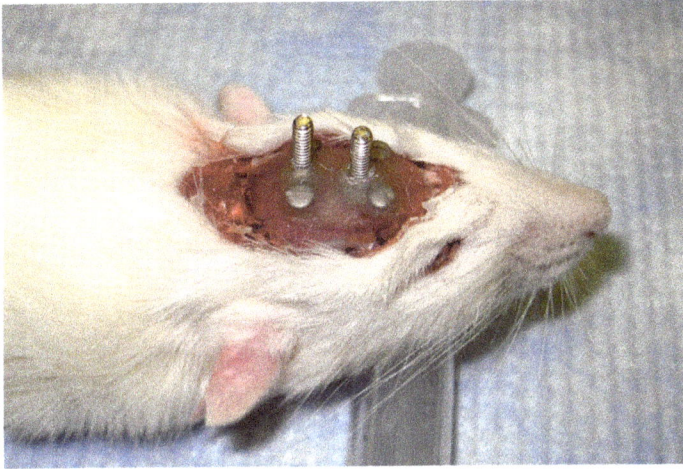

Fig. 2 Acrylic helmet

protocol was adapted from one used by Gordon et al. in the sciatic nerve rat model [6]. Two silver Teflon coated wires were bared of insulation for 2–3 mm (AGT0510, W-P Instruments, Inc.). Following nerve repair, the first wire was looped around the proximal stump of the facial nerve. The second wire was imbedded into muscle tissue adjacent to the facial nerve, at a location just proximal to the first wire. The insulated wires were led to an isostim stimulator (A320D, W-P Instruments, Inc.) which delivered a 1.5 mA current in pulses of 100 microseconds in a continuous 20 Hz train for a period of 1 h. The adequacy of stimulation was verified by the presence of a right ear flutter. At the completion of stimulation, the wires were removed from the animal and the incision closed with interrupted 3-0 vicryl sutures.

Head implant surgery

Following the facial nerve procedure, head implant surgery was then completed without reversing the general anesthetic. A small incision was made using a 15-blade scalpel from the anterior to posterior margin of the cranium. Blunt dissection was employed to fully expose

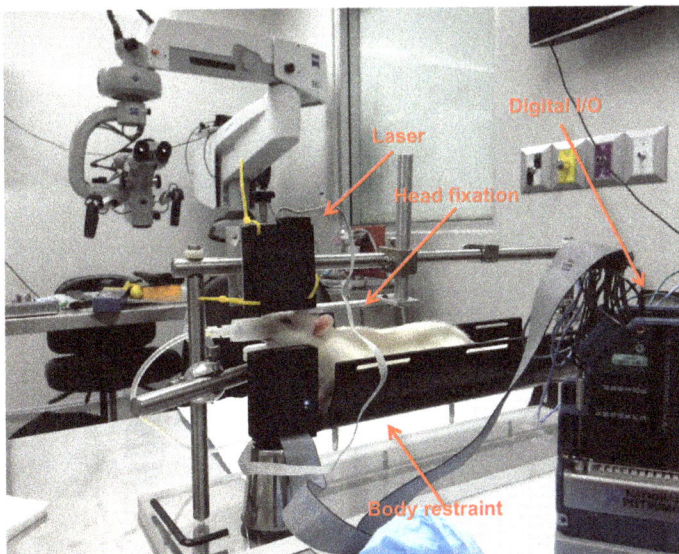

Fig. 3 Whisking model

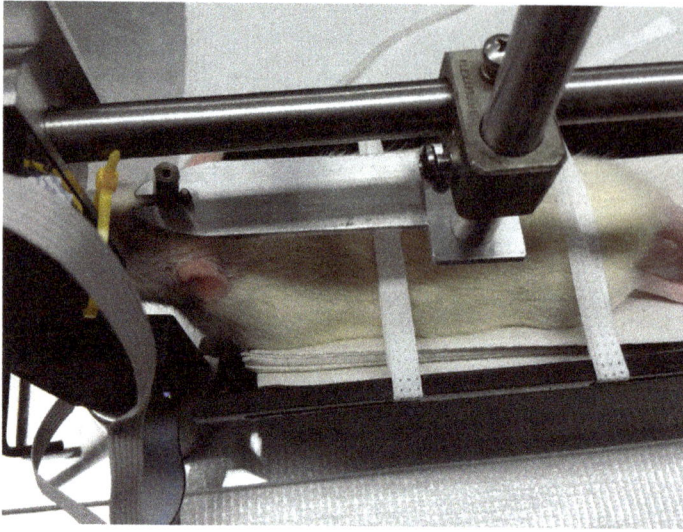

Fig. 4 Head fixation

the underlying bony cranium. Using an electric drill, 4 holes were made in each quadrant of the skull approximately 15 mm apart from each other. 1.6 mm screws were then placed within each drill site (Fig. 2). Dry acrylic resin was then liquefied and placed onto the skull, covering the placed screws. Two larger 5 mm threaded screws were then inverted with the threads directed upwards into the acrylic before it solidified.

Head fixation and body restraint

Two weeks prior to surgery, all animal subject were handled daily for conditioning. After surgery, all subjects were placed in body restraints daily for a week. At post-operative day 14, whisker measurements were started. Subjects were initially given dose low dose isoflurane and transported to the body restraint apparatus described in section 3.2 (Fig. 3). Here they underwent head fixation with bolts applied across the exposed threaded screws (Fig. 4). Whisker markers were then placed on either side of the rat's face as described in section 3.3.

Once this was completed, a scented stimulus was introduced and recording started usually for a period of 5 min. The non-operative left side was used as the

control for each subject. This procedure was completed for each rat at 2, 4, and 6 weeks post-operatively.

Results

All animals tolerated the surgical procedure without perioperative complications. They exhibited normal cage behavior and did not lose weight. Three animals had problems with the head implantation device. In these animals, the device became loose at approximately week 4. This required an addition anesthetic with isoflurane and a new acrylic device to be made and fixed in place on the cranium. No animals had to be removed from the study.

All animals experienced complete ipsilateral loss of whisking amplitude post-operatively. At week 2 the average amplitude observed for group 1 was 4.4° (Table 1). Showing a statistically significant improvement over group 1, the group 2 average was 14.0° at 2 weeks post-operatively ($p = 0.0004$). At week 4, group 1 showed improvement having an average of 9.7°, while group 2 remained relatively unchanged with an average of 12.8°. The week 6 results showed the greatest improvement from baseline for group 1. Group 1 had an average

Table 1 Post-operative whisking amplitudes at week 2, 4, and 6

	Week 2 amplitude (degrees)	Week 4 amplitude (degrees)	Week 6 amplitude (degrees)
Nerve repair (group 1) Right side (operated)	4.4	9.7	13.63
Nerve repair (group 1) Left side (control)	72.1	66.6	71.8
BES (group 2) Right side (operated)	14.0	12.8	15.84
BES (group 2) Left side (control)	71.9	70.9	67.5

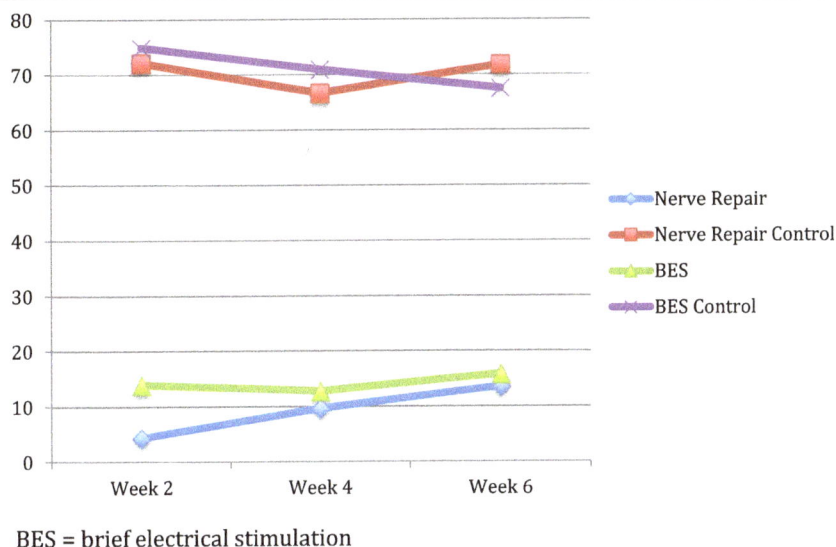

BES = brief electrical stimulation

Fig. 5 Whisking amplitude in degrees at 2, 4, and 6 weeks postoperatively. *BES* brief electrical stimulation

amplitudes of 13.63° at 6-weeks from surgery. Similarly, group 2 showed a slight increase in amplitude with an average of 15.84°. There was no statistically significant difference between the two groups at 4 and 6 weeks after facial nerve surgery (Fig. 5) (Table 2).

Discussion

Our animal study directly compared the facial nerve functional outcome in a group of rats receiving brief electrical stimulation following nerve transection and repair compared to those not receiving stimulation. Our results indicate a significant improvement in whisking amplitude in those animals receiving BES over those that did not in the early weeks following nerve surgery; however, by week 6 post-operatively, the difference between the two groups no longer bore statistical significance. Similarly, Nix et al. detected earlier and larger electromyographic signals in reinnervated rabbit soleus muscles with electrical stimulation after crush injury [12]. Our findings support conclusions made by these earlier rabbit studies, that electrical stimulation can accelerate early axonal regeneration and the rate of recovery of peripheral nerves.

Results of our study are consistent with other reports investigating the effects of electrical stimulation on peripheral nerve regeneration. Gordon et al. were able to demonstrate that electrical stimulation of the sciatic nerve in a rat model accelerated both axonal regeneration and the development of preferential motor reinnervation [6]. The authors also found that electrical stimulation of the sciatic nerve for 1 h was as effective in motor axonal regeneration as electrical stimulation for up to 2 weeks. The stimulation model we employed was based on the methodology described by Gordon et al. [6] Our results showed an initial acceleration in whisking amplitude in the stimulation group over the control group. However, by week 6 this difference had dissipated and both groups were found to have similar whisking measurements. Interestingly, Gordon et al. also found an initial acceleration in the number of motor neurons that regenerated into appropriate muscle in the animals that received electrical stimulation. However, by week 8 both groups showed similar motor neuron numbers [6]. Hadlock et al. also showed similar results in their 2010 rat facial nerve transection study. By week 11, the initial acceleration of whisking amplitude of the electrical stimulation rat group had equalized with the control group [2].

Gordon et al. have hypothesized that preferential motor reinnervation in a nerve injury model begins occurring at

Table 2 Statistics for experimental groups at week 2, 4, and 6

	Week 2 amplitude (degrees)	Week 4 amplitude (degrees)	Week 6 amplitude (degrees)
Nerve repair (group 1) Right side (operated)	4.4 +/− 1.0	9.7 +/− 5.0	13.6 +/− 8.1
BES (group 2) Right side (operated)	14.0 +/− 6.6	12.8 +/− 8.3	15.8 +/− 10.9
P-value	0.039	0.515	0.779

approximately 2 to 3 weeks following injury [6]. Prior to that moment, inappropriate sensory pathways are being created at the same rate as appropriate motor pathways. It appears that electrical stimulation is capable of starting preferential motor reinnervation at an earlier time point compared to non-stimulated nerves. Acceleration of preferential motor regeneration could contribute to counteracting the delay of nerve reinnervation pathways that are known to compromise functional outcome.

Although our study was not designed to detect synkinesis, the results of our study taken together with the findings of other researchers indicate the potential for acceleration of facial nerve function with electrical stimulation in animals. Although there are currently no human trials using BES following facial nerve injury, its application in the human clinical setting appears optimistic. Gordon et al. were able to demonstrate that patients receiving BES following carpal tunnel release surgery increased muscle reinnervation as early as 3 months following surgery [13]. Wong et al. demonstrated slight improvement in functional outcomes in humans receiving BES following digital nerve injury compared to a control group [14]. Rodents are also known to possess a greater ability to regenerate peripheral nerves and therefore modest animal findings may in fact indicate more significant potential results in humans. Future work will include corroborating our whisking findings facial muscle fiber count as well as facial motor neuron studies.

Conclusion

In our study, we have shown that brief electrical stimulation of a rat facial nerve transection model accelerates whisker movement and therefore potentially facial nerve function. If facial nerve function is accelerated, brief electrical stimulation has the potential ability to counteract nerve reinnervation delays that are known to affect overall outcome. This has interesting clinical benefits and potential applications in human facial nerve injuries.

Ethics approval

Prior to commencement of this study ethics approval was obtained from the University of Alberta Health Research Ethics Board.

Abbreviations

ACUC: Animal Care and Use Committee; BES: brief electrical stimulation; HSLAS: Health Sciences Laboratory Animal Services; SMRI: Surgical Medical Research Institute; UAPWC: University Animal Policy and Welfare Committee.

Competing interests

The authors declare that they have no competing interests.

Authors' contributions

AM carried out the rat surgery, whisking testing, study design, data analysis, and drafted the manuscript. HS participated in the study design and helped revise the manuscript. VB participated in the rat surgery and statistical analysis. LZ participated in rat surgery, animal care, and whisking testing. DC participated in study design, data analysis, and manuscript revision. All authors read and approved the final manuscript.

Acknowledgement

We would like to acknowledge Dirk Everaert for his help with this manuscript.

Financial support/Disclosure

Division of Otolaryngology-Head and Neck Surgery, University of Alberta.

Author details

[1]Department of Surgery, Division of Otolaryngology-Head and Neck Surgery, University of Alberta, Edmonton, AB, Canada. [2]Faculty of Medicine and Dentistry, University of Alberta, Edmonton, AB, Canada. [3]1E4 Walter C Mackenzie Centre, 8440-112 Street NW, Edmonton, AB T6G 2B7, Canada.

References

1. Lad D, Sharma N, Wurster RD, Marzo SJ, Jones KJ, Foecking EM. Electrical stimulation facilitates rat facial nerve recovery from a crush injury. Otolaryngol Head Neck Surg. 2008;139(1):68–73. doi:10.1016/j.otohns.2008.04.030.
2. Hadlock T, Lindsay R, Edwards C, Cmitson C, Weingberg J, Knox C, et al. The effect of electrical and mechanical stimulation on the regenerating rodent facial nerve. Laryngoscope. 2010;120(6):1094–102. doi:10.1002/lary.20903.
3. Post R, de Boer KS, Malessy MJ. Outcome following nerve repair of high isolated clean sharp injuries of the ulnar nerve. PLoS One. 2012;7(10), e47928. doi:10.1371/journal.pone.0047928.
4. Fawcett JW, Keynes RJ. Peripheral nerve regenration. Annu Rev Neurosci. 1990;13:43.
5. Griffin JW, Hogan MV, Chhabra AB, Deal DN. Peripheral nerve repair and reconstruction. J Bone Joint Surg Am. 2013;95(23):2144–51. doi:10.2106/JBJS.L.00704.
6. Al-Majed AA, Neumann CM, Brushart TM, Gordon T. Brief electrical stimulation promotes the speed and accuracy of motor axonal regeneration. J Neurosci. 2000;20(7):2602–8.
7. Sunderland S. Nerve and nerce injuries. London: Churchill Livingstone; 1978.
8. Borgens RB, Roederer E, Cohen MJ. Enhanced spinal cord regeneration in lamprey by applied electric fields. Science. 1981;213(4508):611–7.
9. Borgens RB. Electrically mediated regeneration and guidance of adult mammalian spinal axons into polymeric channels. Neuroscience. 1999;91(1):251–64.
10. Foecking EM, Fargo KN, Coughlin LM, Kim JT, Marzo SJ, Jones KJ. Single session of brief electrical stimulation immediately following crush injury enhances functional recovery of rat facial nerve. J Rehabil Res Dev. 2012;49(3):451–8.
11. Heaton JT, Kowaleski JM, Bermejo R, Zeigler HP, Ahlgren DJ, Hadlock TA. A system for studying facial nerve function in rats through simultaneous bilateral monitoring of eyelid and whisker movements. J Neurosci Methods. 2008;171(2):197–206. doi:10.1016/j.jneumeth.2008.02.023.
12. Nix WA, Hopf HC. Electrical stimulation of regenerating nerve and its effect on motor recovery. Brain Res. 1983;272(1):21–5.
13. Gordon T, Brushart TM, Chan KM. Augmenting nerve regeneration with electrical stimulation. Neurol Res. 2008;30(10):1012–22. doi:10.1179/174313208X362488.
14. Wong JN, Olson JL, Morhart MJ, Chan KM. Electrical stimulation enhances sensory recovery: a randomized control trial. Ann Neurol. 2015. doi:10.1002/ana.24397.

20

Upper airway obstruction due to a change in altitude: first report in fifty years

Oleksandr Butskiy[1*] and Donald W. Anderson[1,2]

Abstract

Background: Air travel mostly causes minor ear, nose and throat complaints. We describe a second report in literature of airway obstruction caused by a drop in atmospheric pressure during a routine commercial flight.

Case presentation: A 54-year-old male was referred to a head and neck surgeon with a 2 cm left submandibular mass that would enlarge during commercial flights. As the plane gained elevation, the mass would grow and cause him to become stridorous and short of breath. The shortness of breath and stridor would only resolve upon landing of the plane. A CT scan showed a large air sac extending from the larynx at the level of the true vocal cords up to the angle of the mandible. Based on the history and the CT findings a diagnosis of a laryngocele was made. The laryngocele was excised using an external approach, resolving the patient's difficulty with flying.

Conclusion: This article reports a rare case of upper airway obstruction caused by atmospheric pressure changes during air travel. The reported case is of significance as only a few uncomplicated laryngoceles have been reported to cause airway distress in the literature. This report highlights the epidemiology, presentation, complication and management of laryngoceles.

Keywords: Airway obstruction, Air travel, Neck mass, Laryngocele

Background

With the exception of otic barotrauma, air travel has only been reported to cause minor complaints in the ear, nose and throat [1]. We describe a case of upper airway obstruction during a routine commercial flight. Based on our search of Embase®, Pubmed, Google Scholar, and Web of Science™ databases (last search June 2015), we believe this is to be the second case report of airway obstruction caused by airplane's change in altitude [2].

Case presentation

A 54-year-old male smoker was referred to a head and neck surgeon with a 2 cm left submandibular mass. On history, the patient described a chronic non-painful left neck mass that fluctuated in size over the years. The patient's chief complaint, however, was the problem he experienced during commercial flights. During the plane's ascent, the left neck mass would enlarge, and he would become short of breath and stridorous. These symptoms would only resolve upon the plane's descent. During these episodes he never sought medical attention. However, these episodes were severe enough that he has been avoiding all air travel, and he only pursued surgical consultation to attend his daughter's wedding abroad. On palpation of the neck, no neck mass, swelling, nor lymphadenopathy were appreciated. Flexible laryngoscopy showed an infantile type epiglottis. A CT scan of the neck was ordered and showed a large air-containing sac in the left neck, extending from the level of the vocal cords to the level of the angle of the mandible. The air sac, insinuated between the left strap muscles and left sternocleidomastoid, was causing mass effect on the left submandibular gland and the laryngeal structures (Fig. 1). Based on the history and CT findings, a diagnosis of a laryngocele with internal and external components was made and the patient was counseled regarding its surgical excision.

Discussion and surgical management

A laryngocele is an air filled abnormal dilation of the laryngeal saccule communicating with the laryngeal lumen.

* Correspondence: butskiy.alex@gmail.com
[1]Division of Otolaryngology Head and Neck Surgery, Department of Surgery, Vancouver General Hospital & University of British Columbia, Vancouver, BC, Canada
Full list of author information is available at the end of the article

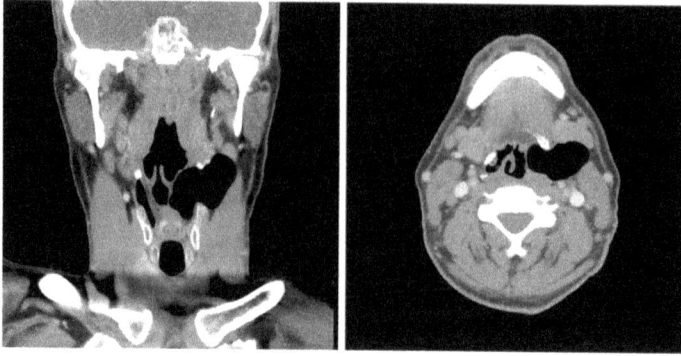

Fig. 1 CT of the neck with contrast demonstrating a laryngocele

The exact etiology of laryngoceles is unknown. Some authors attribute laryngoceles to congenitally present dilation of the saccule exacerbated by factors that increase intra-glottic pressure such as professional trumpet playing [3]. It is important to remember that laryngoceles are know to present in the setting of laryngeal malignancy, secondary to partial of complete obstruction of the saccular orifice [4]. Laryngoceles are rare. Traditionally, the incidence of laryngocele was reported to be approximately 1 in 2.5 million people [5]. The true incidence of laryngoceles is controversial, as more recent report suggest that laryngoceles might be more common than originally thought [6]. Two anatomical variations of laryngoceles have been reported: internal to the thyroid cartilage and a combined type, consisting of external and internal components. The authors of a recent review reported that the treatment of laryngoceles depends on the anatomical variation: internal laryngoceles tend to be treated with microlaryngoscopy with CO_2 laser, while the combined laryngoceles tend to be excised through an external incision [7].

Given the size of the external component of the laryngocele presented in this report, an external approach, to the laryngocele excision was taken. A detailed description of the external surgical approach is available elsewhere [8]. In brief, a lateral thyrotomy without tracheostomy was chosen to resect the laryngocele. Strap muscles were reflected down together with the raised left thyroid ala perichondrium (Fig. 2a). An inverted triangular section of the left thyroid lamina was resected, taking care to stay anterior and parallel to the left oblique line (Fig. 2b). The laryngocele was dissected away from the surrounding paraglottic space down to the laryngeal ventricle (Fig. 2c). The communication between the laryngocele and the laryngeal ventricle was then clamped, tied and cut, delivering the laryngocele out of the neck (Fig. 2d). Following wound closure, the patient was successfully extubated in the operating room. He spent the night in the hospital for

observation, and was discharged home with no changes in his voice, swallowing or breathing.

The patient's follow up consisted of one office visit, 2 weeks after the operation, and one and a half year phone follow up. He was able to return to work 9 days after the operation and had no complaints at any time. He resumed air travel 3 months following his surgery, and he has not experienced airway obstruction or neck swelling during flights again.

The presented case highlights a typical patient who might present with a laryngocele: a male in his fifth or sixth decade referred with a non-tender neck mass that fluctuates in size [7]. The unusual part of the presented case is the airway obstruction caused by the laryngocele during air travel. Uncomplicated laryngoceles rarely cause airway obstruction [3]. Infected laryngoceles, or laryngopyoceles, can on occasion lead to airway distress [7] and can potentially be lethal [9]. The airway obstruction experienced by the patient presented in this case was likely due to the drop in the atmospheric pressure in the cabin of an airplane. If the junction of the laryngocele with the laryngeal saccule was intermittently obstructed, the drop in air pressure during the plane's ascent would have led to laryngocele expansion, explaining the patient's symptoms.

We searched Embase®, Pubmed, Google Scholar, and Web of Science™ databases (last search June 2015) and found one case reports from 50 years ago of airway obstruction during air travel caused by a laryngocele [2]. In addition, we also found a more recent brief communication by an ophthalmologist recounting her experiences from a commercial flight. Twenty minutes into a flight, she was asked to assist a passenger experiencing bulging on the side of the neck. It is unclear if the passenger had symptoms of airway obstruction. This bulge resolved as the plane made an emergency landing. The author of this brief communication did not follow the patient into the hospital, and was writing to request an opinion with

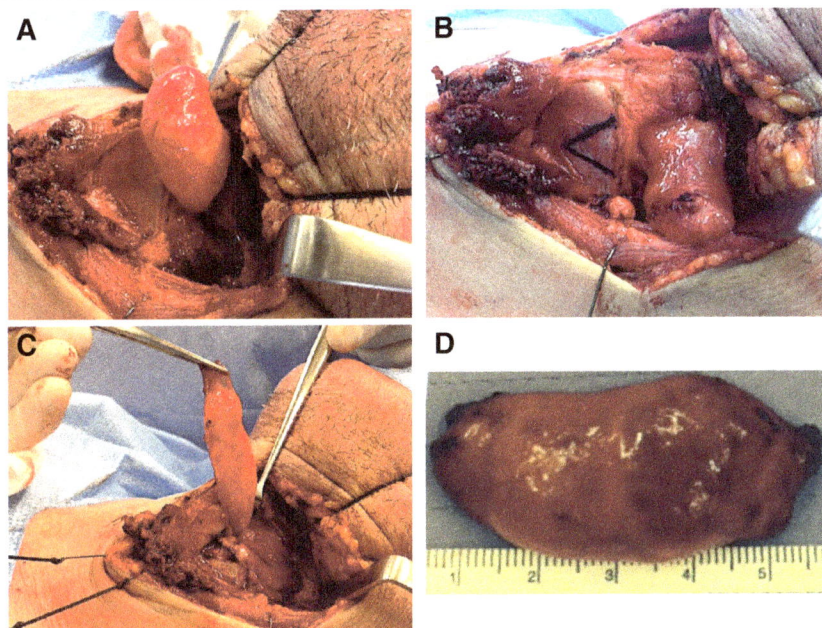

Fig. 2 Resection of the laryngocele. (**a**) Strap muscles reflected inferiorly, bringing the laryngocele into view; (**b**) Planning to resect a portion of left thyroid lamina to gain further exposure; (**c**) Laryngocele dissected away from the paraglottic space down to the laryngeal ventricle; (**d**) Laryngocele delivered out of the neck

regard to what might have caused this unusual presentation [10]. Given the similarities to the presented case, it is likely that the passenger might have had reversible airway obstruction due to a laryngocele.

Conclusions

The presented case is the second case report of upper airway obstruction during air travel. Given the ubiquity of air travel, it is likely that other patients with laryngoceles have experienced at least some worsening of their symptoms during airplane's ascent. We encourage practitioners to question the rare patient that presents with a suspicion of a laryngocele about symptom changes with air travel. As illustrated in this case, a change in symptoms during the ascent and descent of air travel can potentially support the physician's diagnostic suspicion of a laryngocele.

Consent to publish

Patient provided written informed consent for publication of the case report. Editor-in-chief was provided with a copy of the written consent.

Competing interests
The authors declare that they have no competing interests.

Authors' contributions
AD conceived this report and reviewed the manuscript. OB prepared the manuscript. Both authors read and approved the final manuscript.

Acknowledgements
None.

Author details
[1]Division of Otolaryngology Head and Neck Surgery, Department of Surgery, Vancouver General Hospital & University of British Columbia, Vancouver, BC, Canada. [2]Gordon & Leslie Diamond Health Care Centre, 4th. Fl. 4299B-2775 Laurel Street, Vancouver, BC V5Z 1 M9, Canada.

References
1. Morse RP. The effect of flying and Low humidity on the admittance of the tympanic membrane and middle Ear system. JARO J Assoc Res Otolaryngol. 2013;14:623–33.
2. Krekorian EA. Laryngocele in a jet flyer. Laryngoscope. 1966;76:563–71.
3. Vasileiadis I, Kapetanakis S, Petousis A, Stavrianaki A, Fiska A, Karakostas E. Internal laryngopyocele as a cause of acute airway obstruction: an extremely rare case and review of the literature. [Review]. Acta Otorhinolaryngol Ital. 2012;32:58–62.
4. Celin SE, Johnson J, Curtin H, Barnes L. The association of laryngoceles with squamous cell carcinoma of the larynx. Laryngoscope. 1991;101:529–36.
5. Stell PM, Maran AG. Laryngocoele. J Laryngol Otol. 1975;89:915–24.
6. Shandilya M, Colreavy MP, Hughes J, Curran AJ, McShane DP, O'Dwyer T, et al. Endolaryngeal cysts presenting with acute respiratory distress. Clin Otolaryngol Allied Sci. 2004;29:492–6.
7. Zelenik K, Stanikova L, Smatanova K, Cerny M, Kominek P. Treatment of laryngoceles: what is the progress over the last Two decades? BioMed Res Int. 2014;2014:e819453.
8. Rosen CA, Simpson B, Leden H, Ossoff RH. Operative techniques in laryngology. 2008th ed. Berlin: Springer; 2008.
9. Byard RW, Gilbert JD. Lethal laryngopyocele. J Forensic Sci. 2015;60:518–20.
10. Bergkvist MH. Lateral neck cyst as a cause of partial upper airway obstruction? Ugeskr Laeger. 2012;174:2811.

21

Evaluation of the utricular and saccular function using oVEMPs and cVEMPs in BPPV patients

Hui Xu[1†], Fa-ya Liang[2†], Liang Chen[3,6*†] , Xi-cheng Song[3], Michael Chi Fai Tong[4], Jiun Fong Thong[5], Qing-quan Zhang[3] and Yan Sun[3]

Abstract

Background: It is well-known that ocular vestibular evoked myogenic potentials (oVEMPs) predominantly reflect utricular function whilst cervical vestibular evoked myogenic potentials (cVEMPs) reflect saccular function. To date, there are no published reports on the systemic evaluation of utricular and saccular function in benign paroxysmal positional vertigo (BPPV), nor are there any reports on the differences in VEMPs between patients with recurrent and non-recurrent BPPV. The aim of this study was to evaluate the difference in cervical and ocular (c/o)VEMPs between patients with BPPV and normal controls, as well as between patients with recurrent and non-recurrent BPPV.

Methods: Thirty patients with posterior canal BPPV and 30 healthy subjects (as normal controls) were prospectively enrolled. cVEMP and oVEMP testing using 500 Hz tone-burst stimuli were performed on all. VEMP tests were repeated 3 times on each subject to ensure reliability and reproducibility of responses. VEMPs were defined as present or absent. Abnormal VEMP was defined by lack of VEMP response.

Results: In the control group, abnormal cVEMPs responses were detected in 6.67 % and abnormal oVEMPs responses were detected in 3.34 %. In BPPV patients (10 with recurrent BPPV, 20 with non-recurrent BPPV), abnormal cVEMPs responses were detected in 30 % and abnormal oVEMPs responses were detected in 56.7 %. More patients with BPPV showed abnormal responses in c/oVEMPs as compared to the control group ($p < 0.05$). oVEMPs was more often abnormal as compared to cVEMPs in BPPV patients ($p < 0.05$). There was no statistical difference between abnormal cVEMP responses in non-recurrent BPPV patients (25 %) and recurrent BPPV patients (40 %) ($p > 0.05$). Differences in abnormal oVEMP responses (non-recurrent BPPV, 40 %; recurrent BPPV, 90 %) were significant ($p < 0.05$).

Conclusion: An increased occurrence of abnormal c/oVEMP recordings appeared in BPPV patients, possibly as a result of degeneration of the otolith macula. oVEMPs were more often abnormal in BPPV patients as compared to cVEMPs, suggesting that utricular dysfunction may be more common than saccular dysfunction. Furthermore, oVEMP abnormalities in the recurrent BPPV group were significantly higher than those in the non-recurrent BPPV group. Assessment of c/oVEMPs in BPPV patients may therefore be of prognostic value in predicting likelihood of BPPV recurrence.

Keywords: Cervical/ocular vestibular evoked myogenic potentials (c/oVEMPs), Benign paroxysmal positional vertigo (BPPV), Utricular, Saccular

* Correspondence: entchenliang@hotmail.com
†Equal contributors
[3]Otorhinolaryngology Head and Neck Surgery Department, Affiliated Yantai Yuhuangding Hospital of Qingdao University Medical College, Yantai City, Shandong Province, China
[6]Otology Department, Affiliated Yantai Yuhuangding Hospital of Qingdao University Medical College, Yantai City, Shandong Province, China
Full list of author information is available at the end of the article

Background

Vestibular evoked myogenic potential (VEMP) is a short-latency myogenic response which is evoked by brief pulses of air-conducted (AC) sound, bone-conducted (BC) vibration or electrical stimulation and recorded using surface electrodes placed over muscles. Cervical vestibular evoked myogenic potentials (cVEMPs), which are a manifestation of the vestibulo-colic reflex, predominantly the sacculo-collic reflex, are assessed by measuring electromyographic (EMG) activity from surface electrodes placed over the tonically activated sternocleidomastoid (SCM) muscles. In 1992 and 1994, cVEMPs was first described by Colebatch and Halmagyi [1, 2], who measured electromyographic (EMG) activity from the sternocleidomastoid (SCM) muscles following vestibular stimulation with brief pulses of sound (clicks). In 1995, Halmagyi et al. [3]. elicited cVEMPs by tapping the forehead with a clinical reflex hammer. The responses had the same biphasic waveform as the AC cVEMPs and were vestibular-dependent, but were also present in patients with conductive hearing loss as the stimulus bypasses the middle ear conductive mechanism. In 2000, Sheykholeslami et al. [4]. recorded cVEMPs using BC sound delivered to the mastoid bone with a clinical bone conductor.

In 2005 and 2007, Rosengren [5] and Todd [6] recorded the short latency potentials from around the eyes by bone-conducted sound (BCS) and demonstrated that it can also be recorded from the extraocular muscles as part of the vestibulo-ocular reflex (VOR). It was recently reported that ocular VEMPs (oVEMPs) are produced by synchronous activity in the extraocular muscles in response to stimulation, including sound [7]. Assessment of oVEMPs is used as a clinical test for the vestibular system because it provides information on otolith function. A more recent study reported that oVEMPs in response to air-conducted sound (ACS) reflect functions of different parts of the vestibular labyrinth from cVEMPs in response to ACS; that is, oVEMPs predominantly reflect utricular functions while cVEMPs reflect saccular functions [8].

Canalolithiasis and cupulolithiasis have been considered as possible mechanisms in the etiology of benign paroxysmal positional vertigo (BPPV) [9, 10]. In addition to these mechanisms, otolith dysfunction has also been suggested as a possible mechanism of BPPV [11–13]. The detachment of the otoconia from the otolith macula is post-viral or post-traumatic in some cases; however, in many instances it seems to occur without an identifiable cause [14]. The finding that BPPV patients had significantly higher incidence of abnormal amplitudes in cVEMPs compared with controls has been reported [15, 16], suggesting that BPPV patients have more saccular damage than controls. However, the systemic evaluation of utricular and saccular damage in BPPV patients has never been reported. There is a significant rate of BPPV recurrence after initial resolution. The reported recurrence rate during a 1-year follow-up period ranged from 10 % to 18 % [17, 18]. To date, there are no reports on the differences in VEMPs between patients with recurrent and non-recurrent BPPV. The aim of this study is to evaluate the difference in c/oVEMPs between patients with BPPV and controls, as well as between patients with recurrent and non-recurrent BPPV. The other objective of this study is to compare oVEMP and cVEMP results in patients with BPPV.

Methods

Subjects

Ethical approval was received from the Ethics Committee of Affiliated Yantai Yuhuangding Hospital of Qingdao University Medical College. We prospectively enrolled 30 consecutive patients from the Dizziness Clinic, affiliated Yantai Yuhuangding Hospital of Qingdao University Medical College, who were diagnosed with posterior canal BPPV (canalolithiasis, nystagmus duration < 60 s) between January 2013 and June 2014. Follow-up was for 1 year. Patients were divided into two groups according to recurrence - 20 non-recurrent BPPV patients and 10 recurrent BPPV patients. Recurrence was defined as BPPV that occurred more than 1 month after a successful repositioning manoeuvre during the 1 year follow-up period. The diagnosis of BPPV and the affected side was based on the typical nystagmus seen during the Dix-Hallpike maneuver. The control subjects were all volunteers from our normal outpatient clinic who had no otological disease. Patients with a history of hearing loss, other vestibular disorders and >60 years old were excluded. Informed consent was obtained from each subject according to the Declaration of Helsinki.

cVEMPs

Cervical vestibular evoked myogenic potentials (cVEMPs) testing was performed on both sides for all patients and controls. In the cVEMPs test, all subjects were placed in a sitting position and asked to rotate their head away from the stimulated side so as to record electromyographic activity over tonically activated sternocleidomastoid (SCM) muscles. Surface EMG activity was recorded with superficial electrodes placed on the middle third of the SCM, with the reference electrode placed on the upper third of the sternum and the ground electrode on the middle of the forehead. Using a Bio-Logic Navigator Pro, 90 dB nHL 500 Hz tone bursts were presented through headphones, and the EMG signal was amplified and bandpass filtered (30–1500 Hz). The analysis window was 100 ms wide and responses to 120 stimuli were averaged. cVEMP tests were repeated 3 times on each subject to ensure reliability and reproducibility of responses. The amplitude of the first positive–negative peak (P13–N23) was recorded. Absence of a meaningful wave form with p13 and n23 was defined as 'no response'. Abnormality was strictly defined as a cVEMP pattern of 'no response', which meant the absence of a meaningful waveform with P13 and N23.

oVEMPs

Ocular vestibular evoked myogenic potentials (oVEMPs) testing was performed on both sides for all patients and controls. In the oVEMPs test, all subjects assumed a sitting position and the subject was instructed to look superomedially at a small fixed target 1 m from the eyes. The visual angle was approximately 30°, which has been found to elicit the largest responses compared with other eye positions [19]. The active electrodes were placed on the face, oriented vertically and approximately 1 cm below the center of the lower eyelid just inferior to the contralateral eye for sound stimulation. The reference electrode was placed about 1 cm below the active electrode on the cheek, and the ground electrode was placed on the forehead. Each subject's eyes remained fixed on the target throughout the test. Using a Bio-Logic Navigator Pro, 95 dB nHL 500 Hz tone bursts were presented through headphones, and the EMG signal was amplified and bandpass filtered (10–300 Hz). The analysis window was 100 ms wide and responses to 120 stimuli were averaged. oVEMP tests were repeated 3 times on each subject to ensure reliability and reproducibility of responses. The initial negative–positive biphasic waveform comprised peaks N1 and P1. We analyzed the waveforms of N1 and P1 at the maximal intensity of stimulation. Abnormality was strictly defined as an oVEMP pattern of 'no response', which meant an absence of a meaningful waveform with N1 and P1.

Statistical analysis

A Fishers exact or Chi-squared test was used to analyze the statistical significance of the inter-group difference in the number of non- cVEMPs and oVEMPs responders in the BPPV and controls groups. A p value of < 0.05 indicated statistical significance.

Results

The ages ranged from 34 to 55 years (mean 45.5, 12 men and 18 women) in patients with BPPV. The control group consisted of 30 normal subjects (10 men and 20 women; mean age 42.2 years; age range 30–60 years). Demographic data for BPPV and control groups are summarized in Table 1. There were no significant differences in age and sex ratio between the two groups ($p > 0.05$). Testing of VEMPs was performed on both sides in all BPPV patients and controls. Only one patient with BPPV showed bilateral abnormalities, so only ipsilesional data are presented In the control group, abnormal

Table 1 Demographic features of subjects in BPPV and control groups

Group feature	Control	BPPV
Number	30	30
Age*	42.2 ± 8.7	45.5 ± 9.2
Sex (M:F)*	10:20	12:18

BPPV Benign paroxysmal positional vertigo. *$p > 0.05$

cVEMP responses were detected in 2 of 30 (6.67 %) subjects and abnormal oVEMP responses were detected in 1 of 30 (3.34 %) subjects (Table 2).

cVEMP abnormalities in BPPV patients

Abnormal cVEMP responses were detected in 9 of 30 (30 %) BPPV subjects (Table 3). More patients with BPPV showed abnormal responses in cVEMPs as compared to the controls ($p < 0.05$) (Fig. 1). In cVEMPs testing, abnormalities were detected in 5 of 20 (25 %) in the non-recurrent BPPV group and in 4 of 10 (40 %) subjects in the recurrent BPPV group; the difference between the two groups was not significant ($p > 0.05$) (Fig. 2).

oVEMP abnormalities in BPPV patients

Abnormal oVEMP responses were detected in 17 of 30 (56.7 %) subjects in BPPV group (Table 4). More patients with BPPV showed abnormal responses in oVEMPs as compared to the controls ($p < 0.05$) (Fig. 3). In oVEMPs testing, abnormalities were detected in 8 of 20 (40 %) in the non-recurrent BPPV group and in 9 of 10 (90 %) subjects in the recurrent BPPV group; the difference between the two groups was significant ($p < 0.05$) (Fig. 4).

Comparison of oVEMPs with cVEMPs within BPPV patients

Abnormal oVMEPs responses were detected in 17 of 30 (56.7 %) subjects in BPPV group while abnormal cVMEPs responses were detected in 9 of 30 (30 %). The abnormal results for oVEMPs showed a higher percentage than those for cVEMPs in BPPV patients ($p < 0.05$) (Fig. 5).

Discussion

The exact pathophysiology of BPPV remains unclear. Several studies have previously suggested the cause being dislodgement of otoconia from the gelatinous layer of the otolithic membrane [20], which may be associated with osteopenia and osteoporosis [21]. At present,

Table 2 The abnormal c/oVEMP responses details in control group

VEMP test	Abnormal	Normal	Total	Percent
cVEMP	2	28	30	6.67 %
oVEMP	1	29	30	3.34 %

Table 3 cVEMPs abnormalities in BPPV groups

BPPV group	Abnormal	Normal	Total
NG	5 (25 %)	15 (75 %)	20
RG	4 (40 %)	6 (60 %)	10
Total	9 (30 %)	21 (70 %)	30

NG Nonrecurrent group, *RG* Recurrent group, NG VS RG: ($p > 0.05$)

cVEMPs which are evoked by air-conducted sound (ACS), are widely used to evaluate the function of saccule and inferior vestibular nerve by recording the inhibitory potential from the SCM. oVEMPs are also evoked by ACS. Although its origin is controversial, it was recently reported to be involved in the stimulation of the utricular macula. Curthoys et al. [7]. and Shin et al. [22]. reported that the oVEMP evoked by ACS may be predominantly mediated by the superior vestibular nerve due to the activation of the utricular receptors. In BPPV, the degenerative process of otolith not only affects the macula of the utricle and causes detachment of the otoliths, but might also affect the macula of the saccule. Von Brevern et al. [23]. reported that utricular dysfunction, which is associated with idiopathic BPPV, possibly results from degeneration of the utricular macula. Our study results supports this hypothesis with regards to utricular dysfunction in BPPV patients. However, they failed to demonstrate any significant change in saccular function. Our study is in concordance with several other studies that reported on cVEMPs in patients diagnosed with BPPV [15, 24]. Korres S et al. [24]. found an increased occurrence of abnormal cVEMP recordings in BPPV patients and attributed this to possible degeneration of the saccular macula, which is part of the neural VEMP pathway. With regards to the amplitude and latency values of VEMPs, there are many factors that can affect these values such as basic muscle activity, patient's position, and general

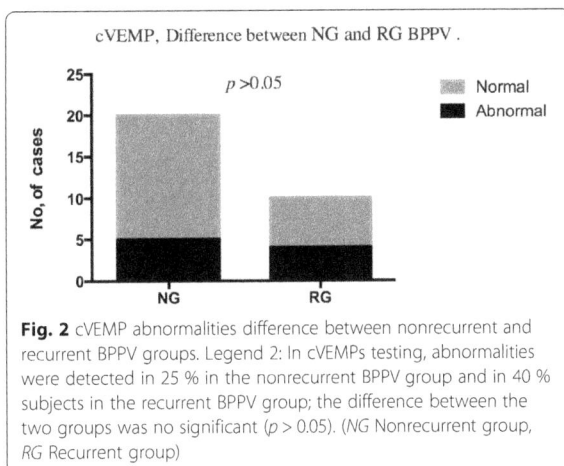

Fig. 2 cVEMP abnormalities difference between nonrecurrent and recurrent BPPV groups. Legend 2: In cVEMPs testing, abnormalities were detected in 25 % in the nonrecurrent BPPV group and in 40 % subjects in the recurrent BPPV group; the difference between the two groups was no significant ($p > 0.05$). (*NG* Nonrecurrent group, *RG* Recurrent group)

conditions [25, 26]. Because of their non-specific value in VEMPs testing, we used a qualitative approach to VEMPs results. Our definition for abnormal VEMP is an absence of VEMP response. The main objective in this study was to report c/o VEMPs findings in BPPV patients and to verify some clinical characteristics of BPPV in VEMPs. We evaluated both the function of utricle and saccule by measuring c/oVEMPs.

In our study, we found that patients with BPPV showed higher rate of abnormal responses in c/oVEMPs by stimulation on their affected side than the controls. Hong et al. 16 reported that 24.5 % of patients with BPPV showed abnormal cVEMP responses, such as P13 latency prolongation and VEMP amplitude asymmetry on the affected side. The incidence of abnormal response of cVEMP in our study was 30 %, which is similar with that reported. Brandt et al. [27]. reported that most recurrences were diagnosed within the first year after treatment. Hence, 1 year was chosen as the follow up period in our study. In cVEMPs testing, abnormalities were detected in 25 % of subjects in the non-recurrent BPPV group and in 40 % of subjects in the recurrent BPPV group. Although there was a higher rate of abnormality in the recurrent BPPV group, the difference between the two groups was not significant ($p > 0.05$). This suggests that BPPV recurrence may not be related to saccular damage, although another possibility may be that larger numbers of patients are needed in the study

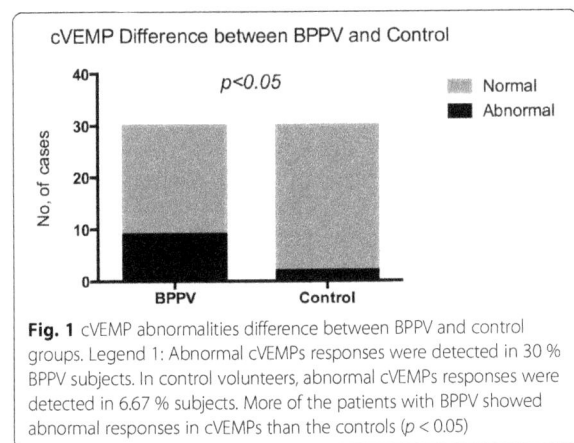

Fig. 1 cVEMP abnormalities difference between BPPV and control groups. Legend 1: Abnormal cVEMPs responses were detected in 30 % BPPV subjects. In control volunteers, abnormal cVEMPs responses were detected in 6.67 % subjects. More of the patients with BPPV showed abnormal responses in cVEMPs than the controls ($p < 0.05$)

Table 4 oVEMP abnormalities in BPPV groups

BPPV group	Abnormal	Normal	Total
NG	8 (40 %)	12 (60 %)	20
RG	9 (90 %)	1 (10 %)	10
Total	17 (56.7 %)	13 (43.3 %)	30

NG Nonrecurrent group, *RG* Recurrent group; NG VS RG: ($p < 0.05$)

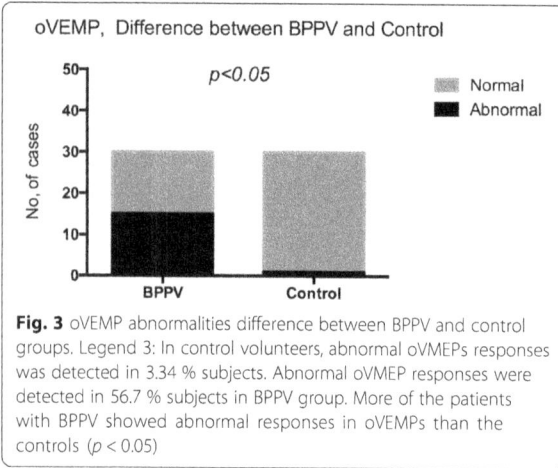

Fig. 3 oVEMP abnormalities difference between BPPV and control groups. Legend 3: In control volunteers, abnormal oVMEPs responses was detected in 3.34 % subjects. Abnormal oVMEP responses were detected in 56.7 % subjects in BPPV group. More of the patients with BPPV showed abnormal responses in oVEMPs than the controls ($p < 0.05$)

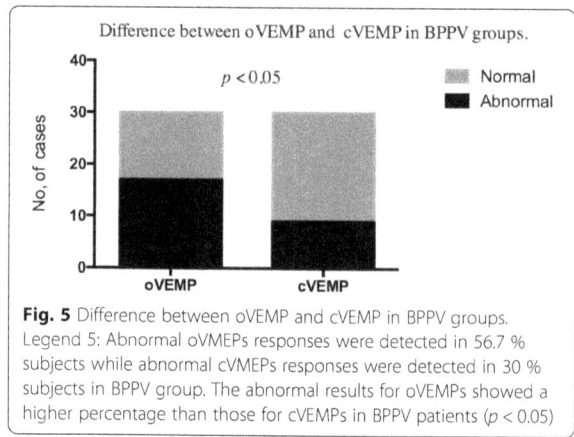

Fig. 5 Difference between oVEMP and cVEMP in BPPV groups. Legend 5: Abnormal oVMEPs responses were detected in 56.7 % subjects while abnormal cVMEPs responses were detected in 30 % subjects in BPPV group. The abnormal results for oVEMPs showed a higher percentage than those for cVEMPs in BPPV patients ($p < 0.05$)

to demonstrate a significant difference. Our findings differ from those of Lee JD et al., who reported a higher incidence (31.25 %) of cVEMP abnormality in recurrent BPPV than non-recurrent BPPV patients [28].

In oVEMPs testing, abnormal response rate was significantly higher in recurrent BPPV patients than non-recurrent BPPV patients, whilst the difference in cVEMPs between the 2 groups was not significant. This suggests that the incidence of utricular dysfunction is higher than saccular dysfunction in recurrent BPPV patients. Clinicians should be aware of the risk of recurrent BPPV in these patients with abnormal oVEMPs and be able to counsel patients appropriately. In our clinical practice, the risk of recurrence is emphasized after the diagnosis of BPPV and strict follow up is recommended for all patients. With our findings, we may now be able to better predict which patients are more likely to have BPPV recurrence.

In our study, there was a higher rate of abnormal oVEMP results than cVEMP results in BPPV patients.

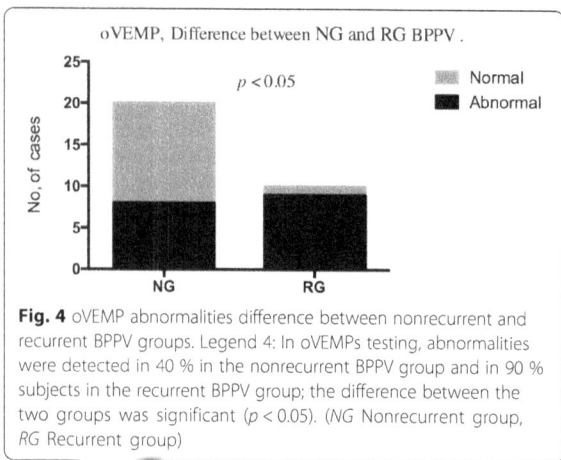

Fig. 4 oVEMP abnormalities difference between nonrecurrent and recurrent BPPV groups. Legend 4: In oVEMPs testing, abnormalities were detected in 40 % in the nonrecurrent BPPV group and in 90 % subjects in the recurrent BPPV group; the difference between the two groups was significant ($p < 0.05$). (*NG* Nonrecurrent group, *RG* Recurrent group)

These findings support the possibility that utricular function in BPPV patients is more heavily damaged than saccular function. Utricular dysfunction seems to play an essential role as an underlying mechanism contributing to BPPV. Bremova T et al. [29]. measured oVEMP amplitudes before and after repositioning manoeuvres in BPPV patients and found significant increase in the amplitudes following the manoeuvres whilst the cVEMPs had no amplitude change.

VEMPs is a good method for evaluation of otolith function; however, this test requires specialized equipment and complicated procedures for separate analyses of utricular and saccular function as the VOR gain reduction is under the influence of both utricular and saccular dysfunction, in addition to semicircular canal-otolith interaction. In the present study, abnormalities in oVEMPs was frequently detected. This finding is consistent with the suggested underlying pathology of BPPV, namely, degeneration of the utricular maculae leading to dislodging of otoconia. Those ears showing abnormal oVEMP as well as cVEMP might have severe changes causing dysfunction of the utricle and the saccule.

Considering the controversy in the stability and repeatability of c/oVEMPs, we defined abnormal c/oVEMPs as absent responses in our study. As a result, we did not analyse the latency and amplitude of the waves in c/oVEMPs. The main limitation of our study is the small number of BPPV patients. As the incidence of BPPV is higher in the elderly and the average age of our study patients was under 60 years, there is a potential bias in the research. In future research, a larger sample size will be obtained such that quantitative analysis of otolith function in BPPV patients can be performed.

Conclusion

An increased occurrence of abnormal c/oVEMP recordings appeared in BPPV patients, possibly as a result of degeneration of the otolith macula. oVEMPs were more often abnormal in BPPV patients as compared to cVEMPs, suggesting that utricular dysfunction may be more common than saccular dysfunction. Furthermore, oVEMP abnormalities in the recurrent BPPV group were significantly higher than those in the non-recurrent BPPV group. Assessment of c/oVEMPs in BPPV patients may therefore be of prognostic value in predicting likelihood of BPPV recurrence in these patients.

Competing interests

The authors declare that they have no competing interests.

Authors' contributions

LC, HX and FYL conceived the study and participated in its design and coordination. They also drafted the manuscript and performed the statistical analysis. XCS, QQZ and YS participated in the study design and collected patient data. MCFT and JFT helped to translated and revised the manuscript. All authors read and approved the final manuscript.

Acknowledgement

Financial disclosure of authors: This work was supported by the Medical and Health Development Plan of Shandong Province, China (No. 2013WS0036) and the Science and Technology Development Project of Yantai City, Shandong Province, China (No. 2013WS202).

Author details

[1]Stomatology Department, Affiliated Yantai Yuhuangding Hospital of Qingdao University Medical College, Yantai City, Shandong Province, China. [2]Otorhinolaryngology Head and Neck Surgery Department, Sun Yat-sen Memorial Hospital of Sun Yat-sen University, Guangzhou, China. [3]Otorhinolaryngology Head and Neck Surgery Department, Affiliated Yantai Yuhuangding Hospital of Qingdao University Medical College, Yantai City, Shandong Province, China. [4]Otorhinolaryngology Head and Neck Surgery Department, The Chinese University of Hong Kong, New Territories, Hong Kong, China. [5]Otorhinolaryngology Head and Neck Surgery Department, Singapore General Hospital, Singapore, Singapore. [6]Otology Department, Affiliated Yantai Yuhuangding Hospital of Qingdao University Medical College, Yantai City, Shandong Province, China.

References

1. Colebatch JG, Halmagyi GM. Vestibular evoked potentials in human neck muscles before and after unilateral vestibular deafferentation. Neurology. 1992;42(8):1635–6.
2. Colebatch JG, Halmagyi GM, Skuse NF. Myogenic potentials generated by a click evoked vestibulocollic reflex. J Neurol Neurosurg Psychiatry. 1994;57(2):190–7.
3. Halmagyi GM, Yavor RA, Colebatch JG. Tapping the head activates the vestibular system: a new use for the clinical reflex hammer. Neurology. 1995;45(10):1927–9.
4. Sheykholeslami K, Murofushi T, Kermany MH, Kaga K. Bone-conducted evoked myogenic potentials from the sternocleidomastoid muscle. Acta Otolaryngol. 2000;120(6):731–4.
5. Rosengren SM, Todd NPM, Colebatch JG. Vestibular-evoked extraocular potentials produced by stimulation with bone-conducted sound. Clin Neurophysiol. 2005;116(8):1938–48.
6. Todd NPM, Rosengren SM, Aw ST, Colebatch JG. Ocular vestibular evoked myogenic potentials (OVEMPs) produced by air- and bone-conducted sound. Clin Neurophysiol. 2007;118(2):381–90.
7. Curthoys IS, Iwasaki S, Chihara Y, Ushio M, McGarvie LA, Burgess AM. The ocular vestibular-evoked myogenic potential to air-conducted sound; probable superior vestibular nerve origin. Clin Neurophysiol. 2011;122(3):611–6.
8. Murofushi T, Nakahara H, Yoshimura E, Tsuda Y. Association of air-conducted sound oVEMP findings with cVEMP and caloric test findings in patients with unilateral peripheral vestibular disorders. Acta Otolaryngol. 2011;131(9):945–50.
9. Hall SF, Ruby RR, McClure JA. The mechanics of benign paroxysmal vertigo. J Otolaryngol. 1979;8(2):151–8.
10. Brandt T, Steddin S. Current view of the mechanism of benign paroxysmal positioning vertigo: cupulolithiasis or canalolithiasis? J Vestib Res. 1993;3(4):373–82.
11. Ushio K, Morizono T, Yagi T. Three-component analysis of benign paroxysmal positional nystagmus. Acta Otolaryngol. 1995;519:107–9.
12. Akkuzu G, Akkuzu B, Ozluoglu LN. Vestibular evoked myogenic potentials in benign paroxysmal positional vertigo and Meniere's disease. Eur Arch Otorhinolaryngol. 2006;263(6):510–7.
13. Sugita-Kitajima A, Azuma M, Hattori K, Koizuka I. Evaluation of the otolith function using sinusoidal off-vertical axis rotation in patients with benign paroxysmal positional vertigo. Neuroscience Lett. 2007;422(1):81–6.
14. Baloh RW, Honrubia V, Jacobson K. Benign positional vertigo: clinical and oculographic features in 240 cases. Neurology. 1987;37(3):371–8.
15. Longo G, Onofri M, Pellicciari T, Quaranta N. Benign paroxysmal positional vertigo: is vestibular evoked myogenic potential testing useful? Acta Otolaryngol. 2012;132(1):39–43.
16. Hong SM, Park DC, Yeo SG, Cha CI. Vestibular evoked myogenic potentials in patients with benign paroxysmal positional vertigo involving each semicircular canal. Am J Otolaryngol. 2008;29(3):184–7.
17. Sakaida M, Takeuchi K, Ishinaga H, Adachi M, Majima Y. Long-term outcome of benign paroxysmal positional vertigo. Neurology. 2003;60(9):1532–4.
18. Prokopakis EP, Chimona T, Tsagournisakis M, Christodoulou P, Hirsch BE, Lachanas VA, et al. Benign paroxysmal positional vertigo: 10-year experience in treating 592 patients with canalith repositioning procedure. Laryngoscope. 2005;115(9):1667–71.
19. Chihara Y, Iwasaki S, Ushio M, Murofushi T. Vestibular-evoked extraocular potentials by air-conducted sound: another clinical test for vestibular function. Clin Neurophysiol. 2007;118(12):2745–51.
20. Welling DB, Parnes LS, O'Brien B, Bakaletz LO, Brackmann DE, Hinojosa R. Particulate matter in the posterior semicircular canal. Laryngoscope. 1997;107(1):90–4.
21. Jeong SH, Choi SH, Kim JY, Koo JW, Kim HJ, Kim JS. Osteopenia and osteoporosis in idiopathic benign positional vertigo. Neurology. 2009;72(12):1069–76.
22. Shin BS, Oh SY, Kim JS, Kim TW, Seo MW, Lee H, et al. Cervical and ocular vestibular-evoked myogenic potentials in acute vestibular neuritis. Clin Neurophysiol. 2012;123(2):369–75.
23. Von Brevern M, Schmidt T, Schönfeld U, Lempert T, Clarke AH. Utricular dysfunction in patients with benign paroxysmal positional vertigo. Otol Neurotol. 2006;27(1):92–6.
24. Korres S, Gkoritsa E, Giannakakou-Razelou D, Yiotakis I, Riga M, Nikolpoulos TP. Vestibular evoked myogenic potentials in patients with BPPV. Med Sci Monit. 2011;17(1):CR42–7.
25. Isaradisaikul S, Navacharoen N, Hanprasertpong C, Kangsanarak J. Cervical Vestibular-Evoked Myogenic Potentials: Norms and Protocols. Int J Otolaryngol. 2012;2012:913515.
26. Felipe L, Kingma H. Ocular Vestibular Evoked Myogenic Potentials. Int Arch Otorhinolaryngol. 2014;18(1):77–9.
27. Brandt T, Huppert D, Hecht J, Karch C, Strupp M. Benign paroxysmal positioning vertigo: a long-term follow-up (6–17 years) of 125 patients. Acta Otolaryngol. 2006;126(2):160–3.
28. Lee JD, Park KM, Lee BD, Lee TK, Sung KB, Park JY. Abnormality of cervical vestibular-evoked myogenic potentials and ocular vestibular-evoked myogenic potentials in patients with recurrent benign paroxysmal postitional vertigo. Acta Otolaryngol. 2013;133(2):150–3.
29. Bremova T, Bayer O, Agrawal Y, Kremmyda O, Brandt T, Teufel J, et al. Ocular VEMPs indicate repositioning of otoconia to the utricle after successful liberatory maneuvers in benign paroxysmal positioning vertigo. Acta Otolaryngol. 2013;133(12):1297–303.

22

Preoperative vocal cord paralysis and its association with malignant thyroid disease and other pathological features

Emily Kay-Rivest[1], Elliot Mitmaker[2], Richard J. Payne[3], Michael P. Hier[3], Alex M. Mlynarek[3], Jonathan Young[3] and Véronique-Isabelle Forest[3*]

Abstract

Background: Vocal cord paralysis (VCP) is found in both benign and malignant thyroid disease. This study was performed to determine if the presence of preoperative VCP predicts malignancy.

Methods: A retrospective analysis was performed on a cohort of 1923 consecutive patients undergoing thyroid surgery. The incidence of preoperative VCP was recorded. Patient and nodule characteristics were correlated with final pathology.

Results: 1.3 % of our cohort was found to have preoperative VCP. Malignant pathology was discovered in 76 % of patients with preoperative VCP. Among these patients, 72 % had a left sided paralysis. 10.5 % of patients with preoperative VCP had perineural invasion (PNI) on final pathology, compared to 1.1 % of patients with normal VC function.

Conclusion: Preoperative VCP appears to be a strong, though not an absolute, indicator of malignancy. Most VCP were on the left side. Assessing for preoperative VCP is crucial in all patients who need thyroid surgery, as even benign nodules can be accompanied by preoperative vocal cord paralysis.

Introduction

In the past, preoperative vocal cord paralysis was thought to be an absolute marker of thyroid malignancy [1]. However, there are several reports in the literature indicating that benign thyroid disease may also lead to vocal cord paralysis [2–5]. The mechanisms that cause vocal cord paralysis are multiple. In malignant disease, recurrent laryngeal nerve (RLN) paralysis can be caused by direct invasion of malignant cells or by nodular compression. In the case of benign thyroid disease, compression, as well as stretching of the nerve, are possible etiologies. Furthermore, idiopathic VCP unrelated to a thyroid process could also be a cause of a preoperative VCP. The importance of preoperative assessment of the vocal cords is being increasingly recognized since the recent publication of the 2013 American Academy of Otolaryngology—Head and Neck surgery guidelines, which highlighted the importance of this evaluation, even for patients without subjective voice complaints. These guidelines note that at the present time, vocal cord assessment is performed in 6.1 to 54 % of patients in the United States prior to surgery. The objective of this study was to evaluate the presence of vocal cord paralysis before thyroid surgery and to better understand its association with malignant thyroid disease.

Methods

The health records of 1923 patients who had preoperative flexible laryngoscopy and underwent thyroid surgery between 2007 and 2014 at the McGill University teaching hospitals were analyzed retrospectively. Every patient undergoing thyroidectomy has undergone pre-operative flexible laryngoscopy in our database, unless they came in with an emergent airway obstruction. We recorded all cases of preoperative vocal cord paralysis and correlated with final pathology. The study recorded the sex, age and side of paralysis among patients with confirmed

* Correspondence: viforest@yahoo.ca
[3]Division of Head and Neck Surgery, Department of Otolaryngology – Head and Neck surgery, Jewish General Hospital, McGill University, Montreal, QC H3T 1E2, Canada
Full list of author information is available at the end of the article

preoperative vocal cord paralysis and final pathology findings; this data was available for all patients. In addition, the size of the largest nodule seen on ultrasound was also recorded, if documented. Furthermore, histopathological subtypes of thyroid cancer, including the presence of extrathyroidal extension (ETE), perineural invasion (PNI), and lymphovascular invasion (LVI) were examined with respect to the presence or absence of preoperative vocal cord paralysis. Data was analyzed using MedCalc 12.0. Chi-square and student's t-test were used to identify differences between groups. A *p-value* of 0.05 or less was considered statistically significant. Ethical review board approval was obtained from our institution (the Jewish General Hospital) for this study. None of the authors have any competing interests in the manuscript.

Results

Preoperative vocal cord paralysis was diagnosed in 25 out of 1923 patients (1.3 %). Within the vocal cord paralysis group, 72 % of patients were women. In the group without VCP, 77 % of patients were women ($p = 0.3644$). The average age of patients with VCP was 59.9 years, compared to 50.7 years in patients without preoperative VCP ($p = 0.0016$). These results are summarized in Table 1.

Upon further analysis of the 25 patients with confirmed preoperative vocal cord paralysis, we found a left cord paralysis in 72 % of cases. Furthermore, 19 patients (76 %) had malignant final pathologies and 6 had benign nodules. Twelve (48 %) out of the 19 patients with cancer were papillary carcinomas, 4 (16 %) were micropapillary carcinomas, one was a medullary carcinoma, one was a poorly differentiated thyroid carcinoma and one was an osteosarcoma. The benign thyroid pathologies

consisted of thyroid follicular adenomas ($n = 2$) and nodular hyperplasia ($n = 4$) (Table 2). In the cohort of patients with normal preoperative vocal cord movement, 1143 (60.2 %) patients had malignant final pathologies ($p = 0.2218$) (Table 3).

When ultrasound results were available, we used the largest-sized nodule on the side of the paralysis for patients with preoperative VCP, and the largest nodule overall in patients without VCP. Patients with malignant final pathology had a mean nodule size of 2.9 cm and those with benign final pathology had an average nodule size of 3.2 cm ($p = 0.0001$). Regardless of pathology results, the mean size of nodule in patients with normal

Table 1 Demographics of all patients who underwent thyroid surgery from 2007 to 2014

| | | Preoperative vocal cord paralysis | |
		Normal mobility	Paralysis
Total		1898 (98.7 %)	25 (1.3 %)
Age	<30	139 (7.3 %)	0 (0 %)
	30–39	285 (15.0 %)	1 (4.0 %)
	40–49	480 (25.2 %)	5 (20.0 %)
	50–59	470 (24.7 %)	5 (20.0 %)
	60–69	327 (17.2 %)	7 (28.0 %)
	70–79	152 (8.0 %)	3 (12.0 %)
	>80	44 (2.3 %)	4 (16.0 %)
			p-value
Mean; range of age (years)		50.7; 15–94	59.9; 36–88	0.0016
Sex	Male	424 (22.35 %)	7 (28 %)	0.3644
	Female	1474 (77.7 %)	18 (72 %)	

Table 2 Demographics and pathology results of 25 patients with preoperative vocal cord Paralysis

Subject	Sex	Side	Largest nodule on U/S (cm) and side	Final pathology	Adverse pathological features
1	F	R	2.4 (right)	Medullary CA	
2	M	L	1 (left)	Micropapillary CA	ETE
3	M	L	1.2 (left)	Micropapillary CA	
4	M	L	1.2 (left)	Papillary CA	
5	F	R	1.4 (right)	Follicular adenoma	
6	M	R	1.6 (left)	Papillary CA	
7	F	L	1.9 (left)	Nodular hyperplasia	
8	F	L	2.15 (left)	Papillary CA	
9	F	R	2.3 (right)	Papillary CA	
10	F	L	2.4 (midline)	Follicular adenoma	
11	F	L	2.7 (left)	Micropapillary CA	
12	F	L	3 (left)	Papillary CA	
13	F	L	1.7 (left)	Papillary CA	
14	F	L	3.5 (left)	Nodular hyperplasia	
15	F	R	Irregular, >3[a]	Papillary CA	ETE, PNI, LVI
16	M	L	5.5 (left)	Papillary CA	
17	F	L	6.5 (left)	Nodular hyperplasia	
18	F	R	7.7[a](right)	Papillary CA	
19	M	L	9.1 (left)	Papillary CA	ETE, LVI
20	F	L	7 (left)	Nodular hyperplasia	
21	M	L	0.7 (left)	Micropapillary CA	
22	F	L	No imaging[c]	Osteosarcoma[b]	
23	F	R	1.5 (right)	Papillary CA	
24	F	L	No imaging[c]	Poorly differentiated CA	
25	F	L	No imaging[c]	Papillary (tall cell variant) CA	ETE, PNI, LVI

(*M* male, *F* female, *U/S* ultrasound, *CA* carcinoma, *ETE* extrathyroidal extension, *PNI* perineural invasion, *LVI* lymphovascular invasion)
[a]Measure obtained from a CT Scan. No U/S available for this patient
[b]See discussion section regarding this finding
[c]These patients did not have preoperative imaging as they arrived in respiratory distress

Table 3 Status of preoperative vocal cord function according to pathology results

	Preoperative vocal cord paralysis n (% of total)		p-value
	+	-	
Malignant pathology	19 (1.0 %)	1143 (59.6 %)	0.2218
Benign pathology	6 (0.3 %)	671 (35.0 %)	
Total	25 (1.3 %)	1814 (98.7 %)	

vocal cord function was 3.0 cm (range of 0.3–13.0 cm) and it was 3.3 cm (0.7–9.1 cm) in patients with preoperative VCP ($p = 0.5916$). Malignant nodules found in patients with normal vocal cords (mean = 2.89 cm) were smaller than the malignant nodules of patients with preoperative VCP (mean = 3.2 cm), but it was not statistically significant ($p = 0.4168$). On the other hand, benign nodules of patients with normal vocal cords (mean = 3.22 cm) were larger than benign nodules found in patients with preoperative VCP (mean = 3.14 cm). However, this finding was also not statistically significant ($p = 0.9651$).

Other known adverse pathological features, such as ETE, LVI and PNI were also examined. Among patients with preoperative VCP, 21.1 % were found to have ETE, whereas 13.2 % of patients with normal vocal cord function had ETE on pathology. This finding was not statistically significant ($p = 0.27$). For LVI, results were comparable between patients with and without preoperative VCP (15.8 % in the VCP group and 10.8 % for patients with normal VC, $p = 0.4837$). However, PNI was significantly more common in patients with preoperative VCP (10.5 %) compared to patients without VCP (1.1 %) ($p = 0.0028$). These results are summarized in Table 4.

Discussion
Vocal cord paralysis can occur in both benign and malignant thyroid disease. The etiology of the paralysis is not always evident, but can often be explained by direct invasion or compression of the recurrent laryngeal nerve by malignant thyroid disease. In the case of benign

Table 4 Comparison of the incidence of adverse pathological features found in thyroid cancers of patients with and without preoperative VCP

Patients with malignant pathology

	Without VCP	With preop VCP	p-value
Perineural invasion	13 (1.13 %)	2 (10.5 %)	0.0028
Lymphovascular invasion	123 (10.76 %)	3 (15.78 %)	0.4837
Extrathyroidal extension	151 (13.21 %)	4 (21.05 %)	0.2700

thyroid disease, the paralysis could be idiopathic or could be caused by compression or stretching of the nerve. Knowledge of preoperative vocal cord paralysis is imperative for appropriate surgical planning and management. In this study, 1.3 % of patients undergoing thyroid surgery were found to have preoperative VCP. The true incidence of VCP in the general population is difficult to ascertain. A study by *Shafkat et al.* looked at 30,262 patients who attended an ENT outpatient clinic during a 2 year period [5]. One hundred ten of these patients were diagnosed with vocal cord paralysis, an incidence of 42 per 10,000 new patients [5]. Several studies have evaluated all causes of VCP and have found them to be idiopathic in 16.3 % [6], 17.4 % [7], 17.6 % [8] and 31.1 % [9] of patients.

Although the majority of patients undergoing thyroidectomy were women, there was no significant difference between men and women in terms of the presence or absence of preoperative VCP. On the other hand, our study found age to be a significant factor; it was considerably higher in patients with preoperative VCP. *Chiang et al.* also noted this finding in a study looking at thyroid tumours with preoperative recurrent laryngeal nerve palsies [10]. One explanation for this result would be that nodules have more time to evolve and develop adverse features with advancing age.

In our cohort, 76 % of patients with preoperative vocal cord paralysis were found to have malignant disease. Several other studies have also shown preoperative vocal cord paralysis to be a robust marker of malignancy [2–5]. However, it is not a perfect marker. Indeed, in our cohort, 24 % of patients with vocal cord paralysis had benign final pathology results. This finding emphasizes the importance of evaluating the vocal cords of all patients scheduled for thyroid surgery, regardless of fine-needle aspiration (FNA) results.

Many techniques are used to assess vocal cord function preoperatively. Presently, the flexible laryngoscope remains the most widely used. Another promising technique to study the vocal cords is transcutaneous laryngeal ultrasound. *Wang et al.* reported that it accurately diagnosed both normal and palsied vocal folds in 90 % of female patients, with a lesser success rate in males over 40 years of age [11]. The rate of false negatives with this technique appears to be one reason why it has not been widely adopted in the adult population [12–13].

The literature shows a preponderance of left-sided paralysis, and data regarding this finding dates back to the 1940's [15]. According to *Meurman et al.*, the left recurrent laryngeal nerve is more likely to be injured because it branches off the vagus nerve more caudally on the left side as compared to the right. In point of fact, after branching off the vagus nerve, the left recurrent laryngeal nerve, unlike the right, loops under the aortic arch.

It then runs upward in the groove between the trachea and esophagus with a more medial course, closer to the thyroid gland than to the right recurrent laryngeal nerve. Our results show that 72 % of patients had a left-sided paralysis, a finding similar to other reported studies by *Benninger et al.*, *Terris et al.* and *Pavithran et al.* Another reason for the preponderance of left-sided paralysis may lie in the length of each nerve [14–16]. On average, the left recurrent laryngeal nerve measures 12 cm, whereas the right one measures 5 to 6 cm [17]. The added length may explain the higher rate of left-sided paralysis, providing more regions of vulnerability along the nerve [17].

We studied the relationship between nodule size and malignancy. The only statistically significant finding was that overall, benign nodules were slightly larger than malignant ones, regardless of the status of vocal cord function. We found no significant correlation between the size of the nodules and the function of the vocal cords. Indeed, some of the largest nodules corresponded to benign pathologies in both VCP and no VCP groups. This finding is consistent with the literature [18–21]. In 2011, *Moon et al.* published a consensus statement and recommendations on ultrasonography and the ultrasound-based management of thyroid nodules [21], concluding that thyroid nodule size was not helpful for distinguishing malignant and benign nodules. Furthermore, *Kamran et al.* reported that above 2 cm, there was a non-linear relationship between nodule size and cancer risk [18]. It is hypothesized that other mechanisms, such as stretching or compression of the recurrent laryngeal nerve, could be the cause of paralysis. However, other reports suggest that increasing size may indeed correspond to a greater risk of malignancy. For example, *Raparia et al.* described a statistically significant increased risk of malignancy in nodules over 2 cm in size [22].

Histopathological tumor characteristics provide crucial information when it comes to prognosis and risk of recurrence. When these characteristics were retrospectively analyzed in our study, in the setting of preoperative VCP, we found perineural invasion to be far more common in patients with preoperative VCP. No such association was found with extrathyroidal extension and lymphovascular invasion. According to our results, when a preoperative VCP is present, a patient had a 76 % chance of harbouring a thyroid malignancy, with a higher chance of finding perineural invasion on final pathology. With this knowledge, the degree of surgical aggressiveness can be planned accordingly.

There are limitations to this study. First, it is a retrospective analysis. Second, despite a large sample size, the incidence of preoperative VCP is very low overall. Therefore, evaluation of the clinical characteristics of thyroid pathologies remains limited.

Conclusion

This study demonstrates that preoperative vocal cord paralysis is a robust marker of malignancy risk, although not an absolute one. It most commonly affects the left vocal cord. It also emphasizes the importance that every patient undergoing thyroid surgery should have a preoperative vocal cord assessment, even in the context of a benign FNA result, as 24 % of patients with preoperative VCP in this study had benign thyroid pathologies, as demonstrated in several other studies [1, 3–5, 23–30].

Competing interests
The authors declare that they have no competing interests.

Authors' contributions
EKR carried out the data collection, statistical analysis and drafted the manuscript. All authors read and approved the final manuscript.

Author details
[1]Department of Otolaryngology – Head and Neck surgery, McGill University, Montreal, QC, Canada. [2]Department of General surgery, McGill University, Montreal, QC, Canada. [3]Division of Head and Neck Surgery, Department of Otolaryngology – Head and Neck surgery, Jewish General Hospital, McGill University, Montreal, QC H3T 1E2, Canada.

References
1. Raza SN, Shah MD, Palme CE, Hall FT, Eski S, Freeman JL. Risk factors for well-differentiated thyroid carcinoma in patients with thyroid nodular disease. Otolaryngol Head Neck Surg. 2008;139:21–6.
2. Collazo-Clavell ML, Gharib H, Maragos NE. Relationship between vocal cord paralysis and benign thyroid disease. Head Neck. 1995;17:24–30.
3. Holl-Allen RTJ. Laryngeal nerve paralysis and benign thyroid disease. Arch Otolaryngol. 1967;85:121–3.
4. Rueger RG. Benign disease of the thyroid gland and vocal cord paralysis. Laryngoscope. 1974;84:897–907.
5. Shafkat A, Muzamil A, Lateef M. A study of incidence and etiopathology of vocal cord paralysis. Indian J Otolaryngol Head Neck Surg. 2000;54:30–2.
6. Ramadan HH, Wax MK, Avery S. Outcome and changing cause of unilateral vocal cord paralysis. Otolaryngol Head Neck Surg. 1998;118:199–202.
7. Yumoto E, Minoda R, Hyodo M, Yamagata T. Causes of recurrent laryngeal nerve paralysis. Auris Nasus Larynx. 2002;29:41–5.
8. Rosenthal LH, Benninger MS, Deeb RH. Vocal cord immobility: a longitudinal analysis of etiology over 20 years. Laryngoscope. 2007;117:1864–70.
9. Toutounchi SJ, Eydi M, Golzari SE, Ghaffari MR, Parvizian N. Vocal cord paralysis and its etiologies: a prospective study. J Cardiovasc Thorac Res. 2014;6:47–50.
10. Chiang F-Y, Lin J-C, Lee K-W, Wang LF, Tsai KB, Wu CW, et al. Thyroid tumors with preoperative recurrent laryngeal nerve palsy: clinicopathologic features and treatment outcome. Surgery. 2006;140(3):140–417.
11. Wang C-P, Chen T-C, Yang T-L, Chen CN, Lin CF, Lou PJ, et al. Transcutaneous ultrasound for evaluation of vocal fold movement in patients with thyroid disease. Eur J Radiol. 2012;81:288–91.
12. Maia FFR, Matos PS, Silva BP, Pallone AT, Pavin EJ, Vassallo J, et al. Role of ultrasound, clinical and scintigraphyc parameters to predict malignancy in thyroid nodule. Head Neck Oncol. 2011;3:17.
13. Meurman OH. Theories of vocal cord paralysis. Acta Otolaryngol. 1950;38:460–72.
14. Benninger MS, Gillen JB, Altman JS. Changing etiology of vocal fold immobility. Laryngoscope. 1998;108:1346–50.
15. Terris DJ, Arnstein DP, Nguyen HH. Contemporary evaluation of unilateral vocal cord paralysis. Otolaryngol Head Neck Surg. 1998;107:84–90.
16. Pavithran J, Menon J. Unilateral Vocal Cord Palsy: An etiopathological Study. Int J Phonosurg laryngol. 2011;1:5–10.
17. Myssiorek D. Recurrent laryngeal nerve paralysis: anatomy and etiology. Otolaryngol Clin North Am. 2004;37:25–44.

18. Kamran SC, Marqusee E, Kim MI, Frates MC, Ritner J, Peters H, et al. Thyroid nodule size and prediction of cancer. J Clin Endocrinol Metab. 2013;98:564–70.
19. Brito JP, Gionfriddo MR, Al Nofal A, Boehmer KR, Leppin AL, Reading C, et al. The accuracy of thyroid nodule ultrasound to predict thyroid cancer: systematic review and meta-analysis. J Clin Endocrinol Metab. 2014;99:1253–63.
20. Sturgeon C. Surgeon-Performed Laryngeal Ultrasound Can Be Used to Screen for Vocal-Cord Palsy before Thyroid. Surgery. 2013;25:113–5.
21. Moon WJ, Jung SL, Lee JH, Na DF, Baek JH, Lee YH, et al. and Thyroid Study Group, Korean Society of Neuro- and head and Neck Radiology. Benign and malignant thyroid nodules: US differentiation-multicenter retrospective study. Radiology. 2008;247:762–70.
22. Raparia K, Sk M, Mody DR, Anton R, Amrikachi M. Clinical outcomes for "suspicious" category in thyroid fine-needle aspiration biopsy: Patient's sex and nodule size are possible predictors of malignancy. Arch Pathol Lab Med. 2009;133:787–90.
23. Coelho DH, Boey HP. Benign parathyroid cyst causing vocal fold paralysis: a case report and review of the literature. Head Neck. 2006;28:564–6.
24. Kenn K, Balkissoon R. Vocal cord dysfunction: what do we know? Eur Respir J. 2011;37:194–200.
25. Merati AL, Shemirani N, Smith TL, Toohill RJ. Changing trends in the nature of vocal fold motion impairment. Am J Otolaryngol. 2006;27:106–8.
26. Randolph GW, Kamani D. The importance of preoperative laryngoscopy in patients undergoing thyroidectomy: voice, vocal cord function, and the preoperative detection of invasive thyroid malignancy. Surgery. 2006;139:357–62.
27. Sayyahmelli M, Alipanahi R, Ghorjanian A, Mousavipanah S. Value of laryngoscopy Before and After Thyroidectomy. RMJ. 2009;34(1):89–91.
28. Schlosser K, Zeuner M, Wagner M, Slater EP, Dominguez Fernandez E, Rothmund M, et al. Laryngoscopy in thyroid surgery–essential standard or unnecessary routine? Surgery. 2007;142(6):858–64.
29. Chandrasekhar SS, Randolph GW, Seidman MD, Rosenfeld RM, Angelos P, Barkmeier-Kraemer J, et al. Clinical practice guideline: improving voice outcomes after thyroid surgery. Otolaryngol Head Neck Surg. 2013;148:S1–37.
30. Farrag TY, Samlan RA, Lin FR, Tufano RP. The utility of evaluating true vocal fold motion before thyroid surgery. Laryngoscope. 2006;116:235–8.

23

Oral corticosteroid prescribing habits of Canadian Otolaryngologist-Head and Neck Surgeons

Saad Ansari[1], Brian W. Rotenberg[1] and Leigh J. Sowerby[1,2]*

Abstract

Background: Oral corticosteroids (OCSs) are widely prescribed in Otolaryngology-Head & Neck surgery (OtoHNS). There is evidence in the literature regarding specific dosing regimens. However, it is not known to what extent these recommendations are being implemented in practice.

Methods: An anonymous online survey was sent to Canadian Society of Otolaryngology-Head and Neck Surgery members ($N = 696$). Dosing, frequency and tapering of OCSs were assessed in acute rhino-sinusitis (ARS), chronic rhino-sinusitis with (CRSwP) and without polyps (CRSsP), sudden sensori-neural hearing loss (SSNHL), and idiopathic facial nerve/Bell's palsy (IFN). Participants were asked to complete for conditions treated and results were compared with current guidelines. Development of prescribing habits and observed complications were also explored.

Results: 124 surveys (18 %) were completed. In CRSwP ($N = 98$), the median dose was 50 mg (Range: 10–100 mg) and the average duration was 8 days (Range: 1–21 days). In CRSsP ($N = 29$), the median dose was 50 mg (Range: 20-80 mg) and the average duration was 8 days (Range: 1–14 days). In SSNHL ($N = 118$), the median dose was 60 mg (Range: 10–120 mg) and the average duration was 10 days (Range: 1–21 days). In IFN ($N = 108$), the median dose was 50 mg (Range: 10–100 mg) and the average duration was 10 days (Range: 1–21 days). Tapering dosages were used in treating CRSwP (64 %), CRSsP (62 %), ARS (44 %), SSNHL (60 %) and IFN (53 %). Respondents most frequently perceived "Mentor/Preceptor Guidance" as a source of their prescribing habits.

Conclusion: There is significant heterogeneity in OCS prescribing habits despite the availability of fairly consistent evidence in the literature for some of the surveyed conditions. Improvements in standardization should be made with the aim of enhancing outcomes and reducing complications.

Keywords: Oral corticosteroids, Otolaryngology, Dosing regimen, Evidence-based medicine, Chronic Rhinosinusitis, Taper, Sudden Sensori-neural Hearing Loss, Facial Nerve Palsy

Background

Oral corticosteroids (OCSs) are commonly used for a variety of different diseases. In 2013, Overman et al. determined that 1.2 % of the US population over age 20 were prescribed OCSs, translating into over 2.5 million people [1]. In the field of Otolaryngology-Head & Neck Surgery (OtoHNS), OCSs are used for several indications, including chronic rhinosinusitis, sudden sensori-neural hearing loss, and idiopathic facial nerve, or Bell's, palsy.

Due to the significant side effect profile, OCSs are often reserved as part of maximal medical therapy when other treatments have not been successful. Complications such as avascular necrosis of the hip, immunodeficiency, weight gain, insomnia, and psychosis have been well described in the literature [2]. While some are idiosyncratic reactions,

* Correspondence: leigh.sowerby@sjhc.london.on.ca

Meeting presentation Poster presentation at the Canadian Society of Otolaryngology-Head and Neck Surgery Annual General Meeting in Winnipeg, Ontario, Canada in June 2015.

[1]Department of Otolaryngology-Head & Neck Surgery, Western University, London, ON, Canada

[2]Department of Otolaryngology-Head & Neck Surgery, St. Joseph's Hospital, Room B2-501, 268 Grosvenor Street, London, ON N6A 4V2, Canada

most side effects have been shown to correlate with increasing doses of OCSs [3]. Therefore, the dosing of OCSs is important to provide maximal benefit while minimizing potential side effects.

A 2013 UK study by Sylvester et al. qualitatively characterized OCS prescribing habits as part of maximal medical therapy in chronic rhinosinusitis, with 66 % rarely or never prescribing OCSs [4]. Of those that did, 42 % utilized a duration of 0-5 days, 29 % for 6–10 days and 29 % for 11–15 days - suggesting that there is significant heterogeneity in prescribing practice in the UK. Kaszuba & Stewart showed that 36 % of Otolaryngologist-Head & Neck surgeons used OCSs in chronic rhinosinusitis [5]. This study also concluded that maximal medical management was influenced mainly by personal clinical experiences rather than evidence in the literature. Similar studies have not been conducted in Canada regarding OCS prescribing habits.

The aim of this study is to characterize OCS prescribing habits of Canadian Otolaryngologist-Head & Neck surgeons for chronic rhinosinusitis, acute rhinosinusitis, sudden sensori-neural hearing loss, and idiopathic facial nerve (Bell's) palsy. While the evidence for dosage is heterogeneous for some conditions, such as chronic rhinosinusitis, a much clearer consensus on dosage exists for others. This study hopes to provide a glimpse into the status of evidence-based practice for prescribing OCSs in Canadian OtoHNS.

Methods

Formal ethics approval was obtained through the Western University Research Ethics Board (Board number 105523)

prior to beginning the study. An anonymous nationwide survey was conducted through an online survey program (QuestionPro.com®) and electronically distributed to all active members of the Canadian Society of Otolaryngology – Head and Neck Surgery's mailing list ($n = 696$) between October and November 2014. A reminder email was sent approximately 3 months after initial distribution and participants were incentivized with a gift card draw at completion of the study. A cover letter accompanied the survey to outline issues of consent and to disclose the study's goal of characterizing prescribing habits of Canadian Otolaryngologist-Head & Neck surgeons. Respondents were notified that no identifying data would be included in the study.

Demographic data collected focused on the nature of respondents' current practices. Indication, initial dose, duration, frequency, and use of taper were described for five common indications of OCSs in OtoHNS. These were chronic rhinosinusitis with polyposis (CRSwP), chronic rhinosinusitis without polyposis (CRSsP), acute rhinosinusitis (ARS), sudden sensori-neural hearing loss (SSNHL), and idiopathic facial nerve (Bell's) palsy (IFN). Respondents were also asked to describe influences that helped to establish personal dosing regimens as well as observed complications with the use of OCSs in practice (Fig. 1).

Results

Out of the 696 survey requests sent to members of the Canadian Society of Otolaryngology-Head and Neck Surgery, 124 surveys were returned fully completed (18 % response rate). The majority of respondents were surgeons

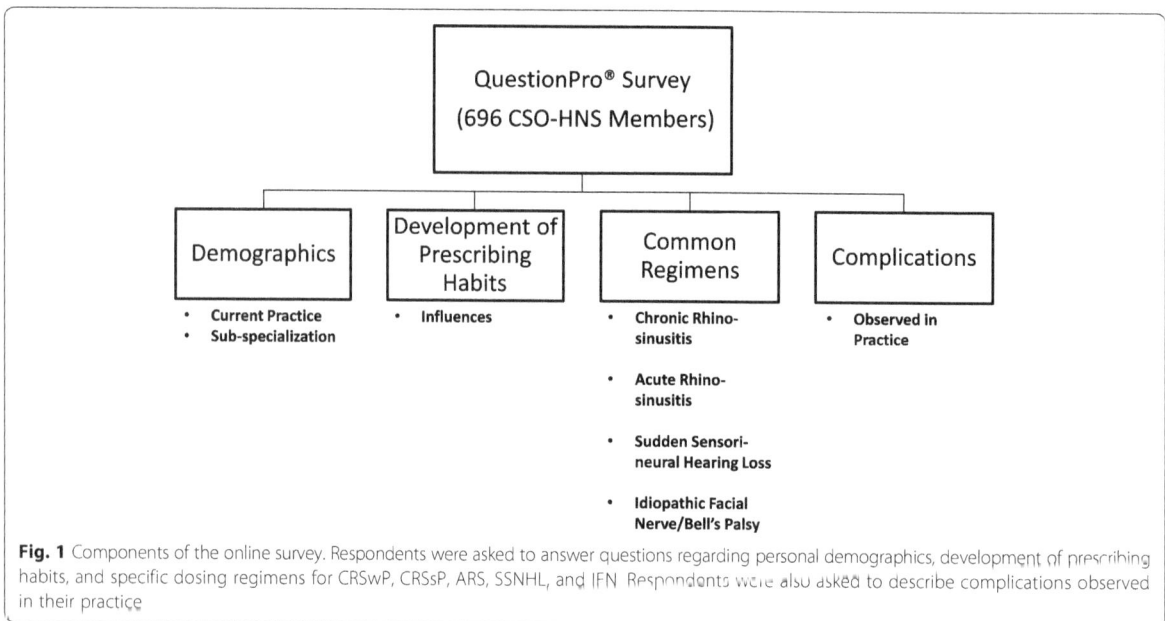

Fig. 1 Components of the online survey. Respondents were asked to answer questions regarding personal demographics, development of prescribing habits, and specific dosing regimens for CRSwP, CRSsP, ARS, SSNHL, and IFN. Respondents were also asked to describe complications observed in their practice

in active practice (87 %). There were slightly more community practitioners (55 %) than academic practitioners (40 %). The remaining 5 % had a mixed academic and community practice. The two most-represented subspecialties were General Otolaryngology (52 %) and Rhinology (27 %). These were followed by Pediatrics (23 %), Head and Neck (20 %), Otology (19 %), Facial Plastic and Reconstructive Surgery (17 %), Laryngology (12 %) and other (4 %). The average number of OCSs prescribed by respondents was 6 prescriptions per month (range: 0–40 prescriptions).

The most common self-described OCS prescribing influence was a respondent's mentor or preceptor (78 %), followed by personal experience (64 %) and clinical guidelines (59 %) (see Fig. 2).

Chronic rhinosinusitis

In chronic rhinosinusitis, 79 % of respondents prescribed OCSs for CRSwP and 23 % for CRSsP. The most common reasons in both cases were "as part of maximal medical therapy" and "symptomatic exacerbation". In CRSwP, there were 12 unique doses described by respondents. The median starting dose was 50 mg with a range between 10 and 100 mg. The average duration was 8 days with a range between 1 and 21 days. In CRSsP, there were 7 unique doses used by respondents. The median dose was 50 mg with a range between 20 and 80 mg. The average duration was 8 days with a range between 1 and 14 days. Tapers were used by approximately two-thirds of those that used corticosteroids for both conditions (Table 1, Figs. 3 & 4).

Acute rhinosinusitis

In acute rhinosinusitis, 7 % of respondents reported prescribing OCSs. All nine respondents had unique dosing regimens. The median dose was 50 mg with a range between 25 and 60 mg. The average duration was 6 days with a range between 2 and 10 days. A total of 44 % used a taper (Table 1, Figs. 3 & 4).

Sudden sensori-neural hearing loss

In SSNHL, an overwhelming majority of respondents used OCSs (95 %). The most common reason to initiate therapy was to improve hearing. There were 11 unique dosing regimens described. The median starting dose was 55 mg with a range between 10 and 100 mg. The most common starting dose was between 40 and 60 mg of prednisone, with 98 (80 %) of respondents doing so. The average duration was 10 days with a range between 1 and 21 days. In this group of respondents, 60 % utilized a taper (Table 1, Figs. 3 & 4). Approximately 80 % (98/123) of respondents used a starting dose between 40 and 60 mg.

Idiopathic facial nerve (Bell's) palsy

For IFN palsy, 87 % of respondents prescribed OCSs. There were 9 unique dosing regimens described. The median dose was 50 mg with a range between 10 and 100 mg. Only 83 (67 %) of respondents used a starting dose of prednisone between 40 and 60 mg. The average duration was 9 days with a range between 1 and 21 days. Of these respondents, 53 % employed a taper (Table 1, Figs. 3 & 4).

Complications

When asked about complications observed in practice, 30 % of respondents had personally managed patients with complications from the use of OCSs (Fig. 5). Insomnia, weight gain and gastrointestinal symptoms were most commonly described. Other rare complications were also mentioned including avascular necrosis, adrenal suppression, and hypoglycaemia (Fig. 6).

Discussion

This study has characterized the corticosteroid prescribing habits of Canadian Otolaryngologist-Head & Neck

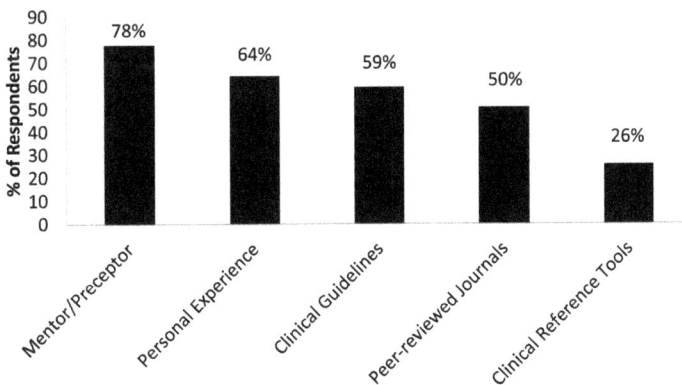

Fig. 2 Influences for current oral corticosteroid prescribing habits of survey respondents

Table 1 Dosing regimens responses for CRS, ARS, SSNHL, and IFN/Bell's Palsy. This table shows the use of OCSs, number of unique dosing regimens reported, median starting dose, average duration, and taper utilization for CRSwP, CRSsP, ARS, SSNHL, and IFN

Indication	Use (% of respondents)	Unique dosing regimens	Median dose with ranges	Duration with ranges	Taper (% of respondents)
CRSwP	79	12	50 (10–100)	8 (1–21)	64
CRSsP	23	7	50 (20–80)	8 (1–14)	62
ARS	7	9	50 (25–60)	6 (2–10)	44
SSNHL	95	11	55 (10–120)	10 (1–21)	60
IFN/Bell's Palsy	87	9	50 (10–100)	9 (1–21)	53

surgeons for five common conditions in OtoHNS. The 18 % response rate, which is similar to previous survey studies of Canadian Otolaryngologist-Head and Neck surgeons, provides a well-balanced representation of community and academic practice respondents [6–9]. The results demonstrate the significant variability in prescribing habits, as evidenced by the high number of unique dosing regimens for each condition. Even greater variation would likely have been seen with a higher response rate, as the findings of this study are in keeping with the heterogeneity seen in previous surveys for OCS usage [4]. This is likely to be expected as mentor and preceptor habits along with personal experience were most commonly selected as being influences on respondents' prescribing habits.

For CRSwP, the 2011 Canadian Society of Otolaryngology-Head and Neck Surgery (CSO-HNS) clinical practice guidelines suggest a two-week course of OCS to aid in treatment [10]. It does not elaborate on dosing regimens. A 2013 International Forum of Allergy & Rhinology review by Poetker et al. provides a more specific regimen of 25–60 mg for 7–14 days with Level A evidence from Level 2–4 studies [11]. The Canadian Family Physician guidelines also provide a dosing regimen of a two-week course of prednisone with a taper [12]. An example regimen was given for 30 mg per day for 4 days, then reduce the dose by 5 mg every 2 days for 10 days. With these guideline recommendations in mind, it is not surprising that this study noted 12 unique regimens and a very wide range of doses (10–100 mg). The guidelines were unable to commit to a specific regimen, as there is significant heterogeneity in the literature. For CRSsP, the same 2011 CSO-HNS guidelines do not provide any dosing or duration suggestions but provide a statement supporting the use of a short course of OCSs in this condition [10]. The 2013 IFAR review by Poetker et al. provide an optional level C recommendation suggesting 40–60 mg for 10–14 days [11]. This heterogeneity and weakness in the literature for CRSsP, as well as CRSwP, may be the reason for wide variety of prescribing habits observed in this study. Regardless, some of the dosing regimens described by respondents fall outside of the broad spectrum of recommendations - either not providing patients with benefit if too low, or exposing them to unnecessary potential risk if too high.

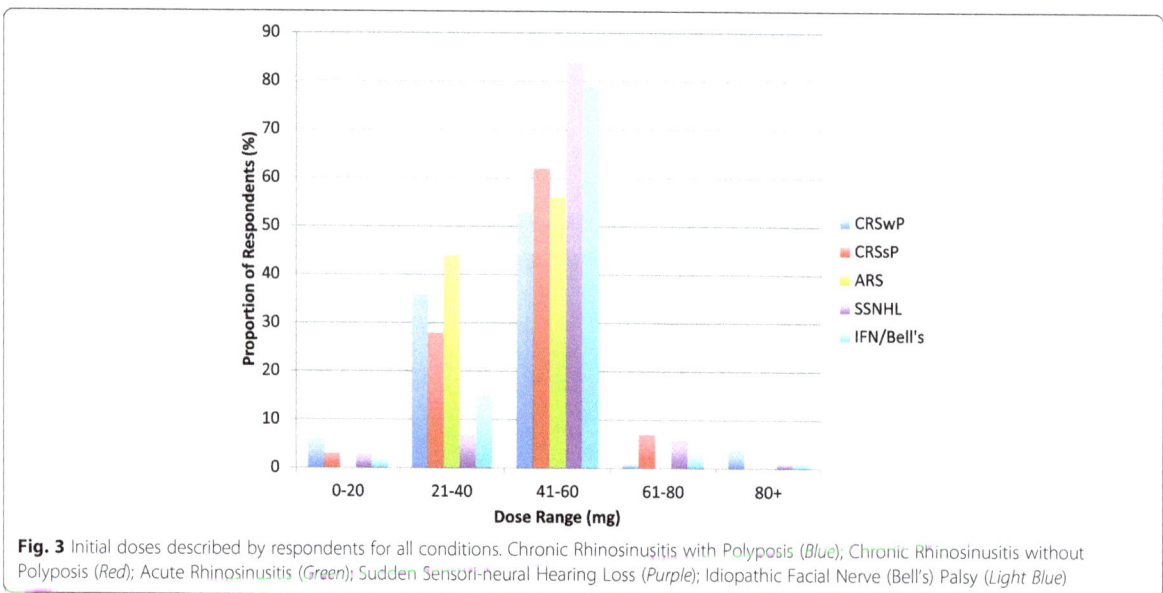

Fig. 3 Initial doses described by respondents for all conditions. Chronic Rhinosinusitis with Polyposis (*Blue*); Chronic Rhinosinusitis without Polyposis (*Red*); Acute Rhinosinusitis (*Green*); Sudden Sensori-neural Hearing Loss (*Purple*); Idiopathic Facial Nerve (Bell's) Palsy (*Light Blue*)

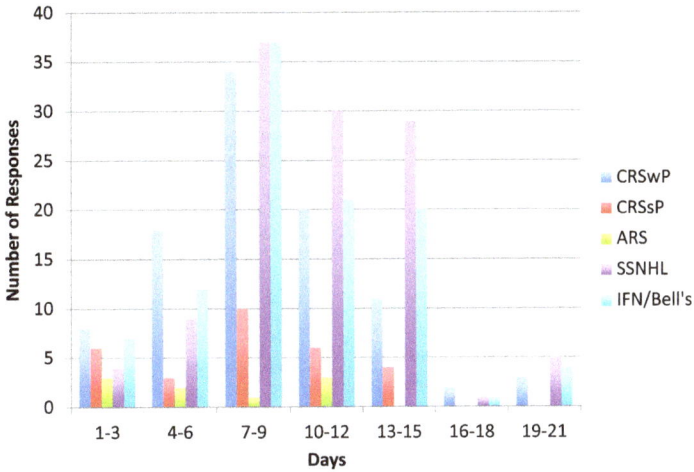

Fig. 4 Durations described by respondents for all conditions. Chronic Rhinosinusitis with Polyposis (*Dark Blue*); Chronic Rhinosinusitis without Polyposis (*Red*); Acute Rhinosinusitis (*Green*); Sudden Sensori-neural Hearing Loss (*Purple*); Idiopathic Facial Nerve (Bell's) Palsy (*Light Blue*)

The dosing and duration recommendations of corticosteroid for SSNHL and IFN palsy, on the other hand, is more granular. For SSNHL, the American Academy of Otolaryngology–Head and Neck Surgery clinical guidelines recommend the use of OCSs at 60 mg for 10–14 days from level B evidence [13]. In IFN palsy, the Canadian Medical Association Journal guidelines provide a strong recommendation for a five-day course of 60 mg per day followed by a five day taper, reducing the previous day's dose by 10 mg per day [14]. It is also suggested that a total dose of over 450 mg is necessary to obtain optimal benefit. Only 37 % of respondents prescribed a dose over this total amount. The evidence supporting these recommendations is stronger than the literature for CRS, and should provide prescribers with greater guidance as to the ideal dose and duration of corticosteroid. The results of this study, in spite of stronger guideline recommendations, demonstrate that there still is a range in doses and duration for both conditions with only 80 and 67 % of respondents using the recommended initial dose in SSNHL and IFN respectively. Prescribing below the guideline

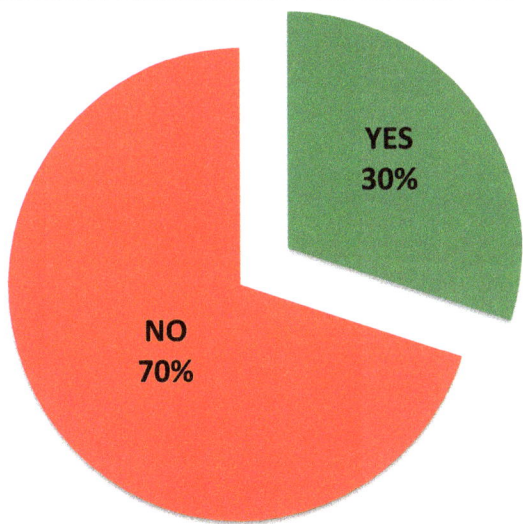

Fig 5 Percentage of respondents who have observed a complication with oral corticosteroids in their practice. Thirty percent of respondents answered "Yes" (*Green*) and 70 % answered "No" (*Red*)

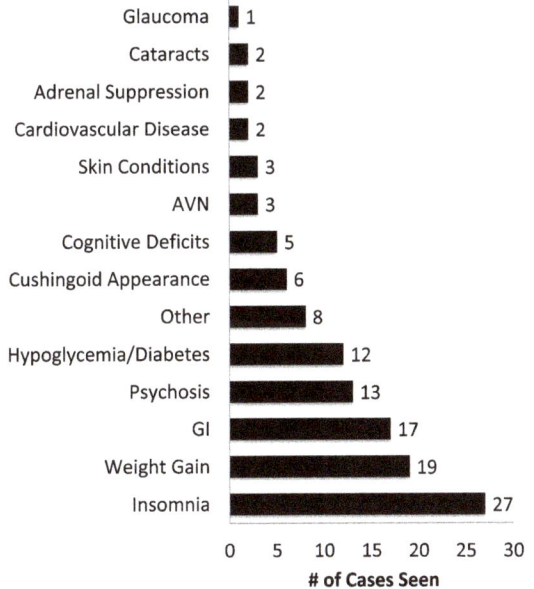

Fig. 6 Complications observed with the use of oral corticosteroids by respondents

recommendations could potentially not provide patients with the intended benefit, while prescribing above could be exposing patients to unnecessary risk without any further additional benefit.

Evidence for corticosteroid use in acute rhinosinusitis is against routine use and not supported by current guideline recommendations [10, 15]. In spite of this, 7 % of respondents in this survey used OCSs in their treatment regimen, likely exposing patients to unnecessary risk without benefit.

Overall, this study was able to characterize current in-practice dosing regimens for five common conditions in which OCSs are used in OtoHNS. Further study needs to be performed to determine the optimal dose and duration for OCSs in CRS. However, there is significant heterogeneity in OCS prescribing habits irrespective of the strength of guideline recommendations regarding dose and duration. Perhaps greater emphasis is needed to encourage adherence to evidence-based practice to optimize medical therapy for patients.

Although this study aids in characterizing the dosing regimens of OCSs used in OtoHNS in Canada, it is self-reported. Hawthorne effect bias is likely present when respondents were completing this survey. Therefore, the results may be an under-estimation of the variability in the prescribing habits. This would further strengthen the conclusions made from this study. Additionally, it was difficult to parse out the reason for respondents to select "Yes" or "No" when replying to questions regarding the use of OCSs in each of the conditions mentioned in the survey. Some may have interpreted it as a question inquiring about the use of OCSs in their practice while others may have understood it as a question of whether they believed in prescribing OCSs for each specific condition. This would have potentially skewed the results of this question for each of the conditions. Further clarification of the question would have been optimal along with a third option of "Do not prescribe in my practice".

Conclusion

OCSs are widely used in OtoHNS. This study provides a glimpse into the in-practice prescription habits of Canadian Otolaryngologist-Head & Neck surgeons for chronic rhinosinusitis with and without polyps, acute rhinosinusitis, sudden sensori-neural hearing loss, and idiopathic facial nerve palsy. As expected, there is a wide range of dosing regimens currently being used – some being within the recommended guidelines and others that are not. Further research to standardize prescribing habits in order to optimize patient outcomes and minimize potential risk from unnecessarily high doses of corticosteroid would be beneficial.

Abbreviations
ARS: acute rhinosinusitis; CRSsP: chronic rhinosinusitis without polyposis; CRSwP: chronic rhinosinusitis with polyposis; IFN: idiopathic facial nerve (Bell's) Palsy; OCS: oral corticosteroid; OtoHNS: Otolaryngology-Head and Neck Surgery; SSNHL: sudden sensori-neural hearing loss.

Competing interests
The authors declare that they have no other competing interests.

Authors' contributions
SA participated in the design of the study, carried out the survey, and drafted the manuscript. LJS conceived the study, participated in the study design, drafting and editing of the manuscript. BWR participated in the study design, drafting and editing of the manuscript. All authors read and approved the final manuscript.

Acknowledgements
This study was funded through the Schulich Research Opportunities Program (SROP) from the Schulich School of Medicine and Dentistry, Western University, London, Ontario. This funding body had no role in the design, collection, analysis, and interpretation of data; in the writing of the manuscript; and in the decision to submit the manuscript for publication.

Confirmation of original material
This material has never been published and is not currently under evaluation in any other peer-reviewed publication.

References
1.   Overman RA, Yeh JY, Deal CL. Prevalence of oral glucocorticoid usage in the United States: a general population perspective. Arthritis Care Res (Hoboken). 2013;65(2):294–8.
2.   Liu D, Ahmet A, Ward L, Krishnamoorthy P, Mandelcorn ED, Leigh R, et al. A practical guide to the monitoring and management of the complications of systemic corticosteroid therapy. Allergy Asthma Clin Immunol. 2013;9(1):30.
3.   Manson SC, Brown RE, Cerulli A, Vidaurre CF. The cumulative burden of oral corticosteroid side effects and the economic implications of steroid use. Respir Med. 2009;103(7):975–94.
4.   Sylvester DB, Carr S, Nix P. Maximum medical therapy for chronic rhinosinusitis: a survey of otolaryngology consultants in the United Kingdom. Int Forum Allergy Rhinol. 2013;3(2):129–32.
5.   Kaszuba SM, Stewart MG. Medical management and diagnosis of chronic rhinosinusitis: a survey of treatment patterns by United States otolaryngologists. Am J Rhinol. 2006;20:186–90.
6.   Madana J, Morand GB, Barona-Lleo L, Black MJ, Mlynarek AM, Hier MP. A survey on pulmonary screening practices among Otolaryngology-Head & Neck surgeons across Canada in the post treatment surveillance of head and neck squamous cell carcinoma. J Otolaryngol Head Neck Surg. 2015;44(1):5.
7.   Williams BA, Trites JR, Taylor SM, Bullock MJ, Hart RD. Surgical management of primary hyperparathyroidism in Canada. J Otolaryngol Head Neck Surg. 2014;43(1):44.
8.   Merdad M, Eskander A, De Almeida J, Freeman J, Rotstein L, Ezzat S, et al. Current Management of papillary thyroid microcarcinoma in Canada. J Otolaryngol Head Neck Surg. 2014;43:32.
9.   Brak M, Moore P, Taylor SM, Trites J, Murray S, Hart R. Expectantly waiting: a survey of thyroid surgery wait times among Canadian Otolaryngologists. J Otolaryngol Head Neck Surg. 2013;42:47.
10. Desrosiers M, Evans GA, Keith PK, Wright ED, Kaplan A, Bouchard J, et al. Canadian clinical practice guidelines for acute and chronic rhinosinusitis. J Otolaryngol Head Neck Surg. 2011;40 Suppl 2:S99–193.
11. Poetker DM, Jakubowski LA, Lal D, Hwang PH, Wright ED, Smith TL. Oral corticosteroids in the management of adult chronic rhinosinusitis with and without nasal polyps: an evidence-based review with recommendations. Int Forum Allergy Rhinol. 2013;3(2):104–20.
12. Kaplan A. Canadian guidelines for chronic rhinosinusitis: clinical summary. Can Fam Physician. 2013;59(12):1275–81.
13. Stachler RJ, Chandrasekhar SS, Archer SM, Rosenfeld RM, Schwartz SR, Barrs DM, et al. Clinical practice guideline: sudden hearing loss. Otolaryngol Head Neck Surg. 2012;146 Suppl 3:S1–S35.

14. de Almeida JR, Guyatt GH, Sud S, Dorion J, Hill MD, Kolber MR. Management of Bell palsy: clinical practice guideline. CMAJ. 2014;186(12):917–22.
15. Venekamp RP, Thompson MJ, Hayward G, Heneghan CJ, Del Mar CB, Perera R, et al. Systemic corticosteroids for acute sinusitis. Cochrane Database Syst Rev. 2014;25(3):CD008115.

24

Submental island flap reconstruction reduces cost in oral cancer reconstruction compared to radial forearm free flap reconstruction: a case series and cost analysis

D. Forner[*] [ORCID], T. Phillips, M. Rigby, R. Hart, M. Taylor and J. Trites

Abstract

Background: In Canada, 4,400 cases of oral cancer are diagnosed yearly. Surgical resection is a key component of treatment in many of these cancers. Reconstruction of defects, with the goal of preserving function, is of utmost importance. Several choices are possible for reconstruction of larger defects, including both free and pedicled flaps. Free flap reconstruction is reliable and effective, but requires additional personnel and peri-operative resources. Pedicled flaps remain an important alternative to free flaps, and are less resource intensive. This paper reviews our inaugural experience with the submental island flap (SIF) and compares costs incurred to a matched cohort of oral cancer patients reconstructed with forearm free flaps.

Methods: Charts of patients who underwent SIF and RFFF reconstruction from January 1st 2013 to April 1st 2015 were retrospectively examined. Associated costs were obtained via online database and previously reported costs at the study institution.

Results: Mean length of ICU stay in glossectomy RFFF reconstruction was 4.7 days. Only one patient required ICU stay for one night in the SIF group. Mean length of hospital stay was not significantly different in SIF patients vs RFFF patients (12.4 vs 15.4 days, $p > 0.05$). Mean operative time was significantly lower in the SIF group compared to the RFFF group (347 vs 552 min, $p < 0.05$). Total mean intraoperative costs were found to be $4780.59 for RFFF operations, versus $2307.94 for SIF. Total mean cost of post-operative stay was $18158.40 in the SIF group and $43617.60 in the RFFF group. Total cost savings were therefore $27931.85 per patient for the SIF group.

Conclusions: We have demonstrated the use of the submental island flap as an alternative to radial forearm free flaps, showing both decreased hospital costs and comparable patient outcomes. Pedicled flaps are making a resurgence in head and neck reconstruction, and the submental island flap offers an excellent alternative to more labour intensive and costly free flap alternatives.

Keywords: Oral cancer, Reconstruction, Submental Island Flap, Radial Forearm Free Flap, Cost, Pedicle Flap, Free Flap

* Correspondence: david.forner@dal.ca
Division of Otolaryngology – Head and Neck Surgery, Department of Surgery, Dalhousie University, Halifax, Canada

Background

Head and neck cancer accounts for over 500,000 cancer diagnoses worldwide [1], with approximately 3 % of new cancer cases in the United States being head and neck in origin [2]. In Canada, 4400 new cases of oral cancer are diagnosed yearly [3]. Surgical resection is typically a key component of treatment in most cancers originating in the oral cavity, pharynx, face, or neck [4]. For larger mucosal defects, primary reconstruction is often pursued to optimize functional outcomes. In addition to its social and esthetic importance, the head and neck region is also fundamental in speech, swallowing, and respiration. Consequently, reconstructive options in head and neck surgery have been studied extensively. Tissue flaps are one such option, and these include both free flaps and pedicled flaps [5]. Free tissue transfer has become a mainstay of reconstruction in recent years, offering improved vascularity and wound healing, potential for innervation, tailoring of the wound defect, and a wide variety of tissue options [5]. These flaps have become the standard against which other means of reconstruction must be evaluated.

However, free flap reconstruction is limited due to increased operative time, and need for specialized equipment and microvascular expertise [6]. A lengthy hospital admission can also be anticipated. In a context of limited health care resources, the indiscriminate use of free tissue transfer allows fewer patients to receive timely surgical care. Not surprisingly, free flap operations have been associated with greater costs in both the intraoperative and immediate post-operative periods [7].

Health care costs in Canada have increased every year since 1975. Between 2000 and 2010, health care costs increased an average of 7 % per year. In the past four years, health care spending has continued to rise, albeit at a slightly slower rate [8]. Together with a modest but steady climb (1.2 %/yr) in the incidence of oral cancer in Canada [9], some of which is likely attributable to human papillomavirus, these realities demand a revisiting of more economical alternatives for reconstruction in head and neck surgery.

Quite independent of these fiscal pressures, pedicled flaps have re-emerged as important alternatives to free flaps. In particular, the submental island flap has recently grown in popularity. Originally reported in 1993 by Martin et al. [10], the submental island flap is a fasciocutaneous flap derived from the submental region, and is supplied by the submental vessels of the facial artery [11]. When mobilized on its vascular pedicle, the flap exhibits great flexibility and can be transposed into a number of locations. The flap is commonly employed in oral reconstruction (tongue, floor-of-mouth, buccal vestibule, palate), but other indications include defects of the oropharynx, hypopharynx and lower face.

The submental island flap offers several advantages. Like all pedicled flaps, it obviates the need for microvascular surgery. This feature alone would be expected to reduce operative time. We hypothesized that it would also reduce the demand on specialized care (ICU) as well as total hospital stay, and, consequently, reduce the overall costs associated with surgical care. Although it is beyond the scope of this paper, this flap has proven to be exceptionally reliable, and to provide plenty of pliable soft tissue up to 75 cm². The donor site is largely obscured by the chin, and older patients or those with significant skin redundancy (jowling) can enjoy a sharpened cervico-mental angle following the procedure. Although some surgeons have been reluctant to embrace the SIF on oncologic grounds, we have found it to afford a comprehensive level I lymphadenectomy, and this has been supported by high volume longitudinal studies [12].

These advantages make the SIF a good option for selected surgical defects which might otherwise have been reconstructed with free flaps. As with all reconstructive modalities, these pedicled flaps are not without potential disadvantages. In the SIF, these include excess tissue bulk and hair (beard)-bearing skin. As with the forearm free flap, these issues may need to be addressed with additional procedures. In most cases, neither bulk nor hair are issues if radiation therapy is required in the adjuvant setting.

In this paper we review a series of submental island flaps used for a broad range of indications. Recognizing the limitations of doing so in a public health system, we also estimate costs associated with this procedure, and compare these with a similar group reconstructed with forearm free flaps. In order to ensure homogeneity among the two groups, enrolment was restricted to patients receiving nearly identical oncologic surgery, including partial (up to 50 %) glossectomy with ipsilateral selective neck dissection. All patients also received a temporary tracheostomy. Costs are compared between those patients whose surgical defects were reconstructed with SIFs and those whose defects were reconstructed with forearm free flaps. We hypothesized that the SIF would offer substantial cost savings when compared to RFFF operations.

Methods
Patient demographics and outcomes
For initial assessment, all patients who received submental island flap reconstruction from January 1st 2013 to April 1st 2015 were examined retrospectively. All patients who received radial forearm free flaps over the same time period were evaluated as potential comparators. Within each of these two groups, those patients who met the inclusion criteria (surgery limited to

tracheotomy, <50 % glossectomy, and ipsilateral neck dissection) were included for the comparison. Cancer staging was based on the sixth edition of the tumor-node-metastasis staging system for head and neck cancer by the American Cancer Society [13]. Comorbidity scoring was based on the American Society of Anesthesiology (ASA) risk stratification score.

Cost analysis

Cost analysis was based on a cost difference method, where modalities similar in both SIF and RFFF reconstruction were effectively negated between the groups. This included pre-operative workup and consultation, intra-operative and post-operative pathology and pathologist costs, post-operative follow-up, and adjuvant therapy. Therefore, only costs associated with the operative procedure and post-operative hospital stay were included in the analysis. This included anesthesia costs, nursing costs, surgeon costs, operative consumable costs, ICU costs, and hospital stay costs. Additionally, an alternative cost difference analysis was completed using an estimation of the cost associated with flap debulking following SIF reconstruction.

Nursing costs were obtained by averaging the minimum and maximum hourly wages, as obtained by www.careerbeacon.com. This average was then included in calculations involving procedure time and number of nurses required for the procedure. Costs associated for remaining areas was obtained by contacting the Queen Elizabeth II Health Science Centre Business Department. Surgeon and anesthesiologist salaries were obtained from a previous publication in the division of otolaryngology – head and neck surgery at our institution [14]. Briefly, billing codes were used to determine the annual salary of Head and Neck Surgeons, which was divided by the average number of hours worked per week to yield an average hourly wage.

Statistical analysis and research approval

Statistical analysis was completed using the commercially available software SPSS (v21; IBM, Chicago, Illinois). Categorical variables were compared using either Chi-square test with or without Monte Carlo procedure (iteration = 10,000 cross tables). Continuous variables were compared using Student's T-Test or Mann–Whitney U-Test.

The Nova Scotia Research Ethics Board has approved this study as a Quality Assurance/Delivery of Care Initiative under Article 2.5 of the Tri-Council Policy Statement 2.

Results

Submental island flap reconstruction series patient demographics

A total of 12 patients were identified within the study period that were scheduled for submental island flap reconstruction. Two of the 12 were converted during the perioperative period to supraclavicular flap reconstruction, and one was converted to primary defect closure. Therefore, nine patients remained who underwent submental island flap reconstruction. All of the procedures were performed by a single surgeon (JT). Follow-up time ranged from 8 days to 746 days (Table 1; mean 272 days).

There was no strong gender predominance (44 % male), and the mean age at time of procedure was 65 years of age. Tumor size was generally large, with 33 % of patients having T3 or greater primary tumor size, and no tumor involvement less than T2. Defects commonly involved the tongue (66 %), floor of mouth (33 %), or palate (22 %). Full defect involvements for all patients are listed in Table 1.

Submental island flap reconstruction series patient outcomes

Flap sizes ranged from 7x4cm to 14x6cm, with a mean area of 37.4 cm (Table 1). All donor sites were closed

Table 1 Submental island flap group details

Patient	Age	Sex	Defect	Pathology	Flap size	Complications
1	53	F	Anterior tongue to base of tongue	Carcinoma in situ	7 x 4	Revision (tethering)
2	80	F	Retromolar trigone, palate, and oropharynx	T4 N0	14 x 6	
3	57	F	Left anterior tongue	pT2 N1 M0 SCC	8 x 5	Debulking, flap dehiscence
4	84	F	Maxilla, Hard palate, retromolar trigone	T4 N0 SCC		
5	68	M	Anterior and mid tongue, floor of mouth	T2 N0 SCC	12 x 4.5	Debulking
6	50	M	Tongue Base, floor of mouth	T2 N0		Depilation, debulking
7	60	F	Osteoradionecrosis of right mandible	N/A		External flap failure
8	74	M	Tongue, oropharynx	T3 N2a	14 x 5	
9	59	M	Tongue, floor of mouth		13 x 4.5	

primarily by local tissue advancements. The most common complications were requirement for debulking (33 %) and depilation (11 %). One patient required revision for reasons other than debulking (sulcus reconstruction). One patient experienced flap failure. This is believed to be the result of draping of the vascular pedicle over a heavy reconstruction plate.

Mean length of hospital stay in submental island flap reconstruction patients for all indications was 12.4 days, with a mean operative time of 346 min.

Submental island flap vs radial forearm flap glossectomy reconstruction comparison

There were nine patients in the SIF glossectomy group, and 12 patients in the RFFF group. The SIF group and the radial forearm free flap (RFFF) did not differ significantly in gender distribution, age, stage distribution, or comorbidity score ($p > 0.05$, Table 2). The RFFF did have significantly larger flap areas (56.9 vs 69.0 cm^2, $p < 0.05$, Table 2). No patients in the RFFF group required debulking or depilation (Table 3). Complications in the RFFF group are outlined in Table 3.

Mean length of ICU stay in glossectomy reconstruction RFFF patients was 4.7 days (Fig. 1). Only one patient required ICU stay for one night in the SIF group, giving a mean length of ICU stay of 0.14 days (Fig. 1). Mean length of hospital stay was not significantly different in SIF patients vs RFFF patients (12.4 vs 15.4 days, $p > 0.05$, Fig. 2). Mean operative time was significantly lower in the SIF group compared to the RFFF group (347 vs 552 min, $p < 0.05$, Fig. 3).

Cost analysis

For this study, mean hourly wage was calculated at $44.72 for nurses, $125 for anesthesiology and $140 for surgeons. One additional nurse is required for six hours in RFFF operations. Similarly, each RFFF operation requires two surgeons. The cost of the extra surgeon was estimated using the time required of the additional nurse.

Intraoperative costs are summarized in Table 4. Using the above salaries, nursing costs for RFFF operations

were 1.9 times greater than the nursing costs for SIF operations, anesthesiologist costs were 1.6 times greater, and surgeon costs for RFFF operations were 3.2 times greater. Total mean intraoperative costs were found to be $4780.59 for RFFF operations, versus $2307.94, yielding a total cost difference of $2472.65. This represents a cost increase of 2.1 times in the RFFF group. The greatest contributor to intraoperative cost savings were the costs of an additional surgeon for an extended operation length, resulting in a difference of $840.00.

One night in hospital was found to be $1404.00 per night, while one night in an ICU bed was calculated to be $6084.00 per night. This equated to a total mean cost of $18158.40 in the SIF group and $43617.60 in the RFFF group, yielding a cost difference of $25,459.20. This represents a cost increase of 2.4 times in the RFFF group for post-operative hospital stay alone, primarily due to the cost of ICU beds. Combining cost differences in both the intraoperative setting and postoperative hospital stay yields a total cost savings of $27931.85 for the SIF group. The greatest contributor to this total difference was the cost of post-operative stay (90.2 %).

The most common post-operative revision required in the SIF group was flap debulking. This is completed in the minor procedure clinic, and requires one nurse and one surgeon for one hour. Analysis shows an estimated cost of $184.72 for this procedure.

Discussion

With rising health care costs in Canada, concerns over the high costs of surgical care is well justified. Historically, the use of pedicled flaps in head and neck reconstruction has been overshadowed by the use of free flaps. However, free flaps are typically associated with longer operative times and increased length of hospital stays. Furthermore, free flaps have a requirement of intensive care monitoring in most centers for part of the post operative period. Due to these factors free flaps are associated with a much higher cost to the medical system and a more cost efficient option should be considered.

In direct comparison to radial forearm free flap reconstruction, submental island flap reconstruction was associated with shorter operative times and length of hospital stay. Furthermore, only a single patient in the SIF group required any intensive care monitoring, and in total spent a single day in the ICU. This is opposed to the RFFF group that required a minimum of one night ICU stay, and had a mean length of ICU stay much greater than this. It is institutional policy that all patients receiving any free flap spend a minimum of one night under intensive care monitoring.

The main objective of this study was to demonstrate the cost effectiveness of submental island flap

Table 2 Comparison of gender, age, tumor staging, and flap size

Variable	SIF	RFFF	Statistic
Gender (%)	43	75	$p > 0.05$
Age (years)	63	65	$p > 0.05$
Stage[a]			$p > 0.05$
ASA	2.4	2.3	$P > 0.05$
Flap Area	56.9	69.9	$p < 0.05$

[a]TNM is tumor (range T2 – T4), node involvement (range N0 – N2c), and distant metastasis (none in this study)
There was no significant difference in gender, age, or tumor stage

Table 3 Radial forearm free flap group details

Patient	Age	Sex	Defect	Pathology	Flap size	Complications
A	55	F	Left lateral tongue, pharynx, floor of mouth	T3N2c SCC	10 x 7	
B	64	M	Left tongue, right pharynx	T3N2b SCC	12 x 10	
C	61	M	Right tongue, right pharynx, right floor of mouth	T3N0 SCC	9 x 6	
D	71	M	Left tongue, left floor of mouth	T2N0M0 SCC	9 x 6	
E	63	M	Tongue, pharynx	T1N0M0 SC	12 x 6	
F	66	M	Tongue, oropharynx	T4aN0M0 SCC	10 x 12	
G	55	M	Tongue, floor of mouth	T3N0M0 ACC	8 x 5	Revision (tracheostomy teathering)
H	55	F	Left tongue, left pharynx, left floor of mouth	T3N2c SCC	10 x 7	
I	80	F	Left tongue, left floor of mouth	T2N0 SCC	8 x 5	
J	64	M	Left tongue, floor of mouth	T2N1 SCC	6 x 5	Hematoma (neck, left forearm), dysphagia, forearm wound infection
K	73	M	Right tongue	T2N1M0 SCC	8 x 4	
L	69	M	Tongue, pharynx, mandible	T4aN1	14 x 9	

reconstruction. It should also be noted, however, that SIF reconstruction does indeed offer excellent functional and cosmetic outcomes, particularly at the donor site. We have demonstrated the use of submental island flaps as a reliable and safe procedure in many forms of head and neck cancer reconstruction. Patients in our case series had very few complications, the majority of which were non life threatening. This is in keeping with previous studies which have shown the low morbidity and mortality rates of submental island flap reconstruction [7, 15–18]. Furthermore, when compared to RFFF reconstruction patients, SIF reconstruction patients had a similar incidence of complications, also with low severity.

Common disadvantages of SIF reconstruction often cited are the need for depilation and potential for recurrence due to submental and submandibular nodal involvement. Hair growth may be an issue in patients with thick, fast growing facial hair. In patients requiring adjuvant radiotherapy, hair growth quickly ceases. Recent studies have begun examining the most effective forms of depilation in SIF reconstruction patients, with electrolysis and laser therapy typically showing preferred results [19]. Finally, should patients not receive radiotherapy and elect to not receive depilation therapy, it has commonly been noted that over time, hair growth in the flap ceases independently (mucosalization) [20]. In terms of recurrence risk, several studies have shown no

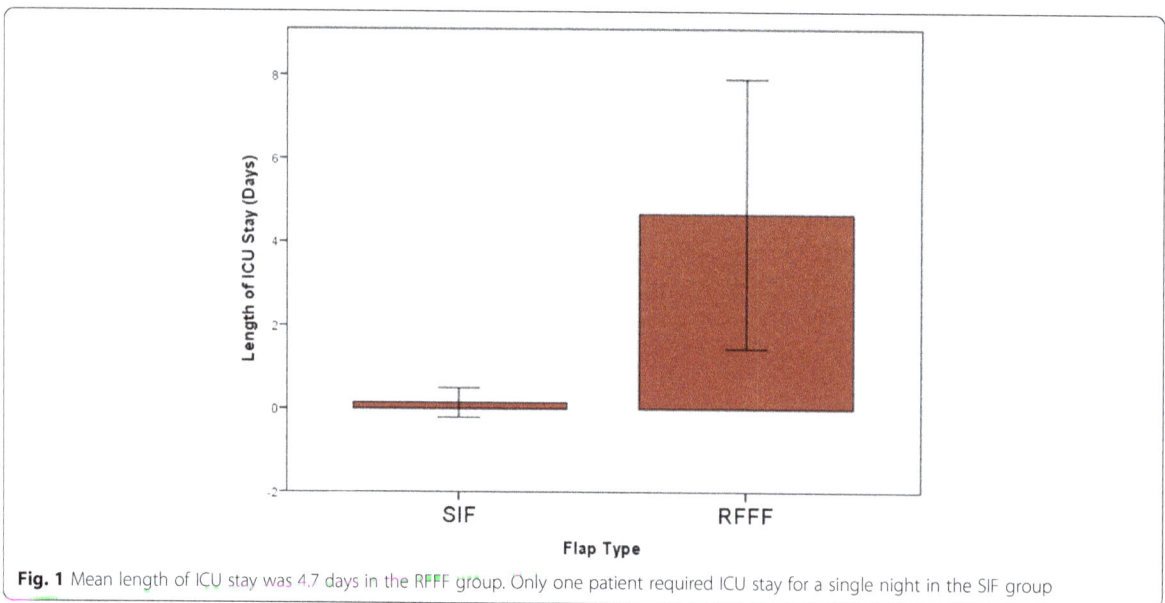

Fig. 1 Mean length of ICU stay was 4.7 days in the RFFF group. Only one patient required ICU stay for a single night in the SIF group

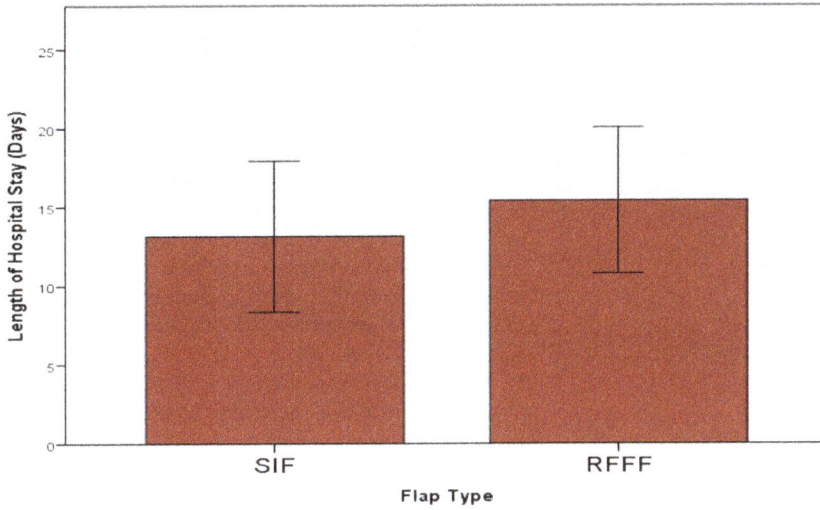

Fig. 2 The mean length of hospital stay was not significantly different between SIF patients and RFFF patients

increased risk of recurrence when there is no obvious nodal involvement [12]. This risk is further decreased with judicious node dissection and thinning of the flap during harvesting. Indeed, we have not yet experienced any recurrence when utilizing the submental island flap for reconstruction of head and neck cancers.

Another possible sequelae of SIF reconstruction is the need for flap debulking in the post-operative period. In this study, 33 % of patients required debulking of their flap. Disposables are also an associated cost of this procedure, but vary according to the patient and specific procedure, and are generally low. We have therefore estimated the cost of flap debulking using only the

associated personnel cost, and found it to be minimal when it is necessary.

The submental island flap also offers excellent cosmetic outcomes. The incision for flap harvesting may be hidden in the submental crease, behind the mandibular arch, and due to the nature of the harvest, many patients express enjoyment of their "neck tightening" procedure. Furthermore, when used for facial reconstruction, the color matching ability of the submental island flap is essentially unparalleled.

Further advantages of the submental island flap are seen with surgeon preferences, in that the submental island flap is a relatively easy and safe dissection. The

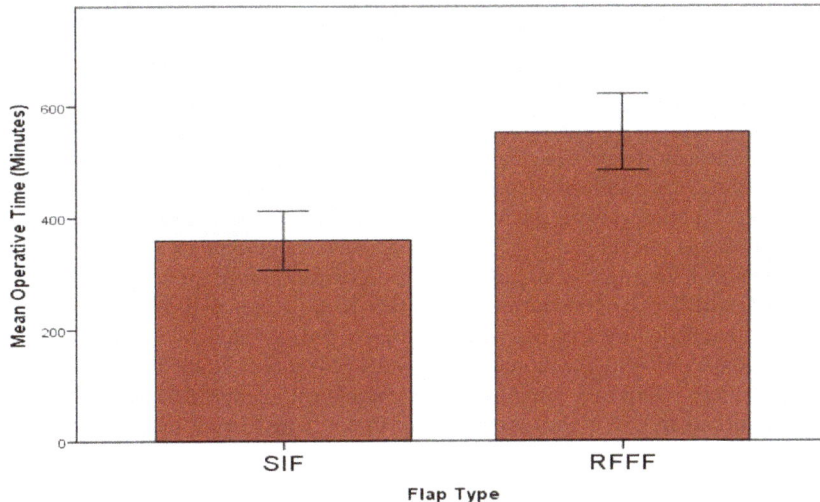

Fig. 3 The mean operative time was significantly lower in the SIF group as compared to the RFFF group

Table 4 Intraoperative cost breakdown

Flap Type	HCP	Number of HCP	Hourly wage ($/h)	Hours	Total Cost ($)
SIF	Nurse	3	44.72	5.78	775.45
	Surgeon	1	140	5.78	809.62
	Anaesthesiologist	1	125	5.78	722.88
RFFF	Nurse	3	44.72	9.2	1234.27
	Extra Nurse	1	44.72	6	268.32
	Surgeon	1	140	9.2	1288.00
	Extra Surgeon	1	140	6	840.00
	Anaesthesiologist	1	125	9.2	1150.00

HCP = Health care professional, SIF = Submental island flap, RFFF = Radial forearm free flap

technique of harvesting the flap has recently been modified to be safe for residents in training [21], potentially offering further widespread use. Tissue from the submental region is also thin, supple, and pliable, giving it ideal characteristics for reconstruction.

Our SIF group findings are comparible in terms of mean flap area and length of hospital stay to a previous study be Paydarfar et al. [17] examining SIF vs RFFF in oral reconstruction. Patients in our study experienced shorter operative times than this previous study, regardless of whether examining the glossectomy subset or full patient population.

The cost differences in this study were found to be in agreement with our hypothesis. Substantial cost differences were observed when comparing SIF reconstructions to RFFF reconstructions. This finding is similar to those reported by Miller et al. whereby submental island flaps were associated with a 40 % cost reduction in reconstruction of temporal bone defects as compared to free flaps [7].

Reduced cost associated with procedures is alluring in itself. However, in dividing the cost differences into their component parts, other advantages of SIF operations have been highlighted.

The majority of cost differences were due to ICU requirement following RFFF reconstruction. Utilizing pedicled flaps in order to reduce the number of patients requiring ICU beds would therefore increase ICU bed availability. Not all institutions include protocols for minimum length of ICU stay following free flap reconstructions. It is debated whether ICU monitoring is required in the post-operative period for free flap reconstruction [22]. However, some authors have supported a minimum ICU stay for patient safety and complication prevention [23]. For institutions in which post operative ICU stay is not required, the cost saving associated with pedicled flaps would be reduced. It is also important to note that institutions that do not require an ICU stay often still require a one-to-one nurse-to-patient ratio in

the immediate post-operative period, which increases costs. Nonetheless, for institutions including post-operative ICU monitoring as part of their free flap protocols, pedicled flaps offer an opportunity to reduce cost and improve bed availability.

Despite contributing a lesser amount to overall cost savings, the cost differences and health care professional requirements are important. Free flap reconstruction in this study required an extra nurse for six hours, and an extra surgeon for those six hours. Pedicled flaps therefore offer the opportunity for hospital staff resources to be used more efficiently, and potentially allow additional procedures to be completed. Regardless of differences in cost, the increased time required for free flap reconstruction potentially covers the time of an additional pedicled flap operation (ie, three SIF operations may take place in the time required for two RFFF operations). Performing pedicled flaps when possible may therefore help reduce patient wait times by increasing the number of potential operations in a given time span. Furthermore, the decreased operative time associated with pedicled flap reconstruction may benefit patients unable to tolerate longer operative times. With relatively few downsides, pedicled flaps clearly offer many potential advantages over free flaps when the case is appropriate. Finally, pedicled flaps allow for treatment of time-sensitive cancer cases that would otherwise be postponed or cancelled if ICU beds were not available.

There are limitations to this study. The sample population was small, although it does represent the majority of submental island flap reconstructions at this institution. The two groups used for comparison were not perfect matches. However, we were able to highlight the lack of statistical significance in gender, patient age, and tumor stage between SIF and RFFF groups. Flap area was larger in the RFFF group. This outlines that RFFF reconstruction may be more appropriate than SIF reconstruction when larger defects are expected. Limitations in the cost analysis portion of the study were also present. Namely, cost difference was completed as opposed to specific cost analysis. Several factors were assumed to be equivalent between RFFF and SIF operations, namely the preoperative work up costs and postoperative requirements unrelated to hospital stay, such as recurrence, follow-up visits, etc. However, we believe this is an accurate picture of the cost differences between pedicled and free flaps, and our analysis offers a valid preliminary study detailing the cost savings that are possible with pedicled flaps.

In summary, rising health care costs in Canada have called into question the utility of expensive surgeries when cheaper alternatives are available. We have demonstrated the use of the submental island flap as an alternative to radial forearm free flaps, showing both decreased hospital costs and adequate patient and cosmetic outcomes. Pedicled flaps are making a return to the field of head and neck reconstruction, and the submental island flap offers an excellent alternative to more intricate and demanding free flap alternatives

Conclusions

Head and neck cancer remains a substantial contributor to total cancer incidence in Canada. Many of these cancers require reconstruction of surgical defects which vary in size. Rising health care costs dictate that more cost effective procedures should be considered where possible. Free flaps have become a staple in head and neck reconstruction, yet pedicled flaps offer shorter operative times as well as potential for faster patient recovery. In this study, we have detailed that the pedicled submental island flap offers adequate patient outcomes compared to the radial forearm free flap in glossectomy reconstruction, and offers substantial cost savings through reduced operative time and decreased length of ICU stay. This offers further support for the recent resurgence of pedicled flap use, specifically the submental island flap.

Abbreviations
ICU: intensive care unit; RFFF: radial forearm free flap; SIF: submental island flap; SPD: shipping, processing, and delivery; TNM: tumor, node, metastasis (staging).

Competing interests
The authors declare that they have no competing interests.

Authors' contributions
DF completed the retrospective chart review, analyzed patient data, drafted the manuscript and jointly completed cost analysis. TP jointly completed cost analysis and contributed manuscript edits. MR performed aspects of select radial forearm free flap surgeries and contributed manuscript edits. RH performed aspects of select radial forearm free flap surgeries and contributed manuscript edits. JT performed aspects of select radial forearm free flap surgeries, performed all submental island flap surgeries, contributed manuscript edits, and approved the final manuscript. All authors read and approved the final manuscript.

Authors' information
JT is a staff Otolaryngologist – Head and Neck surgeon at the Queen Elizabeth II Health Sciences Center (Victoria General Hospital, associated with Dalhousie University), specializing in head and neck oncology and reconstructive surgery. MT is a staff Otolaryngologist – Head and Neck surgeon at the Queen Elizabeth II Health Sciences Center (Victoria General Hospital, associated with Dalhousie University), specializing in head and neck surgery, facial, plastic, and reconstructive surgery; and oncology. RH is a staff Otolaryngologist – Head and Neck surgeon at the Queen Elizabeth II Health Sciences Center (Victoria General Hospital, associated with Dalhousie University), specializing in head and neck oncology, microvascular head and neck reconstruction, and thyroid and parathyroid surgery. MR is a staff Otolaryngologist – Head and Neck surgeon at the Queen Elizabeth II Health Sciences Center (Victoria General Hospital, associated with Dalhousie University), specializing in head and neck surgical oncology, thyroid and parathyroid surgery, rhinology and anterior skull base surgery, and microvascular head and neck reconstruction. TP is a PGY-4 resident in otolaryngology – head and neck surgery at Dalhousie University. DF is a 3rd year medical student at Dalhousie University.

References
1. Jemal A, Bray F, Center MM, Ferlay J, Ward E, Forman D. Global cancer statistics. CA Cancer J Clin. 2011;61(2):69–90. doi:10.3322/caac.20107.
2. Siegel RL, Miller K, Jemal A. Cancer statistics, 2015. CA Cancer J Clin. 2015;65(1):5–29.
3. Society CC, Records NCIoCACo, Registries. Canadian cancer statistics. Canadian Cancer Society's Advisory Committee on Cancer Statistics. Canadian Cancer Statistics 2015. Toronto, ON: Canadian Cancer Society; 2015.
4. Brana I, Siu LL. Locally advanced head and neck squamous cell cancer: treatment choice based on risk factors and optimizing drug prescription. Ann Oncol. 2012;23(10):1780185.
5. Chim H, Salgado CJ, Seselgyte R, Wei FC, Mardini S. Principles of head and neck reconstruction: an algorithm to guide flap selection. Semin Plast Surg. 2010;2(1535–2188):148–54.
6. Smeele LE, Goldstein D, Tsai V, Gullane PJ, Neligan P, Brown DH, et al. Morbidity and cost differences between free flap reconstruction and pedicled flap reconstruction in oral and oropharyngeal cancer: Matched control study. J Otolaryngol. 2006;35(2):102–7.
7. Miller C, Hanley JC, Gernon TJ, Erman A, Jacob A. The Submental Island Flap for Reconstruction of Temporal Bone Defects. Otology and Neurotology. 2015;36(5):879–85.
8. Canadian Institute for Health Information. National Health Expenditure Trends, 1975 to 2014. Ottawa, ON: CIHI; 2014.
9. Nichols AC, Palma DA, Dhaliwal SS, Tan S, Theuer J, Chow W et al. The epidemic of human papillomavirus and oropharyngeal cancer in a Canadian population. Curr Oncol. Vol 20, No 4 (2013). 2013;212-19.
10. Martin D, Pascal JF, Baudet J, Mondie JM, Farhat JB, Athoum A, et al. The submental island flap: a new donor site. Anatomy and clinical applications as a free or pedicled flap. Plast Reconstr Surg. 1993;92(5):867–73.
11. Faltaous AA, Yetman RJ. The submental artery flap: an anatomic study. Plast Reconstr Surg. 1996;97(1):56–60.
12. Howard BE, Nagel TH, Donald CB, Hinni ML, Hayden RE. Oncologic Safety of the Submental Flap for Reconstruction in Oral Cavity Malignancies. Otolaryngol Head Neck Surg. 2014;150(4):558–62. doi:10.1177/0194599814520687.
13. Patel SG, Shah JP. TNM staging of cancers of the head and neck: striving for uniformity among diversity. CA Cancer J Clin. 2005;55(4):242–58.
14. Phillips TJ, Sader C, Brown T, Bullock M, Wilke D, Trites JR, et al. Transoral laser microsurgery versus radiation therapy for early glottic cancer in Canada: cost analysis. J Otolaryngol Head Neck Surg. 2009;38(6):619–23.
15. Chow TL, Chan TT, Chow TK, Fung SC, Lam SH. Reconstruction with submental flap for aggressive orofacial cancer. Plast Reconstr Surg. 2007; 120(2):431–6.
16. Multinu A, Ferrari S, Bianchi B, Balestreri A, Scozzafava E, Ferri A, et al. The submental island flap in head and neck reconstruction. Int J Oral Maxillofac Surg. 2007;36(8):716–20.
17. Paydarfar JA, Patel UA. Submental island pedicled flap vs radial forearm free flap for oral reconstruction: Comparison of outcomes. Arch Otolaryngol Head Neck Surg. 2011;137(1):82–7.
18. Sebastian P, Thomas S, Varghese BT, Iype EM, Balagopal PG, Mathew PC. The submental island flap for reconstruction of intraoral defects in oral cancer patients. Oral Oncol. 2008;44(11):1014–8.
19. Kaune KM, Haas E, Jantke M, Kramer FJ, Gruber R, Thoms KM, et al. Successful Nd:YAG Laser Therapy for Hair Removal in the Oral Cavity after Plastic Reconstruction Using Hairy Donor Sites. Dermatology. 2013;226(4): 324–8.
20. Amin AA, Sakkary MA, Khalil AA, Rifaat MA, Zayed SB. The submental flap for oral cavity reconstruction: Extended indications and technical refinements. Head Neck Oncol. 2011;3:51. doi:10.1186/1758-3284-3-51.
21. Patel UA, Bayles SW, Hayden RE. The submental flap: A modified technique for resident training. Laryngoscope. 2007;117(1):186–9.
22. Arshad H, Ozer HG, Thatcher A, Old M, Ozer E, Agarwal A, et al. Intensive care unit versus non-intensive care unit postoperative management of head and neck free flaps: comparative effectiveness and cost comparisons. Head Neck. 2014;36(4):536–9. doi:10.1002/hed.23325.
23. Ryan MW, Hochman M. Length of stay after free flap reconstruction of the head and neck. Laryngoscope. 2000;110(2):210.

25

Decisional conflict in patients considering diagnostic thyroidectomy with indeterminate fine needle aspirate cytopathology

Benjamin A. Taylor, Robert D. Hart, Matthew H. Rigby, Jonathan Trites, S. Mark Taylor and Paul Hong[*]

Abstract

Background: Fine needle aspiration (FNA) cytopathology is the gold standard work-up for thyroid nodules. However, indeterminate lesions are encountered commonly and can lead to difficult treatment decisions. We sought to determine whether patients experienced decisional conflict surrounding management with diagnostic thyroidectomy in the setting of indeterminate FNA results.

Methods: Patients with indeterminate results of thyroid nodule FNA were prospectively enrolled. All consultations were carried out by three otolaryngologists in a consistent manner. After consultation, participants completed a demographics form and the Decisional Conflict Scale (DCS) questionnaire.

Results: Thirty-five patients (28 female) between the ages of 30 and 88 years (mean age 54.89) participated. The median total DCS score was 10.94 (interquartile range, 4.69–25.0). Twelve patients (34 %) scored at or above 25 on the DCS, indicating clinically significant level of decisional conflict. Patients reported feeling significantly more confident about their decision after the surgical consultation compared to before the consultation ($p = 0.00$). The total DCS score was significantly negatively correlated with self-reported confidence after the consultation ($r = -0.421, p = 0.012$).

Conclusion: Many patients experienced clinically significant decisional conflict when considering thyroidectomy for management of a thyroid nodule with indeterminate cytopathology. Future research should be directed at developing decision support tools for this patient group, and exploring the impact of decisional conflict on health outcomes.

Keywords: Decisional conflict, Thyroid cancer, Thyroidectomy, Fine needle aspiration, Shared decision-making

Background

Thyroid cancer has demonstrated the most rapid increase in incidence of any cancer in North America, and now ranks as the fifth most common cancer in women [1, 2]. Part of the increase is attributed to early detection, often incidentally, through improved diagnostic imaging techniques [3–5].

One of the most important diagnostic tools for suspected thyroid cancer is the fine needle aspirate (FNA).

The FNA is performed for most thyroid nodules greater than 1.5 cm, or smaller in patients with suspicious sonographic features or those with high-risk history [6]. Over 500,000 thyroid nodule FNA procedures are performed annually in the United States [7]. The sample obtained via FNA is analyzed cytopathologically and reported at most institutions with the guidance of the Bethesda Grading System [8]. The Bethesda system describes six categories: nondiagnostic or unsatisfactory, benign, atypia of undetermined significance (AUS) or follicular lesion of undetermined significance (FLUS), follicular neoplasm or suspicious for a follicular neoplasm (SFN), suspicious for malignancy (SFM), or malignant [8].

* Correspondence: Paul.Hong@iwk.nshealth.ca
Division of Otolaryngology Head and Neck Surgery, Department of Surgery, IWK Health Centre, Dalhousie University, 5850 University Avenue, Halifax, NS B3K 6R8, Canada

Indeterminate results include AUS, FLUS, and SFN, which are encountered in about 15–30 % of samples, and carry a 6–32 % risk of malignancy [7, 9, 10]. Practice guidelines have traditionally recommended surgery for indeterminate lesions; however, final pathology yields a benign result in 70–85 % of cases [7].

Patients with indeterminate results on FNA who are considering diagnostic thyroidectomy may face challenges in decision-making because of limited consultation time with surgeons, complexity of information on risks/benefits, and the uncertainty of their diagnosis. As a result, patients may experience *decisional conflict*, which can lead to emotional distress and other negative sequelae [11, 12]. Tools such as decision aids can help patients and practitioners become more involved in decision-making by providing information about treatment options and outcomes, clarifying personal values about the treatment, and providing guidance throughout the decision-making process. The use of decision aids has been shown to result in a range of favorable outcomes including less decisional conflict, improved patient knowledge, and greater concordance between patient values and chosen treatment option [13]. As well, the use of decision aids can lead to reduction in unnecessary variation in care and costs across different healthcare regions [14]. In fact, there is a sleeper provision in the Affordable Care Act (Section 3506) that encourages the use of shared decision-making in healthcare with decision aids. Before a decision aid can be appropriately developed, a decision-needs analysis is first required, which includes measuring the level of decisional conflict in certain procedures.

There is a paucity of data in the literature surrounding decisional conflict and to date, none are available for diagnostic thyroidectomy. The purpose of this study was to assess the level of decisional conflict in patients with an indeterminate result on thyroid nodule FNA who are considering thyroidectomy. We also evaluated the relationship between patient factors and decisional conflict

Methods

All adult patients who received an indeterminate result on thyroid FNA during the study period (January 2014 to June 2014) were invited to participate in this study. The only exclusion criteria was the inability to speak or read English ($n = 0$) or the lack of decision-making authority ($n = 0$). Also, patients who had multiple FNAs of the same thyroid nodule were also excluded ($n = 4$). All patients were being considered for diagnostic hemithyroidectomy.

Patients were approached after the consultation visit with their head and neck surgeon where they were informed of their indeterminate FNA results. Informed consent for inclusion in this study was obtained from all those who agreed to participate. Each patient was asked to complete a Demographic/Condition form and the Decisional Conflict Scale (DCS).

For providers, three head and neck fellowship trained otolaryngologists participated. All used a consistent script to ensure that similar information was shared during the visit.

Local Institutional Review Board approval was obtained for this study.

Demographic/condition form

The demographic information collected on this form included patient age, family composition, employment status, occupation and income. Data was also collected on previous surgical experience, confidence level in their medical decision-making before and after the consultation, how well they usually handle medical appointments, and whether they were aware that surgery was an option before presenting.

Decisional conflict scale (DCS)

This 16-item scale assesses patient uncertainty about medical decisions. It is a Likert scale with ratings of strongly agree, agree, neither agree or disagree, disagree, and strongly disagree. The DCS produces a total score ranging from 0 (no decisional conflict) to 100 (maximal decisional conflict). Five Subscales scores are also produced. The subscales are interpreted as follows: uncertainty subscale [scores range from 0 (extremely certain about best choice) to 100 (extremely uncertain about best choice)], informed subscale [0 (feels extremely informed) to 100 (feels extremely uninformed)], values clarity subscale [0 (feels extremely clear about personal values for benefits and risks) to 100 (feels extremely unclear about personal values)], support subscale [0 (extremely supported in decision making) to 100 (extremely unsupported in decision making)], and effective decision-making subscale [0 (good decision) to 100 (bad decision)] [16].

The DCS is a validated scale that is designed to be context non-specific. It has demonstrated high test-retest reliability and high content validity, as scores on the DCS were higher for patients who delayed or were unsure of their decision in comparison to those who accepted or rejected treatments [16]. Previous research has defined clinically significant decisional conflict as a DCS score at or above 25 [16].

Data analysis

The DCS scores were not normally distributed; therefore, nonparametric statistical tests were used. Descriptive statistics including median, interquartile range (IQR), and standard error (SE) of the total DCS scores are reported. The DCS subscale scores along with the number of patients with total DCS score at or above 25, indicating clinically significant decisional conflict, are also reported. The relationship between baseline factors and total DCS scores were explored using Mann Whitney U tests.

Results

Participants

The study was conducted at a head and neck oncology clinic situated in a tertiary care academic hospital in Eastern Canada. Thirty-five new consecutive patients who met the inclusion criteria were invited to participate in this study. All patients approached agreed to participate. None of the patients had other diagnostic testing (e.g., molecular testing or gene profile analysis).

Patients ranged in age from 30 to 88 years (mean = 54.89, SD = 15.30). Twenty-eight (80 %) patients were female and 7 (20 %) were male. Twenty-eight (80 %) patients had undergone previous surgery in the past, and 19 (68 %) of those had undergone more than one. The most common operations reported were tonsillectomy ($n = 7$), gynecological procedures ($n = 6$), cesarean section ($n = 5$), breast surgery ($n = 5$), and cholecystectomy ($n = 4$). Twenty (57 %) patients had family members who had undergone previous surgery. All patients reported that they had handled previous medical visits well ($n = 9$) or very well ($n = 26$). Most patients ($n = 33$, 94 %) reported that they knew surgery was an option prior to the consultation visit, while one patient was unaware (data was unavailable for one participant).

Three head and neck fellowship trained otolaryngologists, ranging in age from 36 to 46 years, participated. All were male. All were in a salaried academic practice and all trained in North America.

Decisional conflict

The median total DCS score was 10.94 (SE = 3.01, IQR = 4.69–25). Twelve patients (34 %) were found to have clinically significant decisional conflict, as they scored at or above 25 on the DCS (Fig. 1). Three patients (8.5 %) scored zero on the DCS, indicating no uncertainty about their decision. Summary of the DCS results is presented in Table 1.

There were no significant differences in the total DCS scores or subscale scores based on whether the patient had previous surgery or if another family member had previous surgery. As well, no significant correlation existed between DCS scores and patient income, patient gender, or previous awareness of surgery. However, there was a significantly negative correlation between values clarity subscale scores and patients' self-report of how well they tolerated previous surgery ($r = -0.347$, $p = 0.041$). As well, patient age and support subscale scores were significantly positively correlated ($r = 0.382$, $p = 0.023$).

Patients' self-reported confidence levels were significantly higher after surgical consultation (mean = 7.11 out of 10) compared to before consultation (mean = 6.43 out of 10; $p = 0.00$). The total DCS score was significantly negatively correlated with confidence level after consultation ($r = -0.421$, $p = 0.012$).

Discussion

It is estimated that 15–30 % of FNA samples yield indeterminate results, of which 70–85 % are diagnosed to be benign after thyroidectomy [3, 4]. In light of this uncertainty, patients may experience decisional conflict when faced with the decision to proceed with diagnostic surgery. In the current study, the median total DCS score was 10.94. However, 12 (34 %) individuals scored at or above the cutoff score of 25, indicating the presence of clinically significant decisional conflict. This level of decisional conflict is similar to previous studies that have assessed other elective surgical procedures [12, 15, 18–23]. Given the high prevalence of indeterminate thyroid lesions, the number of patients experiencing decisional conflict may be substantial. Decisional conflict is associated with negative outcomes such as emotional distress, cancelled surgeries, and non-adherence to treatment plans [12]. To overcome this problem, an approach is needed to help both healthcare providers and their patients in surgical decision-making.

Shared decision-making is a strategy that could be used in the current patient population. This is an approach that requires collaboration between healthcare providers and their patients to understand the treatment options and have knowledge of the risks and benefits of these options. At the same time, shared decisions should consider the patients' own preferences and values in decision-making [17]. The importance of shared decision-making goes well beyond reducing decisional conflict and the associated negative outcomes. This includes improved quality of care and reduced variation in care and costs across different regions since there is a more consistent decision-making process and better compliance with clinical guidelines [15]. As mentioned above, there is a provision in the Affordable Care Act that encourages the use of shared decision-making in healthcare [24]. Unfortunately, the concept of shared decision-making in medicine is in its infancy at this time.

To date, no studies have assessed the level of decisional conflict in patients considering diagnostic thyroidectomy. However, a decisional conflict analysis was performed on patients considering adjuvant radioactive iodine treatment for early stage papillary thyroid cancer as part of a randomized control trial assessing the utility of a decision aid. The mean total DCS score was very high (52.1, SD = 21.9) in those patients deciding on whether to accept or reject the radioactive iodine treatment [18]. Clearly, significant

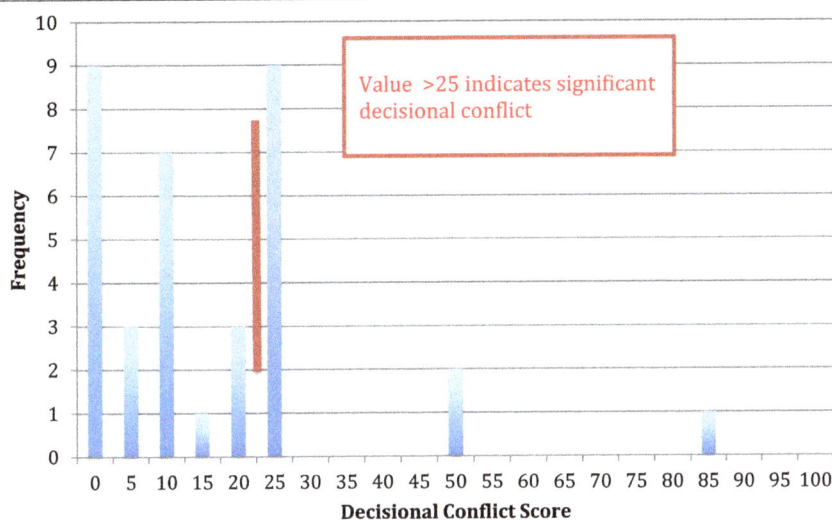

Fig. 1 Frequency of total Decisional Conflict Scale scores. Scores to the right of the red line (≥25) indicate clinically significant decisional conflict

decisional conflict is prevalent in patients who are undergoing work-up and treatment of thyroid nodules and malignancies.

There are other studies reporting decisional conflict in patients undergoing work-up and treatment of malignancies. Women diagnosed with ductal carcinoma in situ of the breast were found to have a mean total DCS score of 20.5 with 47 % reporting clinically significant decisional conflict when considering various treatment options [19]. Another study with breast cancer patients faced with surgical decisions reported a mean total DCS score of 19.9 [20]. Studies in patients dealing with prostate cancer screening and pre-treatment decisions found a mean total DCS score of 25 [21] and 53 [22], respectively. Again, these data indicate that decisional conflict is common in patients with common malignancies.

Subscale analysis of the DCS showed that the uncertainty and values clarity subscales had the highest levels of decisional conflict. The informed and support subscales had the lowest levels of decisional conflict. Patient age and support subscale scores were significantly positively correlated, indicating that older patients were more likely to have less support in their decision-making. This is an important finding as older patients without adequate social or family support may be at higher risk of having significant

decisional conflict. Therefore, clinicians may need to provide additional decision support to some older patients.

A significant negative correlation existed between values clarity subscale scores and patients' self-report on how well they handled previous surgeries. This indicates that patients were more likely to feel clearer about personal values for the benefits and risks of surgery if they did not handle previous operations well. One would expect that a patient with positive previous surgical experience would be more familiar and perhaps more insightful to their personal values regarding surgery. However, the converse was noted in the current study. The explanation for this finding is unclear but the modest nature of the correlation should be iterated ($r = -0.347$, $p = 0.041$).

Patients were significantly more confident in their decision-making after the surgical consultation, compared to before. This was a reassuring finding that consultation with surgeons, which involved a detailed discussion of the risks and benefits of the diagnostic surgery, had a positive effect on the decision-making process. However, it is to be noted that the change in confidence level (6.43 to 7.11 out of 10) was small and the clinical significance remains unclear. Therefore, effect size calculation with increased sample size is required to make a more definitive conclusion.

Table 1 Median total decisional conflict scale and subscale scores

	Total	Uncertainty	Informed	Clarity	Support	Effective
Median	10.94	25.00	8.33	25.00	8.33	12.50
SE	3.01	3.23	2.32	2.57	2.08	2.27
IQR	4.69–25	8.33–25	0.00–25	0.00–25	0.00–25	0.00–25

Abbreviations: SE standard error, *IQR* interquartile range

Unsurprisingly, the total DCS score was significantly negatively correlated with self-reported confidence level after the consultation visit. Although causation cannot be proven, this suggests that most individuals felt more confident after the consultation, which may have contributed to lower levels of decisional conflict.

Decision aids are evidence-based tools used to support patients in challenging medical decision-making situations (i.e., when there isn't one superior treatment option). Decision aids have been shown to improve patient knowledge, enhance shared decision-making, increase the number of patients with realistic ideas about the risks and benefits of a medical procedure, and reduce decisional conflict [23]. They can also empower the patient with information to facilitate a more meaningful and informed discussion with their physician [24]. Decision aids usually include three sections: 1) a description of the health condition and management options being considered; 2) a summary of the evidence for each of these options including risks and benefits; 3) and an element to help the patient consider this information in the context of their personal values [25].

In oncology, decision aids have been used in cancer patients considering surgical intervention with good success. In a meta-analysis, O'Brien et al. found that the use of decision aids in cancer related illness leads to significantly improved knowledge about screening, treatment, and preventative measures compared to usual practice [26]. Overall, the use of well-developed decision aids led to reduced decisional conflict and no increase in general anxiety [26]. Further support for decision aids comes from randomized controlled trials in patients with thyroid, breast, and prostate malignancies. Decisional conflict was significantly reduced in patients given decision aids, compared to those who underwent conventional consultation [18, 19, 21, 22]. Although there are many positive aspects, no comprehensive evidence-based decision aids exist in otolaryngology at this time [25]. Clearly, decision support tools, such as decision aids, would benefit patients with indeterminate thyroid nodule FNA results.

There has been a recent call for the development of decision aids in otolaryngology as there are many elective surgical procedures within this specialty (e.g., tonsillectomy, sinus surgery, rhinoplasty) [25, 27]. Although there are numerous processes reported for developing decision aids [28], the most rigorous and well-received method is best practices recommended by the International Patient Decision Aid Standards (IPDAS) Collaboration [29]. The IPDAS framework outlines an iterative process, which allows multiple stakeholders (e.g., patients, clinicians, decision experts) to define their needs so that the decision aid will be feasible and useful to all potential users. Even though there are a number of decision aids currently available, many have been developed without following a specific methodology, which can lead to poor quality and information presented in a biased manner [28]. Therefore, decision aids in otolaryngology and beyond should be created following the method outlined by the IPDAS Collaboration.

Limitations of this study include the involvement of multiple head and neck surgeons. This caused an inherent variability of approach to patients and counseling style, perhaps resulting in different experiences for patients. To control for this, the surgeons used a semi-structured interview script to keep the delivered information consistent (i.e., same risks and benefits discussed). Unfortunately, the sample size did not allow for direct statistical comparison of the DCS scores between surgeons. The use of multiple providers does, however, allow for a more broad perspective of the decisional conflict that exists across the patient population. The second limitation of this study is the consideration of only indeterminate thyroid lesions. More information regarding decisional conflict could be gleaned from comparison of all FNA results. Third, the long-term influence of clinically significant decisional conflict is unknown in our study population. That is, some patients with decisional conflict may have been less satisfied with their overall experience or may have changed their decision over time. Fourth, some demographic information was not measured (e.g., education levels, ethnicity) that may have influenced the level of post-consultation decisional conflict. Finally, the sample size of the participants was small, but was comparable to other studies assessing decisional conflict [12, 15, 18–22, 30].

To advance research in this area, future studies should consider incorporating observations of consultation visits (e.g., video-recording) of a larger number of providers across multiple healthcare centers. Moreover, research should assess long-term outcomes of decisional conflict including knowledge about the procedure and postoperative care. Finally, as mentioned above, future research should aim to identify strategies that could improve the decision making process for patients (and providers) with the potential aim of developing decision support tools, such as decision aids.

Conclusion

Many patients with indeterminate thyroid FNA results experienced clinically significant decisional conflict and therefore were uncertain about their decision to proceed with diagnostic thyroidectomy. Decisional conflict has been associated with many negative outcomes, and therefore future research should aim to find methods to reduce decisional conflict.

Competing interests
The authors declare that they have no competing interests.

Authors' contributions

BAT participated in the design of the study, data collection and analysis, and wrote the first draft of the manuscript. RDH, MHR, JT, and SMT participated in data collection and analysis, and revised the all versions of the manuscript. PH participated in the design of the study, data analysis, and revised all versions of the manuscript. All authors read and approved the final manuscript.

Acknowledgements

We thank all patients who participated in this study. We also thank the clinical staff that assisted in patient recruitment and data collection. Finally, we are grateful to Dr. Ayala Gorodzinsky for her help with statistical analyses.

References

1. Nguyen QT, Lee EJ, Huang MG, Park YI, Khullar A, Plodkowski RA. Diagnosis and treatment of patients with thyroid cancer. Am Health Drug Benefits. 2015;8:30–40.
2. Hoang JK, Nguyen XV, Davies L. Overdiagnosis of thyroid cancer. Acad Radiol. 2015;22:1024–9.
3. Aspinall SR, Ong SG, Wilson MS, Lennard TW. How shall we manage the incidentally found thyroid nodule? J Surge. 2013;11:96–104.
4. Sosa JA, Hanna JW, Robinson KA, Lanman RB. Increases in thyroid nodule fine-needle aspirations, operations, and diagnoses of thyroid cancer in the United States. J Surg. 2013;154:1420–7.
5. Hegedus L. Clinical practice: the thyroid nodule. N Engl J Med. 2004;351: 1764–71.
6. Cooper DS, Doherty GM, Haugen BR, Kloos RT, Lee SL, Mandel SJ, Mazzaferri EL, McIver B, Pacini F, Schlumberger M, Sherman SI, Stweard DL, Tuttle RM. Revised american thyroid association management guidelines for patients with thyroid nodules and differentiated thyroid cancer. Thy. 2009;19:1167–214.
7. Duick DS, Klopper JP, Diggans JC, Friedman L, Kennedy GC, Lanman RB, McIver B. The impact of benign gene expression classifier test results on the endocrinologist-patient decision to operate on patients with thyroid nodules with indeterminate fine-needle aspiration cytopathology. Thy. 2012; 22:996–1001.
8. Cibas ES, Ali SZ. The Bethesda system for reporting thyroid cytopathology. Am J Clin Pathol. 2009;132:658–65.
9. Terris DJ, Snyder S, Carneiro-Pla D, Inabnet WB, Kandil E, Orloff L, Shindo M, Tufano RP, Tuttle RM, Urken M, Yeh MW. American thyroid association surgical affairs committee writing task force american thyroid association statement on Outpatient thyroidectomy. Thy. 2013;23:1193–120.
10. Williams BA, Bullock MJ, Trites JR, Taylor SM, Hart RD. Rates of thyroid malignancy by FNA diagnostic category. J Otolaryngol Head Neck Surg. 2013;42:61.
11. LeBlanc A, Kenny DA, O'Connor AM, Légaré F. Decisional conflict in patients and their physicians: a dyadic approach to shared decision making. Med Decis Making. 2009;29:61–8.
12. Graham ME, Haworth R, Chorney J, Bance M, Hong P. Decisional conflict in patients considering bone-anchored hearing devices in children with unilateral aural atresia. Ann Otol Rhinol Laryngol. 2015;124:925–30.
13. Légaré F, O'Connor AC, Graham I, Saucier D, Côté L, Cauchon M, et al. Supporting patients facing difficult health care decisions. Use of the Ottawa decision support framework. Can Fam Physician. 2006;52:476–7.
14. Oshima Lee E, Emanuel EJ. Shared decision making to improve care and reduce costs. N Engl J Med. 2013;368:6–8.
15. Lorenzo AJ1, Braga LH, Zlateska B, Leslie B, Farhat WA, Bägli DJ, Pippi Salle JL. Analysis of decisional conflict among parents who consent to hypospadias repair: single institution prospective study of 100 couples. J Urol. 2012;188:571–5.
16. O'connor AM. Validation of a decisional conflict scale. Med Decis mak. 1995; 15:25–30.
17. O'Connor AM. User manual—Decisional Conflict Scale. Available at https://decisionaid.ohri.ca/docs/develop/User_Manuals/UM_Decisional_Conflict.pdf. Updated 2010. Accessed August 20, 2014.
18. Swaka AM, Stratus S, Rotstein L, Brierley JD, Tsang RW, Asa S, C, Zahedi A, Freeman J, Solomon P, Anderson J, Thorpe KE, Gafni A, Rodin G, Goldstein DP. Randomized controlled trial of a computerized decision Aid on adjuvant radioactive iodine treatment for patients with early-stage papillary thyroid cancer. J Clin Oncol. 2012;30:2906–11.
19. De Morgan S, Redman S, D'Este C, Rogers K. Knowledge, satisfaction with information, decisional conflict and psychological morbidity amongst women diagnosed with ductal carcinoma in situ (DCIS). Patient Educ Couns. 2011;84:62–8.
20. Lam WW, Chan M, Or A, Kwong A, Suen D, Fielding R. Reducing treatment decision conflict difficulties in breast cancer surgery: a randomized controlled trial. J Clin Oncol. 2013;31:2879–85.
21. Taylor KL, Williams RM, Davis K, Luta G, Penek S, Barry S, Kelly S, Tomko C, Schwartz M, Krist AH, Woolf SH, Fishman MB, Cole C, Miller E. Decision making in prostate cancer screening using decision aids vs usual care. JAMA Intern Med. 2013;173:1704–12.
22. Chabera C, Zabalequi A, Bonet M, Caro M, Areal J, Gonzalez JR, et al. A decision aid to support informed choices for patients recently diagnosed with prostate cancer: a randomized controlled trial. Cancer Nurs. 2015;38:42–50.
23. O'Connor AM, Légaré F, Stacey D. Risk communication in practice: The contribution of decision aids. BMJ. 2003;327:736–40.
24. Drake RE, Deegan PE. Shared decision making is an ethical imperative. Psychiatr Serv. 2009;60:1007.
25. Pynnonen MA, Randolph GW, Shin JJ. Evidence-based medicine in otolaryngology, part 5: patient decision aids. Otolaryngol Head Neck Surg. 2015;153:357–63.
26. O'Brien MA, Whelan TJ, Villasis-Keever M, Gafni A, Charles C, Roberts R, Schiff S, Cai W. Are cancer-related decision aids effective? a systematic review and meta analysis. J Clin Oncol. 2009;27:974–85.
27. Boss EF, Mehta N, Nagarajan N, Links A, Benke JR, Berger Z, Espinel A, Meier J, Lipstein EA. Shared decision making and choice for elective surgical care: A systematic review. Otolaryngol Head Neck Surg. 2015; Epub ahead of print.
28. Elwyn G, O'Connor A, Stacey D, Volk R, Edwards A, Coulter A, et al. Developing a quality criteria framework for patient decision aids: online international Delphi consensus process. BMJ. 2006;333:417.
29. Volk RJ, Llewellyn-Thomas H, Stacey D, Elwyn G. Ten years of the international patient decision Aid standards collaboration: evolution of the core dimensions for assessing the quality of patient decision aids. BMC Med Inform Decis Mak. 2013;13(Suppl2):S1.
30. Arterburn D, Wellman R, Westbrrok E, Rutter C, Ross T, McCulloch D, Handley M, Jung C. Introducing decision aids at group health was linked to sharply lower hip and knee surgery rates and costs. Health Aff (Millwood). 2012;31:2094–104.

26

Cochlear implant and congenital cholesteatoma

J. Mierzwinski[1*], AJ Fishman[1], T. Grochowski[1], S. Drewa[1], M. Drela[1], P. Winiarski[2]
and I. Bielecki[3]

Abstract

Background: The occurence of cholesteatoma and cochlear implant is rare. Secondary cholesteatomas may develop as a result of cochlear implant surgery. Primarily acquired cholesteatoma is not typically associated with congenital sensorineural hearing loss or cochlear implant in children. The occurrence of congenital cholesteatoma during cochlear implant surgery has never been reported before, partly because all patients are preoperatively submitted to imaging studies which can theoretically exclude the disease.

Case presentation: We have reported a rare case of congenital cholesteatoma, found during sequential second side cochlear implantation in a 3-year-old child. The child underwent a computed tomography (CT) scan and magnetic resonance imaging (MRI) at 12 months of age, before the first cochlear implant surgery, which excluded middle ear pathology. The mass was removed as an intact pearl, without visible or microscopic violation of the cholesteatoma capsule. All the areas where middle ear structures were touching the cholesteatoma were vaporized with a laser and the cochlear implant was inserted uneventfully. Further follow-up excluded residual disease.

Conclusion: We believe that primary, single stage placement of a cochlear implant (CI) with simultaneous removal of the congenital cholesteatoma can be performed safely. However, to prevent recurrence, the capsule of the cholesteatoma must not be damaged and complete laser ablation of the surface, where suspicious epithelial cells could remain, is recommended. In our opinion, cholesteatoma removal and cochlear implantation should be staged if these conditions are not met, and/or the disease is at a more advanced stage. It is suspected, that the incidence of congenital cholesteatoma in pediatric CI candidates is much higher that in average pediatric population.

Keywords: Congenital cholesteatoma, Cochlear implantation, Cochlear implant candidacy, Laser surgery

Background

Cholesteatoma is an uncommon condition that has been rarely associated with cochlear implantation. Primary acquired cholesteatoma is not typically associated with congenital sensorineural hearing loss (SNHL) or CI in children. In case of secondary acquired cholesteatomas – they can develop as the result of cochlear implant surgery due to a breach of the posterior wall of the ear canal from drilling the posterior tympanotomy [1]. The identification of congenital cholesteatoma during CI surgery is unlikely because of thorough pre-operative imaging studies, most commonly involving high-resolution computed tomography (HRCT) and MRI of the temporal bone, which can theoretically exclude congenital cholesteatoma. The incidence of congenital cholesteatoma in the overall population is 0.00012 % and 1–3 % of childhood cholesteatomas are congenital [2, 3]. Chung et al. reported that congenital cholesteatoma was identified in 2 out of 794 pediatric CI patients during their pre-operative evaluations for CI (incidence, 0.25 %) [4]. The authors suggest that the incidence was much higher than expected of this rare condition.

Congenital cholesteatoma was initially described by Cawthorne and Griffith [5]. In 1965, Derlacki and Clemis defined congenital cholesteatoma as an embryologic residue of epithelial tissue behind a normal

---

* Correspondence: jmierzw@gmail.com
[1]Department of Otolaryngology, Audiology and Phoniatrics, Children's Hospital of Bydgoszcz, Chodkiewicza 44, 85-667 Bydgoszcz, Poland
Full list of author information is available at the end of the article

tympanic membrane in the absence of a history of infection or ear surgery [6]. Levenson added that the presence of uncomplicated acute otitis media does not exclude congenital cholesteatoma [7].

Congenital cholesteatoma usually grows slowly as a spherical-shaped keratin-filled cyst in the middle ear with a long asymptomatic period. When early detected, they are located deep to the antero-superior part of the tympanic membrane in two-thirds of the cases. The diagnosis is made at an average age of 4.5 years with a male to female ratio of 1:3. There are two types of congenital cholesteatoma, defined according to their location in the middle ear. The first is an isolated pearl located deep to the anterior part of the eardrum, which is believed to result from arrested epidermal formation at 10 weeks' gestational age. It is suggested that these formations atrophy at approximately 33 weeks of gestational age, or are evacuated through the Eustachian tube. Failure of this mechanism results in this type of congenital cholesteatoma [8]. The second type is located in the posterior part of the middle ear and causes more rapid ossicular destruction and hearing impairment. The origin of this type is thought to be amniotic fluid cells that migrate in the neonate [9]. The theory of congenital cholesteatoma origin assumes that the pathology is present before birth and the diagnosis is most often made by a combination of otoscopy and HRCT. In a completely aerated tympanic cavity absent of any associated soft tissue, HRCT has a high negative predictive value when excluding cholesteatoma [10]. Microsurgical excision is the accepted treatment and associated laser vaporization of contact points has been shown to limit the rate of recurrence [11]. We present a case of congenital cholesteatoma found this time not during diagnostic procedure before CI, but during sequential second side cochlear implantation in a 3-year-old child in spite of prior imaging studies.

Case presentation

The patient was a female child diagnosed with bilateral SNHL of genetic origin at the age of 8 months. Genetic testing identified a deletion - 35delG in gene GJB2. The patient failed the newborn hearing screen at birth with subsequent diagnostic auditory brainstem responses demonstrating bilateral, severe to profound SNHL. The child initially received hearing aids but presented significant speech delay despite conventional amplification. Referred for consideration for CI, the patient underwent thorough diagnostic testing by a multidisciplinary team as well as imaging evaluation with HRCT and MRI. HRCT of the temporal bones was performed with a standard protocol using a bone algorithm with a slice thickness of 0.625 mm and collimation of 0.3 mm.

Preoperative 1.5 Tesla MRI (Fig. 1) and HRCT (Fig. 2) studies showed implantable inner ear spaces, present

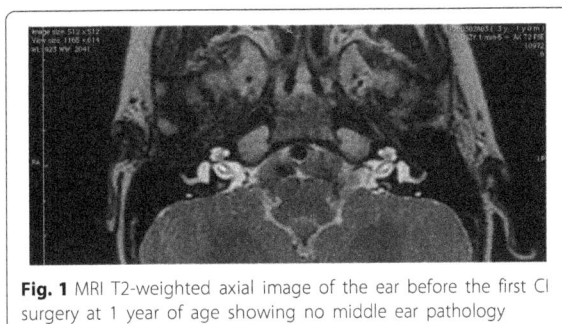

Fig. 1 MRI T2-weighted axial image of the ear before the first CI surgery at 1 year of age showing no middle ear pathology

cochlear nerves, and no suggestion of additional middle ear pathology. A decision was made to implant the right ear and surgery was performed when the child reached 1 year of age. The surgery on this side was uneventful and without complications or findings of associated middle ear diseases. At the same time, the left ear was equipped with an updated hearing aid. The Integration Scale of Development was used to assess the development of hearing and speech, which is our routine protocol for children between 1 and 4 years of age. The results showed that the child achieved excellent speech and language outcomes comparable to age-appropriate normal hearing subjects. The patient was subsequently evaluated for sequential implantation of the left ear, showing unremarkable otoscopy and a normal tympanic membrane. Normal appearance of the tympanic membrane was also confirmed during otomicroscopy intraoperatively at the time of the second CI surgery. The second implantation was performed two years after the first CI surgery when the child was 3 years old. In our clinic, in cases of sequential implantation, we do not routinely re-image the temporal bones if the first examination showed no pathology. The second CI surgery was performed as per our routine protocol using a posterior tympanotomy approach to the round window and promontory. After opening the facial recess, an approximately 3-mm pearl-appearing cholesteatoma was identified between the facial ridge, incudostapedial joint, and cochleariform process (Fig. 3). To remove the pathology en bloc, the ossicles were disarticulated and the cholesteatoma was removed together with the incus. All tissues contacting the cholesteatoma were vaporized superficially with a diode laser at a setting of 2 W with single short pulses of 0.05 s (Fig. 4) delivered through a 0.6-mm fiber. In surgery for isolated cholesteatoma pearls, we routinely use a laser to minimize the risk of recurrence. The CI was then inserted uneventfully through an extended round window approach.

One year after, a CT of the temporal bone was performed to exclude residual disease and suspicious opacification in the facial recess area was revealed.

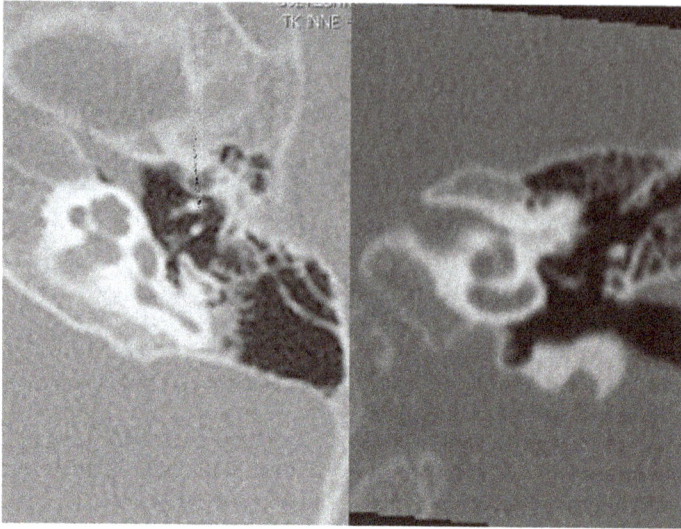

Fig. 2 HRCT image (axial-left and coronal-right) of the left temporal bone before the first CI surgery at 1 year of age showing no middle ear pathology

The residual disease was excluded by the endoscopy of the middle ear through anterior tympanotomy approach. The opacification turned out to be connective tissue used for obliteration of posterior tympanotomy during the CI surgery.

Discussion

Imaging before cochlear implantation is used to confirm the presence of an implantable inner ear space and intact cochlear nerve, as well as to provide important information about the surgical anatomy of the ear [12]. Both MRI and HRCT can potentially diagnose a pathologic mass such as cholesteatoma in the middle ear space. HRCT has excellent sub-millimeter spatial resolution, which provides accurate delineation of even very

small cholesteatomas, as long as there is a well-aerated middle ear cavity. HRCT in this setting offers high sensitivity and excellent negative predictive value [13]. In our case, the conditions for evaluation of the middle ear were excellent. The middle ear was completely free of effusion (Fig. 2), however HRCT has poor specificity because the nature of the soft tissue density cannot be differentiated.

MRI using the conventional sequences (T1-weighted image, T2-weighted image, post-contrast T1-weighted image) provides additional information enabling distinguishment of different pathologic entities, as well as accurate diagnosis of primary and residual/recurrent cholesteatomas. Even higher diagnostic specificity is achieved with diffusion-weighted (DW) echo-planar

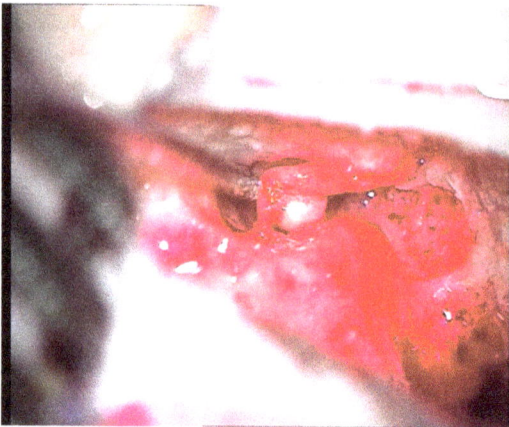

Fig. 3 Cholesteatoma, microscopic view

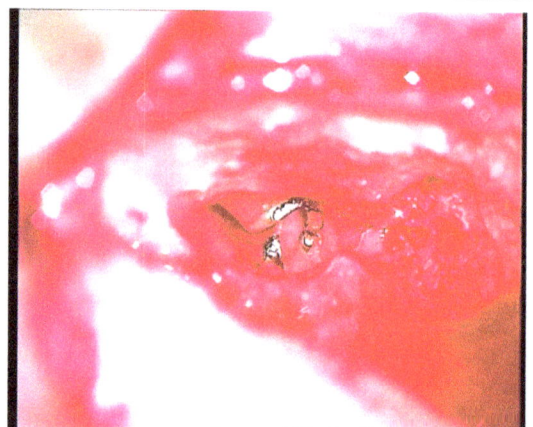

Fig. 4 Diode laser treatment of the operated field, microscopic view

imaging, delayed post-contrast imaging, DW-non-echo-planar imaging, and DWI-PROPELLER techniques. We used a 1.5 Tesla MRI with conventional sequences in our patient, following our routine protocol, which was focused primarily on assessing the anatomical implant feasibility in young children. However, even with conventional proto-cols, a pathological mass greater than 2 mm in size and surrounded by air can be identified on the T2-weighted sequence. In conventional MRI, the diagnosis of sub-millimeter anatomical structures is also possible provided that there is good signal contrast between the structure and its surroundings, as in our case. For temporal bone diagnosis in clinical practice, we use a 1.5 Tesla MRI. With the development of new models, MRI at 3 Tesla or higher is becoming more common and widely avail-able. The main advantage is shorter acquisition time but because of artifacts specific to this anatomic region, diffusion-weighted sequence acquisition is paradoxically longer, which increases the risk of motion artifacts, es-pecially in children, making interpretation more diffi-cult, even for experienced radiologists [14].

Except for paper of Chung et al., to date, there has been no literature published on the incidence of con-genital cholesteatoma found prior to implantation [4]. The authors found this incidence (0,25 %) much higher than expected of this rare condition in general popula-tion (0.00012 %). It is surprisingly common, given the absence of any cases of primarily acquired cholesteatoma in the reported group of patients, which is considerably more common in the pediatric population. Our case, as well as both reported by Chung et al. of congenital cho-lesteatoma patients, most likely had an inherited form of hearing loss and, as they suggested, genetic contribution to the presence of congenital cholesteatoma cannot be excluded [4]. A correlation between the formation of congenital cholesteatoma and abnormal cochleovestibu-lar anatomy and SNHL have also been reported by Propst et al. and Jackler et al. [15, 16].

It has been suggested that if congenital cholesteatoma is found during diagnostic procedures for CI, the choles-teatoma should be removed and implantation delayed to the second stage [4]. In our patient, we made the deci-sion to remove the cholesteatoma and insert an implant in a one-stage procedure because the disease was re-moved as an intact pearl, without visible or microscopic violation of the cholesteatoma capsule, and the areas of contact between the cholesteatoma and middle ear structures were vaporized with a laser. The risk of recur-rence was very unlikely. Such a protocol has been used in our clinic for several years in numerous ear opera-tions, in cases of limited congenital cholesteatoma and small cholesteatoma pearls found during second-look procedures. We consider the procedure safe and do not hesitate to proceed with ossicular reconstruction in such

cases. What is more, revision surgery is also not planned in such situations.

Although the laser is not universally utilized in the treatment of cholesteatoma, Hamilton concludes that the appropriate use of the laser during cholesteatoma surgery facilitates significantly the complete removal of the disease and presents no extra risk to the vital struc-tures within the temporal bone [11]. Also James et al. stated that current technological advances such as laser and middle ear endoscopy contribute to better outcomes in the treatment of cholesteatoma [17]. As it has been mentioned we routinely use laser during cholesteatoma surgery in our clinic.

It has long been recognized that a second-look pro-cedure in cases of congenital cholesteatoma is required less often than in acquired pediatric cholesteatoma [18]. James et al. suggested that when the cholesteatoma cyst is removed intact, complete eradication can be almost guaranteed, and recommended a second-look procedure when cholesteatoma extends into hidden regions such as the mastoid, or with concerns about the completeness of matrix removal [17]. We also follow this strategy. In our case, the cholesteatoma did not extend into hidden spaces; it was a closed capsule and we had no concerns about incomplete removal. It should be emphasized that the decision to proceed with CI requires careful consid-eration on a case-by-case basis. Particularly with a larger congenital cholesteatoma, a damaged capsule, or wide-spread pathology, delaying CI is the most reasonable and safest option [4].

According to Derlacki and Clemis' criteria the patient's cholesteatoma met the definition of a congenital choles-teatoma - it was totally asymptomatic and behind an in-tact tympanic membrane [6]. Cholesteatoma was not seen at otoscopy before the first and second surgery. Be-fore the first surgery it was most probably so small that it was not within the limits of visibility even for CT and MRI. The cholesteatoma was not seen at otoscopy at the second surgery either because it was located medially to the long crus of the incus and the handle of the malleus. Middle ear pathology located in the posterior mesotym-panum is practically invisible until it touches the tym-panic membrane and can be easily overlooked.

The growth rate of this particular cholesteatoma had to be relatively dynamic.

The original size of the cholesteatoma is important. According to the first theory of origination of congenital cholesteatoma, the diameter of the epidermoid forma-tions frequently found in human fetuses that proceed to congenital cholesteatoma if not absorbed or evacuated through the Eustachian tube, is already known. Huang et al. reviewed 49 fetuses, ranging from 12 weeks to full term. In 16 they found epidermoid formation, which was always located at the anterosuperior edge of the eardrum

[19]. The width and height of the epidermoid formations was 60.82 ± 5.68 microns and 45.87 ± 6.82 microns, respectively. In our case, the cholesteatoma was located in the posterior mesotympanum, and met the second theory of origination, which says that amniotic fluid cells migrate through the Eustachian tube to the middle ear and then form the cholesteatoma. In this case, the cholesteatoma might have arisen from a single cell, or group of cells, also microns in diameter.

Assuming a linear growth for congenital cholesteatoma, James et al. calculated that closed cholesteatoma cysts enlarge by approximately 1 mm in diameter per year, based on CT measurements ([20] James). We can assume in our case that the growth was linear because it was a closed round capsule; therefore, in the first year of life, theoretically, the cholesteatoma would have been approximately 1 mm in diameter, enlarging to approximately 3 mm in diameter at 3 years of age. A 1-mm pearl would be visible by imaging studies and the negative predictive value of CT in such a case is excellent [6].

The explanation for the lack of identification of the cholesteatoma on the initial HRCT is that the pathology was too small to be visualized. The most likely it was a very small sub-millimeter "sleeper" congenital cholesteatoma with no growth between birth and the first year, but with subsequent rapid growth between 1 and 3 years of life.

Bilateral cochlear implantation in young children is increasingly common in clinical practice. Among the benefits of bilateral cochlear implantation is the restoration of some of the advantages of binaural hearing such as localization, improved listening in noise, directional hearing, binaural summation, and squelch. Typically, young hearing-impaired children are being provided with two implants either at the same time (simultaneous implantation) or at different times in early childhood as in our case (sequential implantation) [21]. Our local public funding policy enables children to receive initially unilateral cochlear implant due to economic limitations. In our clinic, excluding the post meningitis deafness, when bilateral implants are put simultaneously, the CI candidates are implanted unilaterally as quickly as possible, starting from the age of 12 months. Only when we are able to provide all candidates with one implant and meet the economic limitations, do we consider giving another implant to prior pediatric CI users.

Examining the findings in this patient, the obvious question arises whether to perform another imaging study which could preclude the existing, newly formed cholesteatoma before the subsequent CI surgery, and how much time should elapse between the first and second implantation, to perform such a study most effectively?

We believe that the rarity of our particular case does not justify the additional cost and burden of repeating the standard HRCT and/or MRI in so young children. Also, our case presented with limited pathology that was controlled by a single-stage procedure. We emphasize the importance of continued follow-up and advise considering staging in either known disease or more extensive disease as a reasonable and safe option.

Conclusions

To our knowledge, this is the first report of an incidental finding of congenital cholesteatoma during CI surgery despite presurgical imaging studies. Primary excision en bloc with the removal of associated ossicular elements and laser surface ablation is the recommended treatment for limited congenital cholesteatoma. Primary placement of an implant during cholesteatoma removal is warranted as long as there is insignificant risk of recurrence, provided that no damage of the capsule has occurred and complete and safe surface contact of epithelial laser ablation was observed. There should be a low threshold for staging the implant if any of these conditions are not met, and/or the disease is found to be more extensive. Follow-up should include regular microscopic ear examination and HRCT.

There is suspicion that the incidence of congenital cholesteatoma in pediatric CI candidates is much higher than in normal pediatric population (4).

Consent

The written consent was obtained from the patient's parents to publish the details of their child's case.

Abbreviations

CT: Computed tomography; MRI: Magnetic resonance imaging; CI: Cochlear implant; SNHL: Sensorineural hearing loss; HRCT: High resolution computed tomography; DW: Diffusion-weighted.

Competing interests

The authors declare that they have no competing interests.

Authors' contributions

JM: otosurgeon, discovered pathology, made recordings and initiated the paper, final manuscript check. AJF: manuscript revise, took part in the discussion on the patient management. TG: collected and proceeded the recordings and imaging data, first draft. SD: radiologist - helped to interpret data and wrote a section regarding interpretation of imaging data regarding congenital cholesteatoma. MD: audiologist, participated in its design and coordination and helped to draft the manuscript. PW: participated in its design and coordination and helped to draft the manuscript. IB: reference review and preparation, decisions regarding the management strategy of the patient. All authors read and approved the final manuscript.

Acknowledgements

We thank language editor Kumiko Shimogami from Edanz Group Global Ltd who has made significant revision of the manuscript. All costs incurred were paid by the first author.

No additional funding was necessary for this publication.

Author details
[1]Department of Otolaryngology, Audiology and Phoniatrics, Children's Hospital of Bydgoszcz, Chodkiewicza 44, 85-667 Bydgoszcz, Poland. [2]Department of Otolaryngology, Head and Neck Surgery, University Hospital of Bydgoszcz, Ujejskiego 52, 85-168 Bydgoszcz, Poland. [3]Department of Pediatric Otolaryngology, University Children's Hospital of Katowice, ul Medyków 16, 40-752 Katowice, Poland.

References
1. Bhatia K, Gibbin KP, Nikolopoulos TP, O'Donoghue GM. Surgical complications and their management in a series of 300 consecutive pediatric cochlear implantations. Otol Neurotol. 2004;25(5):730–9.
2. Tos M. A new pathogenesis of mesotympanic (congenital) cholesteatoma. Laryngoscope. 2000;110(11):1890–7.
3. Koltai PJ, Nelson M, Castellon RJ, Garabedian EN, Triglia JM, Roman S, et al. The natural history of congenital cholesteatoma. Arch Otolaryngol Head Neck Surg. 2002;128(7):804–9.
4. Chung J, Cushing SL, James AL, Gordon KA, Papsin BC. Congenital cholesteatoma and cochlear implantation: Implications for management. Cochlear Implants Int. 2013;14(1):32–5.
5. Cawthorne T. Griffith A Primary cholesteatoma of the temporal bone. Arch Otolaryngol. 1961;73:252–61.
6. Derlacki EL, Clemis JD. Congenital cholesteatoma of the middle ear and mastoid. Ann Otol Rhinol Laryngol. 1965;74(3):706–27.
7. Levenson MJ, Parisier SC, Chute P, Wenig S, Juarbe C. A review of twenty congenital cholesteatomas of the middle ear in children. Otolaryngol Head Neck Surg. 1986;94(5):560–7.
8. Levenson MJ, Michaels L. Parisier S Congenital cholesteatomas of the middle ear in children: origin and management. Otolaryngol Clin North Am. 1989;22(5):941–54.
9. Northrop C. Histological observation of amniotic fluid cellular content in the ear of neonates and infants. Int J Pediatr Otorhinolaryngol. 1986; 11(2):113–27.
10. Vercruysse JP, De Foer B, Somers T, Casselman J, Offeciers E. Magnetic resonance imaging of cholesteatoma: an update. B-ENT. 2009;5(4):233–40.
11. Hamilton JW. Efficacy of the KTP laser in the treatment of middle ear cholesteatoma. Otol Neurotol. 2005;26(2):135–9.
12. Fishman AJ. Imaging and anatomy for cochlear implants. Otolaryngol Clin North Am. 2012;45(1):1–24.
13. Dhepnorrarat RC, Wood B, Rajan GP. Postoperative non-echo-planar diffusion-weighted magnetic resonance imaging changes after cholesteatoma surgery: implications for cholesteatoma screening. Otol Neurotol. 2009;30(1):54–8.
14. Nevoux J, Lenoir M, Roger G, Denoyelle F, Ducou Le Pointe H, Garabédian EN. Childhood cholesteatoma. Eur Ann Otorhinolaryngol Head Neck Dis. 2010;127(4):143–50.
15. Propst EJ, Blaser S, Trimble K, James A, Friedberg J, Papsin BC. Cochleovestibular anomalies in children with cholesteatoma. Laryngoscope. 2008;118(3):517–21.
16. Jackler RK, Luxford WM, House WF. Congenital malformations of the inner ear: a classification based on embryogenesis. Laryngoscope. 1987;97(3 Pt 2 Suppl 40):2–14.
17. James AL, Papsin BC. Some considerations in congenital cholesteatoma. Curr Opin Otolaryngol Head Neck Surg. 2013;21(5):431–9.
18. Friedberg J. Congenital cholesteatoma. Laryngoscope. 1994;104(3 Pt 2):1–24.
19. Huang JM. Epidermoid formation in the developing middle ear and its relationship to congenital cholesteatoma]. Zhonghua Er Bi Yan Hou Ke Za Zhi. 1993;28(4):228–30. 252–3.
20. James AL, Papsin BC, Blaser S, Determining the growth rate of congenital cholesteatoma In Ozgirgin ON Editor, Surgery of the ear current topics, Ankara, Turkey. Rekmay Publishing Ltd. 2009, pp 40–43.
21. Lammers MJ, van der Heijden GJ, Pourier VE, Grolman W. Bilateral cochlear implantation in children: a systematic review and best-evidence synthesis. Laryngoscope. 2014;124(7):1694–9.

27

Age dependent normal horizontal VOR gain of head impulse test as measured with video-oculography

Benjamin Mossman[1†], Stuart Mossman[1*†], Gordon Purdie[2] and Erich Schneider[3]

Abstract

Background: The head impulse test (HIT) is a recognised clinical sign of the high frequency vestibulo-ocular reflex (VOR), which can be quantified with video-oculography. This measures the VOR gain as the ratio of angular eye velocity to angular head velocity. Although normative data is available for VOR gain with video-oculography, most normal studies in general include small numbers of subjects and do not include analysis of variation of VOR gain with age. The purpose of our study was to establish normative data across 60 control subjects aged 20 to 80 years to represent a population distribution.

Methods: Sixty control subjects without any current or previous form of brain disorder or vertigo participated in this study and form the basis for future comparison to patients with vestibular lesions. The relationship between the horizontal vestibulo-ocular reflex (HVOR) velocity gain and age was analysed using a mixed regression model with a random effect for subjects. Differences in testing technique were assessed to ensure reliability in results.

Results: The mean HVOR velocity gain of 60 normal subjects was 0.97 (SD = 0.09) at 80 ms and 0.94 (SD = 0.10) at 60 ms. The 2 SD lower limit of normal HVOR velocity gain was 0.79 at 80 ms and 0.75 at 60 ms. No HVOR velocity gain fell below 0.76 and 0.65 at 80 ms and 60 ms respectively. The HVOR velocity gain declined by 0.012 and 0.017 per decade as age increased at 80 ms and 60 ms respectively. A non-physiologically high horizontal HVOR velocity gain was found to occur in tests where passive HITs were predictable in direction and time and where target distance was below 0.70 m.

Conclusions: Normative data with respect to HVOR velocity gain decreases slightly with age, but with careful attention to methodology the 2 SD lower limit of normal is relatively robust across a wide age range and into the eighth decade, without requirement for adjustment with age.

Keywords: Head impulse test, Horizontal vestibulo-ocular reflex, Semicircular canal, Eye movements

Background

The horizontal head impulse test (HIT) is a well recognised clinical tool to test the horizontal vestibular ocular reflex (HVOR). The subject maintains fixation on an object straight ahead while sudden head impulses are applied in the horizontal angular plane and eye movements are observed for catch up saccades [1]. If a subject's vestibular ocular reflex (VOR) is normal, the eyes should remain focused on the fixation target during head rotation. However, if there is a significant semicircular canal deficit on the side corresponding to rotation, the ipsilateral VOR response will be inadequate and a significant catch up saccade(s) may be seen.

Video-oculography (VOG) goggles allow quantitative recording of the eye and head movements during the HIT. Covert saccades (occurring during the head movement, usually undetectable clinically) and overt saccades (occurring after the head movement and detectable clinically) are both recorded by the camera. VOG also provides a quantitative measure of the VOR deficit, distinguishing

* Correspondence: stuart.mossman@ccdhb.org.nz
†Equal contributors
[1]Department of Neurology, Wellington Hospital, Riddiford Street, Private Bag 7902, Wellington South, Wellington, New Zealand
Full list of author information is available at the end of the article

abnormal from normal subjects. An advantage of the video HIT (vHIT) over search coils [2] is that it is less invasive, has simple setup and is readily available for clinicians. This relatively new technology uses a high speed compact camera (220 Hz sampling rate) that is attached to lightweight goggles (EyeSeeCam HIT) [3]. The system is used in conjunction with computer software to track pupil movement. Head movement is recorded through a motion sensor attached to the goggles [3–5]. A velocity gain is calculated by dividing instantaneous eye velocity by instantaneous head velocity. The objective was to obtain HVOR velocity gain data to represent a population distribution of normal subjects.

Methods
The study used quantitative recordings with VOG to measure the HVOR velocity gain during the high frequency horizontal HIT. Sixty three normal subjects were tested (10 per decade, ranging from 20 to 80 years). Exclusion criteria, ascertained at the time of recruitment were no previous form of brain disorder, vertigo, or restricted neck movement.

Before testing, each subject was given verbal and written information regarding the test procedure and rationale. This outlined the risks and exclusion criteria, with signed consent required. As the study established normative data, approval was not required by our Central Regional Ethics Committee.

Experimental procedure
Before formal testing, we ensured that the subject managed an adequate range of unrestricted, painless angular head rotation. The subject was seated 1.5 m directly in front of a fixation target at eye level. VOG goggles were fitted tightly to the subject's head to reduce goggle slippage. The camera was focused on the eye while the subject fixated on the target. The subject was instructed to keep his/her eyes open widely so as not to obscure the pupil. If the palpebral fissure remained unduly narrowed, including from ptosis with redundant skin folds or long eye lashes, the eyelids were held open by the rims of the goggles. Even though this procedure can alter the vertical offset of the calibration parameters, it has no effect on the scaling of the calibration. The HVOR velocity gain therefore remains unaffected.

The system was calibrated with the subject altering fixation around five dots, 8.5° apart, projected onto the wall in front of them. The dots were emitted from a goggle-mounted laser and a diffraction grating [6]. The fixation sequence was arbitrary and the subject was instructed to spend no more than one second fixating on each dot. If errors occurred, the operator could repeat the calibration procedure.

The testing method outlined to the subjects included that they should:

- clench their teeth during the HIT to reduce jaw movement and facilitate a more direct force transfer to the head and reduce movement artefact
- maintain a relaxed neck musculature and not anticipate or aid in head movements
- not move the goggles once calibration was completed
- keep their eyes open wide and minimise blinking to allow the software to keep precise track of pupil movements
- maintain gaze on the fixation target throughout the testing procedure of angular head rotation

Eye and head rotations were measured during the HIT while the examiner manually applied rapid unpredictable (in direction and time) angular head rotations (peak head velocity 150 °/s to 300 °/s) [7]. Instantaneous HVOR velocity gains were calculated by the EyeSeeCam VOG software at 80 ms and 60 ms [8]. Head accelerations were manually controlled so that peak head velocity would occur at 80 ± 15 ms into each rotation [9]. This was achieved with angular head displacements of small amplitude (6° – 12°) and rapid rotation. Rotation of the subject's head was performed with the examiner standing behind the seated subject. Six to ten unpredictable head rotations in both directions were performed from a central head position. This sequence was repeated twice to ensure adequate data collection and a check for data consistency, but more frequently if a subject needed additional training or if results were affected by artefact. Head rotations were achieved by the examiner firmly holding the mandible with three fingers clasped below and a thumb and forefinger above the jaw line (Fig. 1). This reduced skin movement and thus goggle slippage, decreasing the amount of artefact. Care was taken to avoid touching the goggles strap during head rotation. A single examiner[BM] performed all tests throughout the study.

Data analysis
Data with undue technical artefact (with blinks and obscured pupils) was discarded. This selection was unbiased and not determined by HVOR velocity gain. The graphed HIT sequences for each subject were assessed and the test with the least artefact was selected for analysis of HVOR velocity gain (Figs. 2 and 3 exemplify reliable and artefactual data). Only one of the HIT sequences was used in order to achieve similar properties to those expected from real-world clinical examinations. An average of 3.2 (range 2–6) HIT sequences for each subject were used to calculate repeatability of the test. This method took a pooled standard deviation for the left and right and used a definition for a repeatability coefficient adopted by the British Standards Institution [10].

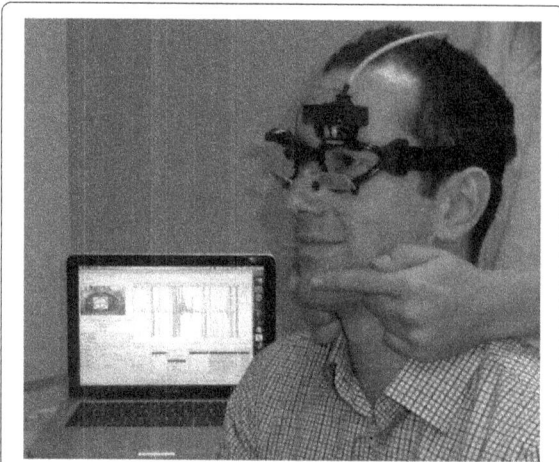

Fig. 1 Method of testing, where the subject's head is firmly held by the mandible, with three fingers clasped below and a thumb and forefinger above the jaw line

HVOR velocity gain at 80 ms and 60 ms for both left and right rotations were used to assess the normative range. The 80 ms time analysis was used in case of artefact occurring in the early stages of head rotation (and attributed to goggle slip) and the 60 ms time analysis because of the frequent occurrence of covert catch up saccades seen in some patients with vestibular deficits. Two analysis intervals obviate these potential problems and provide an internal check for reliability. Analysis for each head impulse was performed over a 10 ms window centred at 80 ms and 60 ms. The median of these values was calculated in order to lessen the weighting from any outliers. Data was manipulated using the EyeSeeCam VOG software backed by Matlab scripts for data analysis. The same scripts were used in another study with search coils [8]. This analysis over a short time window has been recognised as the gold standard [2].

The main purpose of the study was to assess the relationship between HVOR velocity gain and age with analysis using a mixed regression model with a random effect for subjects. Differences between time of HVOR velocity gain analysis (80 ms or 60 ms) and sides were compared with analysis of variance with

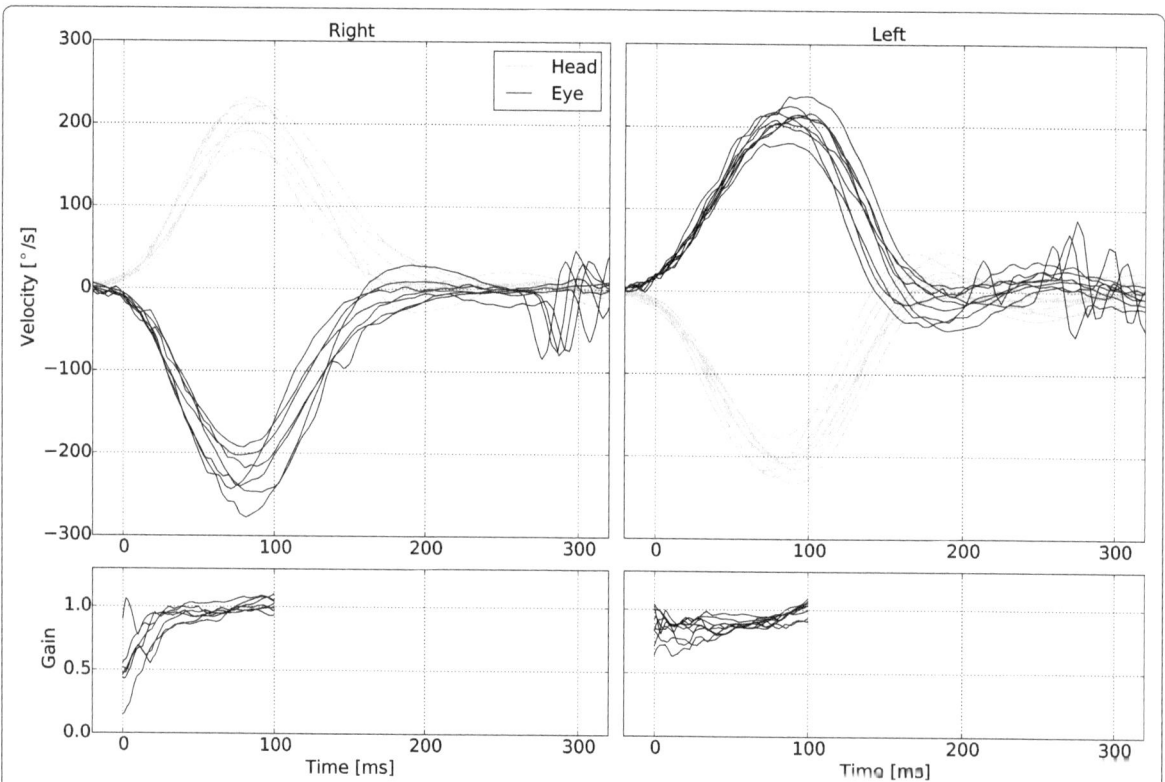

Fig. 2 Example of selected data of HVOR velocity gain vs time, with no artefact

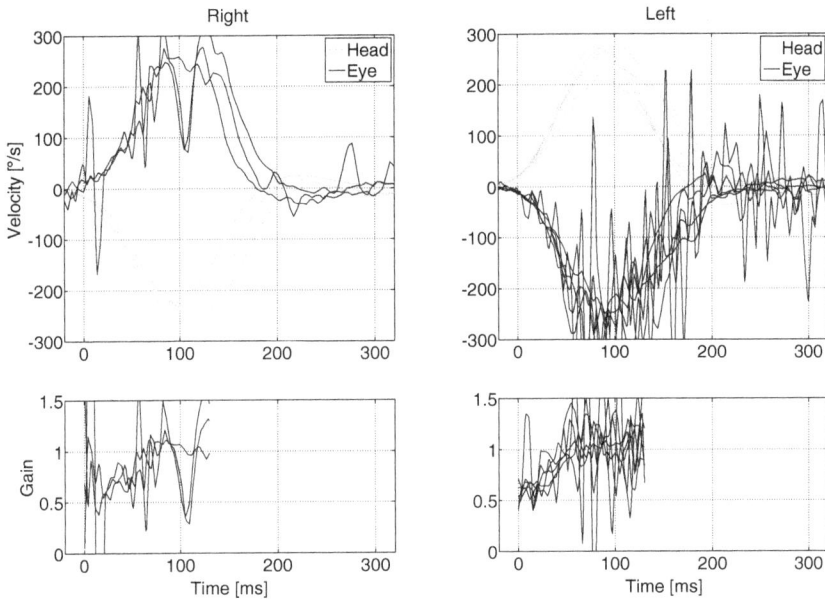

Fig. 3 Example of omitted data of HVOR velocity gain vs time with artefact. In this subject, too few head rotations were plotted, and a narrow palpebral fissure lead to artefact. Nevertheless, the examiner can determine from the observation of the eye and head velocity traces that the vestibular function of this subject is normal. Despite the artefacts, one can observe that peak eye velocity corresponds with peak head velocity

terms for time of velocity gain analysis, side, their interaction and their random terms with subjects.

Additional testing was also performed to assess the effect of fixation distance and predictable versus unpredictable head impulses on data reliability.

Five normal subjects were tested at a series of fixation distances (0.23, 0.40, 0.70, 1.00, 1.30, 1.60 and 1.90 m) to assess the dependence of the HVOR velocity gain on distance. This was analysed using a mixed linear regression with a random term for subject and autoregressive errors with distance.

Eighteen of the normal subjects were tested using both predictable and unpredictable head rotations (in direction and time). Predictable head impulses in direction alternated sequentially between the right and left at a regular time interval. The effect of predictable testing was analysed for variance with terms for side, whether or not the rotation was predictable, a random term for subjects, and interaction terms.

Results

HVOR velocity gains were obtained for 63 subjects over the six decades from age 20 to 80. Horizontal head impulses were carried out with peak head velocities ranging from 150 °/s to 300 °/s (corresponding to peak head accelerations of 2300 °/sec^2 to 5900 °/sec^2). Results in three subjects (5 %) were discarded due to neck stiffness limiting angular head velocity, and

artefact attributed to narrowed palpebral fissures (aged > 60 years). The remaining 60 subjects' left and right HVOR velocity gains were plotted showing a frequency distribution. This included subjects with and without overt saccades as occur in normal subjects clinically. This gave a combined total of 120 HVOR velocity gains at both 80 ms and 60 ms, as displayed in Fig. 4a and b.

The distributions of HVOR velocity gain at 80 ms and 60 ms were not significantly different from normal distributions (Shapiro-Wilk test, $W = 0.988$, $p = 0.39$ and $W = 0.990$, $p = 0.54$ respectively) around mean values of 0.97 (SD = 0.09) and 0.94 (SD = 0.10), $n = 120$. The mean (95 % confidence intervals (CI)) HVOR velocity gains to the left and right are both 0.97 (0.94 – 0.99) at 80 ms, and 0.94 (0.92 – 0.96) to the left and 0.94 (0.92 – 0.97) to the right at 60 ms. The lower limit of the normal HVOR velocity gain (2SD below mean) was 0.79 at 80 ms and 0.75 at 60 ms. The lowest and highest values of the normal HVOR velocity gain were 0.76 and 1.18 at 80 ms and 0.65 and 1.17 at 60 ms.

The interaction of the time of analysis (80 ms or 60 ms) and side was not significant ($p = 0.91$). The HVOR velocity gains were significantly different between 80 ms and 60 ms (0.02; 95 %CI 0.04–0.01; SD 0.05; $p = 0.0004$). The HVOR velocity gains were not significantly different between the sides (0.00; 95 %CI -0.02–0.02; SD 0.08; $p = 0.93$). The HVOR velocity gain repeatability coefficients

a)
**Frequency of normal HVOR velocity gain
at 80 ms in 60 subjects (n=120)**

HVOR velocity gain

b)
**Frequency of normal HVOR velocity gain
at 60 ms in 60 subjects (n=120)**

HVOR velocity gain

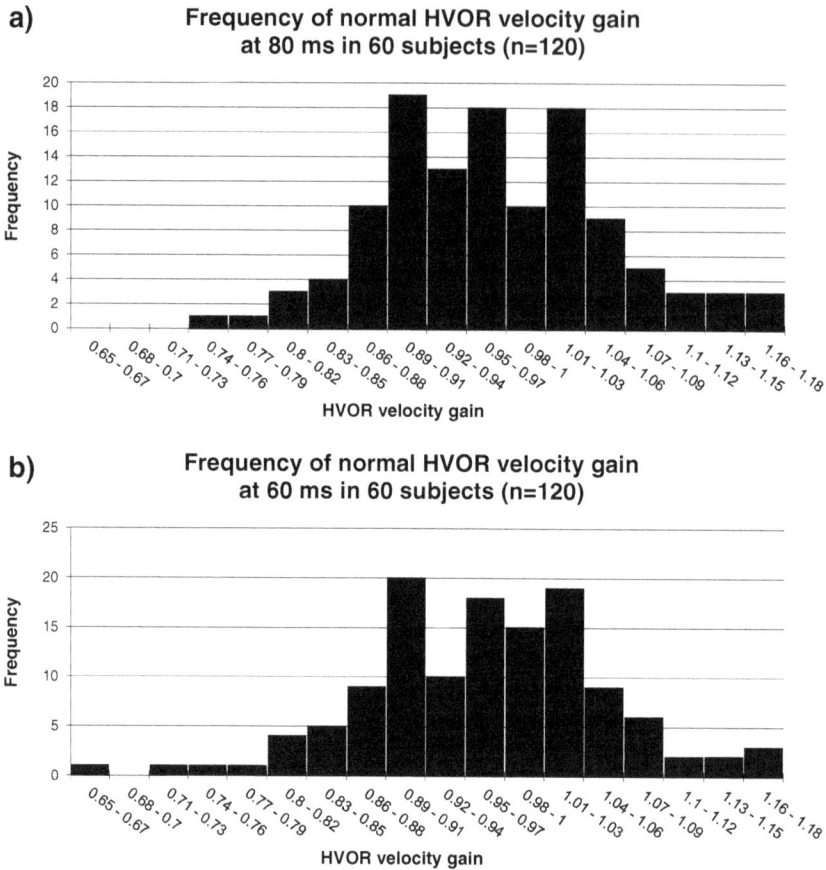

Fig. 4 a: Normal HVOR velocity gain frequency at 80 ms across the second to eighth decades during left and right head rotations. Results show a normal distribution (Shapiro - Wilk test for normality, $p = 39$). HVOR velocity gain is the ratio of angular eye velocity to angular head velocity. **b**: Normal HVOR velocity gain frequency at 60 ms across the second to eighth decades during left and right head rotations. Results show a normal distribution (Shapiro - Wilk test for normality, $p = 0.54$). HVOR velocity gain is the ratio of angular eye velocity to angular head velocity

were 0.12 at 80 ms and 0.10 at 60 ms (95 % of differences are expected to be less than these).

The HVOR velocity gain at 80 ms declined by 0.012 (95 % CI 0.001 – 0.022) per decade as age increased ($p = 0.028$), and at 60 ms declined by 0.017 (95 % CI 0.006 – 0.029) per decade as age increased ($p = 0.005$) (Fig. 5a, b). In patients younger than 70 years, the HVOR velocity gain was always above 0.80 at 80 ms and always above 0.76 at 60 ms.

The normalised HVOR velocity gain asymmetry was the absolute difference between left and right divided by the sum × 100 [11]; the 95th percentile for 80 ms is 9.2 with a maximum of 12.5 and for 60 ms is 8.8 with a maximum of 16.7. There was no significant correlation with age at 80 ms or 60 ms with Spearman correlation coefficients of 0.12 ($p = 0.36$) and 0.11 ($p = 0.42$) respectively. The un-normalised gain asymmetry, or absolute value of the gain difference between the two sides [12, 13], was zero; the 95th

percentile for 80 ms is 0.17 with a maximum 0.26 and for 60 ms is 0.18 with a maximum 0.26.

During testing the direction and time of head rotation was unpredictable. In addition, eighteen of the subjects were also tested using a predictable HIT. The mean HVOR velocity gain at 80 ms was 0.06 (95 % CI 0.01 – 0.10; $p = 0.014$) higher when testing was carried out in a predictable manner (as high as 1.35). HVOR velocity gain between the left and the right increased similarly with predictable rotations ($p = 0.55$).

Five subjects were also tested for target fixation dependence of the HVOR velocity gain at 80 ms over increasing distance (0.23, 0.4, 0.7, 1.0, 1.3, 1.6 and 1.9 m). There was an inverse relationship between HVOR velocity gain and distance, with no significant difference between the rate of HVOR velocity gain change for the left and right ($p = 0.12$). With a common slope, the HVOR velocity gain decreased by 13 % (95 % CI 9 % – 17 %; $p = 0.002$) per metre.

a) Age dependent HVOR velocity gain at 80 ms in 60 subjects (n=120)

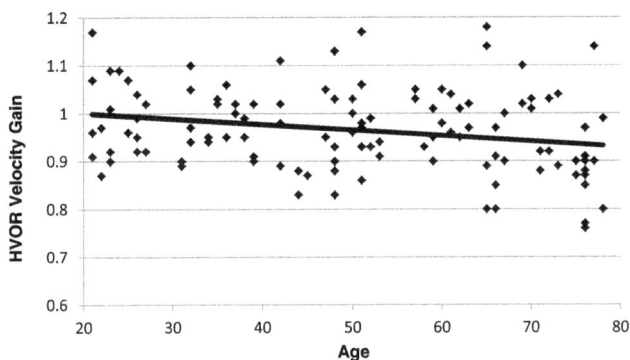

b) Age dependent HVOR velocity gain at 60 ms in 60 subjects (n=120)

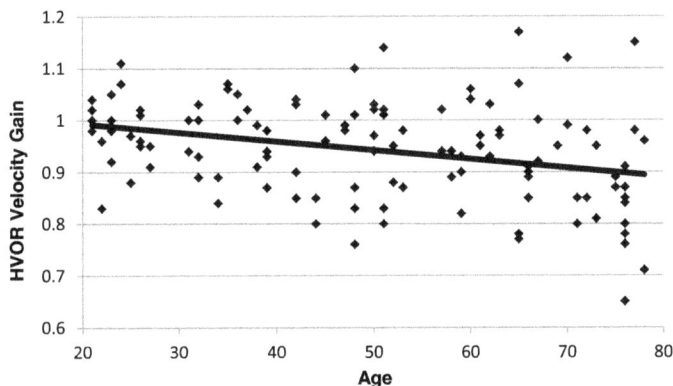

Fig. 5 a: Normal HVOR velocity gain at 80 ms decline with age. HVOR velocity gain was found to decline by 0.012 per decade with increasing age (95 % CI 0.001 to 0.022; $p = 0.028$). HVOR velocity gain is the ratio of angular eye velocity to angular head velocity. **b**: Normal HVOR velocity gain at 60 ms decline with age. HVOR velocity gain was found to decline by 0.017 per decade with increasing age 95 %CI 0.006 – 0.029; $p = 0.005$). HVOR velocity gain is the ratio of angular eye velocity to angular head velocity

Discussion

In 60 normal subjects aged 20–80 years, the mean HVOR velocity gain at 80 ms of 0.97 was little different from that at 60 ms of 0.94. The 2 SD lower limit of the HVOR velocity gain at 80 ms was 0.79 and at 60 ms was 0.75. Although statistically significant, the difference in mean HVOR velocity gain, rounded to 0.02 (95 % CI 0.04–0.01) between 80 ms and 60 ms is not clinically important. Nevertheless, in patients with an impaired HVOR velocity gain, we think 60 ms is a more accurate point of measure in the presence of covert saccades than 80 ms. Nonetheless, using both points of measure provides a check on the consistency of results, and the flatness of the gain trajectory in normal subjects confirms the absence of slip (see lower half of Fig 2).

The lowest and highest values of HVOR velocity gain at 80 ms (0.76 and 1.18 respectively) were very close to those found in another study using a similar VOG camera system, with eight normal subjects (HVOR velocity gains of 0.75 and 1.2 respectively). Comparable results were found in the same eight subjects using search coils with a lowest and highest HVOR velocity gain of 0.70 and 1.00 [14]. That study analysed HVOR velocity gain over a 40 ms window centred at peak acceleration, while our analysis is over a 10 ms window. The mean HVOR velocity gain at 80 ms of 0.97 (SD = 0.09) and at 60 ms of 0.94 (SD = 0.10) for the 60 subjects also sits within a range of HVOR velocity gains observed using the search coil method with comparable accelerations [15].

Earlier studies using vHIT had not referenced the variation of normal HVOR velocity gain with respect to age [14], though recently VOR gain was found to decrease significantly in subjects older than 70 years [16] or 80 years [17]. In our study, HVOR velocity gain at 80 ms and 60 ms declined by 0.012 and 0.017 respectively per decade as age increased. This decline in HVOR velocity gain with age is consistent with the decline shown in a previous study of the HVOR velocity gain with head impulses using the search coil method [18]. At a practical level, the variation of the HVOR velocity gain with age both with vHIT and search coils was small, justifying the inclusion of our 10 subjects in the eighth decade in normative data, despite a statistically significant decrease in HVOR velocity gain with age. Unlike vestibular evoked myogenic potentials which may be lost with age, our results suggest that the vHIT HVOR velocity gain stands up relatively well with age.

Our highest HVOR velocity gain of 1.18 is not physiological and is likely to relate to goggle slip. This was minimised through firm placement of the examiner's hands, clear from the goggle straps, holding the mandible to reduce slip. However, in the elderly who have looser skin and people with different facial structures or long hair, goggle slippage may still occur. We did not attempt to reduce slippage by using band aids across the nose, or placing dental paste on the nose [19], though these approaches might be considered if an individual subject's slippage affects the interpretation of results.

An adequate head acceleration of 2300 °/sec^2 to 5900 °/sec^2 was achieved in each HIT to ensure the detection of a high frequency vestibular deficit [13, 18]. This was monitored in real time by ensuring a peak head velocity of 150 °/s to 300 °/s at 80 ms with low amplitude head movements.

Repeatability at 80 ms and 60 ms revealed consistent results across all four tests carried out on each subject. This verifies that in the absence of artefact, only one sequence of 6 – 10 sets of rotation in each direction is necessary for clinical interpretation of the HVOR.

It is important to ensure that the method of the HIT is unpredictable in direction and time. Testing in a predictable method confirmed a non-physiological abnormally high HVOR velocity gain. This may result from pre-programming which can augment the VOR and enhance the HVOR velocity gain [20, 21].

Analysis was carried out at a fixation target distance of 1.50 m. HVOR velocity gain depends on target distance. As target distance was decreased, HVOR velocity gain increased, consistent with findings during search coil testing [22, 23]. In our study, the major influence of target distance on HVOR velocity gain appeared to occur at distances of less than 0.70 m. Comparable HVOR velocity gains were found between our study (testing at a 1.50 m fixation target distance) and another study (testing at a 0.91 m fixation target distance) [14]. The dependency of the HVOR velocity gain on target distance is due to the different topography of the axes of rotation of the eyes and head [23].

VOG overcomes the clinical problem of a false negative HIT due to covert saccades and allows discrimination

between physiological and pathological overt saccade(s). A clinical application is that in acute vertigo with clear impairment of HVOR velocity gain and the absence of CNS symptoms or signs, neuroimaging is not required; while the acutely vertiginous subject with a normal HVOR velocity gain needs consideration of a CNS cause or inferior vestibular neuritis [24]. The results of this study allow a comparison to be drawn between normal subjects and patients with vestibular lesions, across adult age groups to 80 years.

Conclusions

The mean HVOR velocity gain of 60 normal subjects was 0.97 (SD = 0.09) at 80 ms and 0.94 (SD = 0.10) at 60 ms. Despite a significant variation in the HVOR velocity gain with age, these changes are minor, declining by 0.012 and 0.017 per decade as age increased at 80 ms and 60 ms respectively, justifying the same normative data for the second to the eighth decades. Normative data at 60 ms provides an opportunity for assessment when the 80 ms time interval result may be affected by the appearance of catch-up covert saccades.

Abbreviations
HIT: Horizontal head impulse test; HVOR: Horizontal vestibulo-ocular reflex; vHIT: video HIT; VOG: Video-oculography; VOR: Vestibulo-ocular reflex.

Competing interest
The development of EyeSeeCam vHIT was supported by funds from the German Federal Ministry of Education and Research under the Grant code 01 EO 0901. Erich Schneider is a salaried member of the Brandenburg University of Technology Cottbus - Senftenberg. He also acts as an unpaid consultant and has received funding for travel from Interacoustics, distributor of EyeSeeCam. He is the general manager and a shareholder of EyeSeeTec GmbH, manufacturer of EyeSeeCam.
Dr Stuart Mossman's and Benjamin Mossman's research project salaries were paid through research funds from Wellington Hospital.
Gordon Purdie is a salaried member of Dean's Department, University of Otago, Wellington.

Authors' contributions
Study design, analysis, interpretation, drafting or revising of the paper involved all authors. Data was collected by BM alone. Statistical advice and analysis was performed by GP. All authors have given final approval of the version to be published and agree to be accountable for all aspects of the work in relation to accuracy or integrity of the paper.

Acknowledgements
Thank you to all the Wellington Hospital staff and members of the public who participated as normal subjects in the study.

Author details
[1]Department of Neurology, Wellington Hospital, Riddiford Street, Private Bag 7902, Wellington South, Wellington, New Zealand. [2]Dean's Department, University of Otago, Wellington, New Zealand. [3]Institute of Medical Technology, Brandenburg University of Technology Cottbus, Senftenberg, Germany.

References
1. Halmagyi GM, Cuthroy IS. A clinical sign of canal paresis. Arch Neurol. 1988;45:737–9.
2. Aw S, Haslwanter T, Halmagyi G, Curthoys I, Yavor R, Todd MM. Three-dimensional vector analysis of the human vestibuloocular reflex in

response to high-acceleration head rotations. I. Responses in normal subjects. J Neurophysiol. 1996;76(6):4009–20.

3. Bartl K, Lehnen N, Kohlbecher S, Schneider E. Head impulse testing using video-oculography. Ann NY Acad Sci. 2009;1164:331–3.

4. Hofmann P, Kellig A, Hoffmann H-U, Dara RG. Vestibular equipment onboard MIR. Acta Astronaut. 1998;43(3–6):313–9.

5. Strupp M, Glasauer S, Jahn K, Schneider E, Krafczyk S, Brandt T. Eye movements and balance. Ann NY Acad Sci. 2003;1004:352–8.

6. Pelz JB, Canosa R. Oculomotor behavior and perceptual strategies in complex tasks. Vision Res. 2001;41:3587–96.

7. Halmagyi GM, Weber KP, Aw ST, Todd MJ, Curthoys IS. Impulsive testing of semicircular canal function. Prog Brain Res. 2008;171:187–94.

8. Glasauer S, Lindeiner H, Siebold C, Buttner U. Vertical vestibular responses to head impulses are symmetric in downbeat nystagmus. Neurology. 2004;63:621–5.

9. Weber KP, MacDougall HG, Halmagyi GM, Curthoys IS. Impulsive testing of semicircular-canal function using video-oculography. Ann NY Acad Sci. 2009;1164:486–91.

10. Bland JM, Altman DG. Statistical methods for assessing agreement between two methods of clinical measurement. Lancet. 1986;327:307–10.

11. Schmid-Priscoveanu A, Boehmer A, Obzina H, Straumann D. Caloric and search-coil head impulse testing in patients after vestibular neuritis. J Assoc Res Otolaryngol. 2001;2:72–8.

12. Heuberger M, Saglam M, Todd N,Klaus Jahn K, Schneider E, Lehnen N. Covert Anti-Compensatory Quick Eye Movements during Head Impulses. PLoS ONE. 9(4): e93086. doi:10.1371/journal.pone.0093086

13. Weber KP, Aw ST, Todd MJ, McGarvie LA, Curthoys IS, Halmagyi GM. Horizontal head impulse test detects gentamicin vestibulotoxicity. Neurology. 2009;72:1417–24.

14. MacDougall HG, Weber KP, McGarvie LA, Halmagyi GM, Curthoys IS. The video head impulse test, diagnostic accuracy in peripheral vestibulopathy. Neurology. 2009;73:1134–41.

15. Weber KP, Aw ST, Todd MJ, McFarvie LA, Curthoys IS, Halmagyi GM. Head impulse test in unilateral vestibular loss, vestibulo-ocular reflex and catch up saccades. Neurology. 2008;70:454–63.

16. Matiño-Soler E, Esteller-More E, Martin-Sanchez JC, Martinez-Sanchez JM, Perez-Fernandez N. Normative data on angular vestibulo-ocular responses in the yaw axis measured using the video head impulse test. Otol Neurotol. 2015;36(3):466–71.

17. Li C, Layman AJ, Geary R, Anson E, Carey JP, Ferrucci L, et al. Epidemiology of Vestibulo-Ocular Reflex Function: Data from the Baltimore Longitudinal Study of Aging. Otol Neurotol. 2015;36(2):267–72.

18. Brzenzy R, Glasauer S, Bayer O, Siebold C, Buttner U. Head impulses in three orthogonal planes, influence of age. Ann NY Acad Sci. 2003;1004:473–7.

19. Versino M et al. Artifact avoidance for head impulse testing. Clin Neurophysiol. 2014;125:1071–3.

20. Della Santina CC, Cremer PD, Carey JP, Minor LB. Comparison of head thrust test with head autorotation test reveals that the vestibulo-ocular reflex is enhanced during voluntary head movements. Arch Otolaryngol Head Neck Surg. 2002;128:1044–54.

21. Black RA, Halmagyi GM, Thurtell MJ, Todd MJ, Cuthroys IS. The active head-impulse test in unilateral peripheral vestibulopathy. Arch Neurol. 2005;62(2):290–3.

22. Viirre E, Tweed D, Milner K, Vilis T. A reexamination of the gain of the vestibuloocular reflex. J Neurophysiol. 1986;56(2):439–50.

23. Collewijn H, Smeets JBJ. Early components of the human vestibulo-ocular response to head rotation: latency and gain. J Neurophysiol. 2000;84:376–89.

24. Halmagyi GM, Aw ST, Karlberg M, Curthoys IS, Todd MJ. Inferior vestibular neuritis. Ann NY Acad Sci. 2002;956:306–13.

28

Correction of severe columella and tip retraction in silicone implanted Asian short noses

Serkan Sertel[1,2*], Ioana Irina Venara-Vulpe[1] and Philippe Pasche[1]

Abstract

Background: Silicone Implants and other alloplastic materials are frequently used in rhinoplasty to augment Asian short noses. However, nasal deformities as a result of implant-related infections are increasing in incidence. The resulting tissue scarrings hinder the application of traditional techniques of lengthening short noses. The following paper presents a technique to correct severe postoperative retractions of the tip and columella caused by silicone implants.

Methods: We present a retrospective case study of two Asian patients with recurrent acute infections, secondary to silicone dorsum implants, leading to chronic inflammation of the tip and columella. The treatment consisted of implant removal and the immediate nasal reconstruction by combining uni- or bilateral gingivobuccal flaps along with L-shaped costal cartilage grafting.

To evaluate the surgical results, various anthropometric measurements, particularly the nasal length (NL) and nasal tip projection (NTP) of pre- and postoperative profile photographs, were analyzed.

Results: Successful nasal lengthening and correction of columellar retraction were achieved. In case I, postoperative NTP and NL increased by 34.7 % and 21.1 %, respectively. In case II, NL and NTP increased by 23.8 % and 10.6 %, respectively. However, case II presented necrosis of the distal extremity of one gingivobuccal flap without rib graft resorption, which later healed by secondary intention.

Conclusion: Pronounced columellar retraction in severe short noses can be successfully managed with a combination of gingivobuccal flaps along with L-shaped costal cartilage grafting. The use of autologous materials decreases the risk of long-term extrusion through the tip. The gingivobuccal flap provides vascularity to the exposed rib cartilage on the columella and prevents its resorption.

Keywords: Augmentation rhinoplasty, Nasal lengthening, Silicone implant, Gingivobuccal flap, L-shaped rib cartilage graft, Short nose, Anthropometric measurement

Background

There is an increasing desire in Asian patients to have the same esthetical nasal features of Caucasians with a high and narrow nasal bridge, long columella and projected nasal tip. Rhinoplasty in Asian patients differs significantly from that of Caucasians. Thus, rhinoplasty in Asian patients mainly involves augmentation with grafts or implants, in contrast to resection, reduction, or refinement, which are typical for Caucasian patients. Nasal augmentation can be achieved with either autologous (bone or cartilage) or alloplastic material. Alloplastic materials such as silicone are frequently applied for dorsal augmentation rhinoplasty [1], due to their relative ease of insertion and the rapidity of the procedure.

However, due to implant-related complications subsequent removal of the silicone implant becomes often necessary [1, 2]. In fact, chronic inflammation and shifting of the implant in the subcutaneous tissue, resulting in a cephalic displacement towards the nasion and protrusion through the vestibular skin, are the most frequent problems

* Correspondence: serkan.sertel@chuv.ch
[1]Department of Otorhinolaryngology, Head & Neck Surgery, University Hospital CHUV, Rue du Bugnon 46, 1011 Lausanne, Switzerland
[2]Department of Otorhinolaryngology, Head & Neck Surgery, University of Heidelberg, Heidelberg, Germany

after silicone implantation. The incidence of such complications is reported to be up to 36 % [1]. The consequences are skin contour deformities of the tip and columella, e.g. retraction and severe overrotation of the tip. The removal of the alloplastic material results in scar contracture of the dorsal and of the tip soft tissue [3].

The primary intentions of the reconstruction are to lengthen the overrotated nose and to correct the retracted columella. The latter is often challenging due to the lack of soft tissue in the membranous columella. First of all, a lack of tissue can be observed between the upper lateral cartilage (ULC) and the cephalic part of the lower lateral cartilage (LLC), which might not allow a caudal replacement of the tip. Moreover, soft tissue contracture along mucosal or external tissues can resist lengthening.

The applied lengthening techniques depend on the severity of the short nose. As Asian noses are generally shorter than Caucasian ones, a combination of maneuvers is necessary for their lengthening. Here, we present an innovative technique combining a wire-stabilized L-shaped rib cartilage graft with a uni- or bilateral gingivobuccal flap, which serves as a well-vascularized cover that also prevents the exposure of the L-shaped cartilage graft into the vestibule.

Methods

This is a retrospective case study of two patients who underwent a revision augmentation rhinoplasty at the Centre Hospitalier Universitaire Vaudois (CHUV) in Lausanne. The Human Research Ethics Committee of the Canton Vaud approved the study protocol and the written informed consent.

Case I: WM, ♀, * 16.06.1974

Initially the patient had an augmentation rhinoplasty with a silicone implant carried out in Thailand. Seven years later, she had a revision rhinoplasty because of a thickening of the right vestibule. Later she had recurrent infections of the right vestibule and the dorsum. In addition, she suffered from a renal insufficiency secondary to a glomerulonephritis and was listed for kidney transplantation. For this reason, it was decided to remove the silicone implant to prevent further infection considering her immunocompromised state. In the following years, she noticed an increasing retraction of the columella and infra-tip lobule as well as a synechia of the upper part of the right vestibule (Figs. 1 and 2). Laboratory findings could exclude Wegeners granulamatosis. Preoperatively, we administered a pathogen sensitive intravenous antibiotic treatment for five days, which was continued intraoperatively. During surgery new biopsies were collected around the silicone implant for an antibiogram to adapt the postoperative antibiotic therapy for 48 h intravenously and then for 15 days orally. The

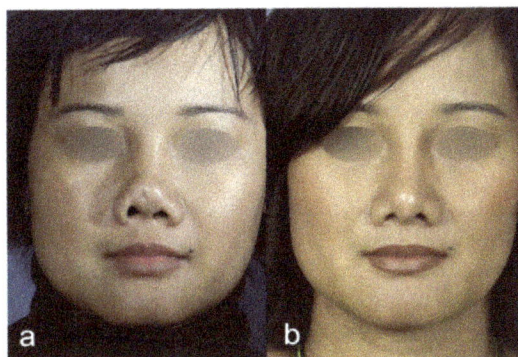

Fig. 1 a Preoperative and b 9 months postoperative frontal views of case I

patient was followed-up 9 months after surgery, because she then moved back to Thailand.

Case II: SL, ♀, * 29.12.1961

This patient underwent an augmentation rhinoplasty with a silicone implant, followed by two revision rhinoplasties and finally the removal of the silicone implant because of a chronic infection. All operations were performed in Thailand. By the time she came to our clinic she had progressively developed a severe columellar retraction as well as a significant overrotation of the tip

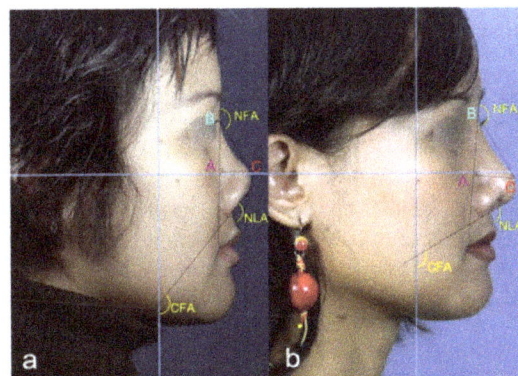

Fig. 2 a Preoperative and b 9 months postoperative lateral views of case I with anthropometric measures. Reference points consisted of the tip-defining point (C), the nasion (B) and the projection of C onto the nasion-alar line (A). Nasal length (NL) was measured as the distance between B and C in centimeters (cm) according to the Goode's method. Nasal tip projection (NTP) was measured as the distance from A to C in cm. The naso-frontal angle (NFA) was measured as the angle in degrees (°) formed between the proximal nasal dorsum and the anterior surface of the forehead below the glabella. The columellar-facial angle (CFA) was measured as the angle between the line drawn from the anterior columella to the subnasale and the line perpendicular to the Frankfurt horizontal plane (blue horizontal line). Postoperative NTP and NL increased by 34.7 % and 21.1 %, respectively due to a lack of cartilaginous support. The distal border of the columella was severely retracted 3–4 mm behind the lateral part of the nostrils. Both soft triangles were also severely retracted, and synechia had reduced the height of the nostrils (Figs. 3 and 4). This patient was followed-up 3 years after surgery.

Operative techniques

Gingivobuccal flap

Several authors have described the transfer of the gingivobuccal flap into the nose [4–6]. In this case, its main indications were the closure of septal perforation and ozena. The flap was harvested according to Meyer's method, without reinforcing the flap with ear cartilage [7, 8]. The vascularization of the gingivobuccal mucosa mainly depends on branches of the superior labial, infraorbital and buccal arteries [9]. In the case of a unilateral gingivobuccal flap, the pedicle is based 5 mm paramedian to the nasal spine. The main blood supply comes from the superior labial artery. However, when the gingivobuccal flap is harvested bilaterally, 2 cm of the untouched mucosa should be left between the two pedicles to preserve the vascularization of both flaps by the branches of the superior labial artery (R. septi nasi).

The flap was transferred to the nasal cavity through a tunnel next to the anterior nasal spine. The entire mucosa of the flap in the tunnel was also left intact. The two flaps covered the anterior septal cartilage on both sides, which in our cases consisted of the L-shaped rib cartilage graft (Figs. 5 and 6). The oral donor site was closed with resorbable sutures (Vicryl 4–0).

L-shaped rib cartilage graft

Severe short noses require an augmentation of the dorsum as well as the retracted columella projection and show. The donor site for the L-shaped costal cartilage graft was the cartilaginous costal arch at the 8th and the 9th rib.[7] Modeling the shape of this graft is crucial for ideal and individual positioning and thus sticks to exact

angles to the dorsum and the caudal septum. The L-shaped graft was carved out in the middle of the rib to avoid warping. A 10 mm wire was inserted in the middle of the horizontal and vertical part of the L-shaped graft to prevent long-term bending of the cartilage and to secure the fixation on the anterior nasal spine (Fig. 7b, c). The shape of the graft can be adapted precisely to the individual anatomy by performing a chondrotomy of the graft, which maintains its stability due to the wire (Fig. 7b).

In order to relieve postoperative pain at the costal cartilage donor site we placed an intravenous canula and administered 5 ml of bupivacaine (2.5 mg/ml) right after closure of the wound and four hours postoperatively.

Patients were advised to do antiseptic mouth rinses with chlorhexidine for 10 days.

Standardized photography

The patient photographs were taken in a standardized fashion with a digital single-lens-reflex (DSLR) camera (Nikon D5100) and a lens of 90 mm focal length by a professional photographer in the Department of Otorhinolaryngology, Head & Neck Surgery of CHUV. Patients were seated in a fixed position with a standardized distance of 1 m to the camera, and were asked to look at designated points for different views. The camera height was adjusted according to the patient's height. Patients were asked to keep their eyes fully open with direct gaze and lips closed and not smiling.

Anthropometric measurement

Photography analysis was performed using the Adobe[R] Photoshop CS5 measuring tool (Adobe Systems, Inc., San Jose, CA, USA). Surgical results were analyzed by anthropometric measurements of pre- and postoperative profile photographs in the Frankfurt horizontal plane. Anthropometric measurements included the nasal length (NL), columellar-facial angle (CFA), nasal tip projection (NTP), naso-frontal angle (NFA) and the nasal tip

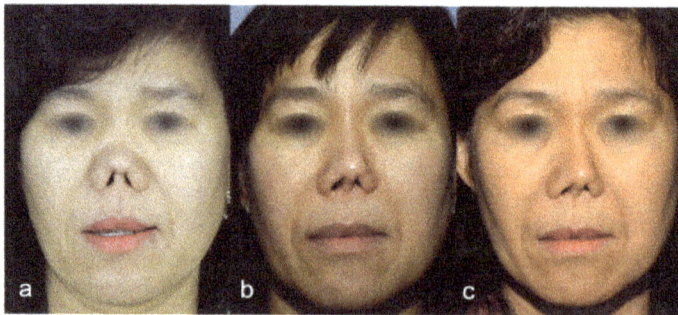

Fig. 3 a Preoperative frontal view of case II with the columella severely retracted into the nose, **b** 8 months postoperative and (**c**) 3 years postoperative frontal views

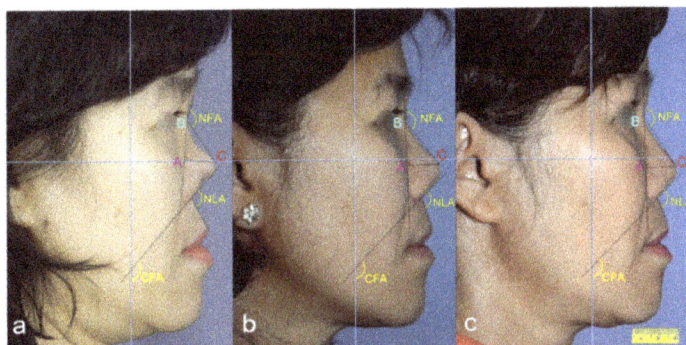

Fig. 4 a Preoperative, **b** 8 months postoperative and (**c**) 3 years postoperative lateral views of case II with NL and NTP increased by 23.8 % and 10.6 %, respectively

projection ratio (Figs. 2 and 4). Reference points consisted of the tip-defining point (C), the nasion (B) and the projection of C onto the nasion-alar line (A) [10]. NL was measured as the distance in centimeters (cm) between B and C according to Goode's method [11]. NFA was measured as the angle in degrees (°) formed between the proximal nasal dorsum and the anterior surface of the forehead below the glabella. NTP was measured as the distance in cm from A to C. The CFA was measured as the angle between a line drawn from the anterior columella to the subnasale and the line perpendicular to the Frankfurt horizontal plane. The nasal tip projection was determined according to Goode's index [11] using the ratio: AC/BC. All anthropometric values were listed and compared pre- and postoperatively, expressed in differences (Δ) and percentage differences (Δ [%]) of different time intervals (Table 1 and 2).

Results

Surgical management

Case I (WM, ♀, *16.06.1974)

We performed an open rhinoplasty to remove the silicone implant. Chronic infection had destroyed the anterior septum and severely damaged the ULC and LLC.

The right vestibular skin was destroyed with granulation tissue over a distance of 1.5 cm. The implant was displaced laterally towards the tip and protruded through the right vestibular skin (Fig. 1a). The silicone implant was removed. The previous implant site was cleaned of granulation tissue with a curette and then irrigated with a betadine/saline solution. Extensive subperiostal undermining of the nasal skin up to the nasion and the anterior wall of the maxilla was performed, in order to maximally mobilize the skin envelope. In addition, scarred tissue between the ULC and LLC was removed for mobilize the tip downwards. Despite mobilizing the septo-mucoperichondral flaps, a gap of 1.5 cm was observed in the right vestibule that was covered with a right gingivobuccal flap (Fig. 6). A spoon-shaped flap from the mucous membrane of the oral vestibule, next to the frenulum above the upper row of teeth was prepared and then passed into the nose through an oronasal tunnel (Fig. 5) [7, 8]. The flap was long enough to add mucosal tissue between the ULC and LLC. A sponge soaked with betadine was left in place in the previous silicone site during the preparation of the graft.

Cartilage was harvested from the 8th rib and carved to an L-shaped form with a tip extension to recreate the

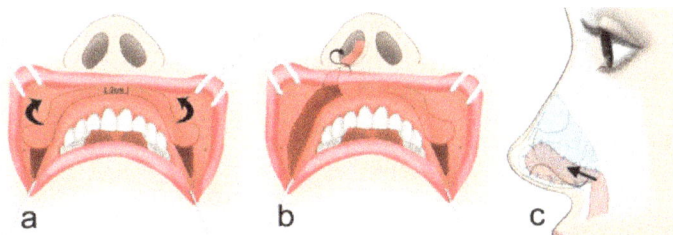

Fig. 5 a Harvest of bilateral gingivobuccal flaps with 2 cm of untouched mucosa between the two pedicles in order to preserve vascularization of both flaps. Each flap is blood supplied by small midline branches of the superior labial artery. **b** Each flap is transferred into the nasal cavity through a tunnel beside the anterior nasal spine. **c** The two flaps cover the anterior septal cartilage on both sides (Modified drawing according to Meyer)

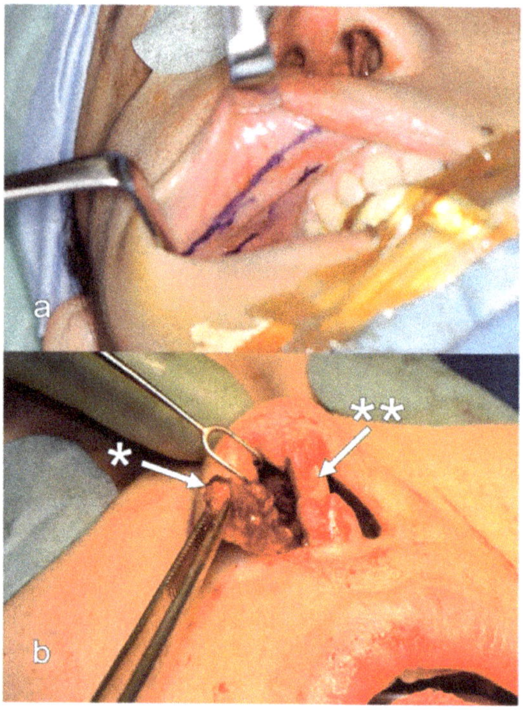

Fig. 6 a Spoon-shaped gingivobuccal flap prepared from the mucosa and submucosa of the oral vestibule next to the frenulum above the upper row of teeth. The superior incision of the flap is done inferior to the stenon duct. **b** Flap passed through an oronasal tunnel into the nose (* Gingivobuccal flap; ** L-shaped graft)

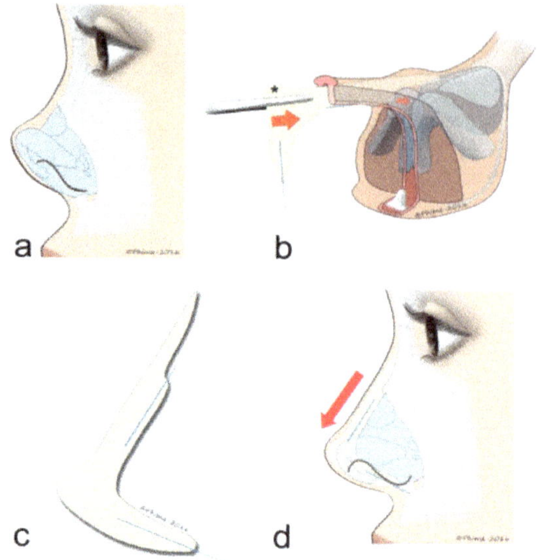

Fig. 7 a Schematic aspect of a preoperative short nose. **b** L-shaped rib cartilage graft with caudal tip extension design (*), inserted with two wires into the cartilage to avoid its bending and to allow its fixation. Fixation with a vertical wire in a hole drilled into the nasal spine. **c** Design of the L-shaped graft with a notch to improve the stability over the dorsum. **d** Successful nasal lengthening and correction of columellar retraction

dome according to the form of the silicone implant. The remaining LLC were sutured to the tip.

Two wires were inserted into the graft to avoid bending of the cartilage and to fixate the rib graft in a hole drilled into the anterior nasal spine. For the dorsum, a notch was created on the cartilage that was embedded into the nasal bone with an extension over the nasal bone (Fig. 7b–d). The second wire can also be placed under the nasal bone to support the stability of the fixation but it is not mandatory. The well-vascularized gingivobuccal flap covered the graft and additionally avoided exposure of the L-shaped cartilage into the vestibule.

Case II (LS, ♀, *29.12.1961)

The same technique as described in case I was used. The main difference was the pronounced skin retraction in the columella-dorso-tip unit, which allowed minimal downward mobilization despite maximal undermining of the skin. The columella was retracted into the nose behind the nostrils. Additional lengthening of the nose would have required a paramedian forehead flap, which was initially refused by the patient. During our first

surgery, we removed the scarred tissue between ULC and LLC and replaced it with an auricular composite graft. The reconstruction of the membranous columella and the vestibule required a bilateral gingivobuccal flap. The L-shaped rib cartilage was inserted as in case I. Ten days later the patient developed a limited distal necrosis of the left gingivobuccal flap without resorption of the rib graft, which later healed by secondary intention. During this time, a minor tip deviation to the left was noted. Within 5 months we performed a reduction of the contralateral flap to improve the nasal breathing.

Anthropometric measurement
Case I

The postoperative NTP increased by 34.7 % from 1.9 cm to 2.56 cm within 9 months. Nasal length (NL) increased by 21 % from 3.64 cm to 4.41 cm. NTP ratio according to Goode's method increased by 11.5 %. All measured angles, NFA, CFA and NLA decreased postoperatively by 3.6 %, 14.7 % and 16.5 %, respectively (Table 1).

Case II

The first postoperative values of NL, NTP and NTP ratio, measured after 8 months increased by 13 %, 22.5 % and 8.5 % respectively. NFA and CFA decreased postoperatively by 1.4 % and 4.9 %, respectively. In contrast, NLA increased by 2.6 % (Table 2). The second

Table 1 Anthropometric values (Nasal tip projection (NTP), Nasal length (NL), NTP ratio equals NTP / NL, Columellar-facial angle (CFA), Naso-frontal angle (NFA)) of preoperative and postoperative results as well as their differences (Δ) and percentage differences (Δ [%]) of case I

		NTP (cm)	NL (cm)	NTP ratio	NFA (°)	CFA (°)	NLA (°)
Pre-OP		1.9	3.64	0.52	145	140.5	118
Post-OP (9 months)		2.56	4.41	0.58	139.7	119.8	98.5
9 months post-op	Δ	+0.66	+0.77	+0.06	- 5.3	- 20.7	- 19.5
	Δ [%]	+34.73	+21.15	+11.53	- 3.65	- 14.73	- 16.52

postoperative measurement after 3 years revealed an increase of NL and NTP of 23.8 % and 10.6 %, respectively. Within the same time period, NTP ratio decreased by 10 %. NFA increased by 1.2 %, whereas CFA and NLA increased postoperatively by 7.5 % and 4.3 %, respectively (Table 2).

Discussion

Augmentation rhinoplasty using alloplastic materials to correct short noses is a relatively common practice in Asia. Several materials are used for augmenting the height of the nose, e.g. silicone, Gore-Tex® and Medpor® [1]. However, alloplastic implant-related complications occur with an incidence of 4 % - 36 % [1, 12, 13] including infections, capsular contractures, extrusions, implant shifts, and calcifications.

The main problem in revision rhinoplasty after the extrusion of alloplastic-implanted material in short noses is the enormous scarring of the skin and inner lining, which hinders the application of traditional techniques. The skin can be mobilized by extensive undermining. If this is insufficient, a regional flap is an alternative. The disadvantage of the regional flap is scarring, which occurs even when nasal subunits are respected. This flap must cover the complete dorsal subunit as well as the dorsum and the tip subunit.

The surgical management of implant-related complications of short noses typically consists of two stages: (I) removal of the alloplastic implant and (II) reconstruction 10 days later in order to eradicate the infection and decrease the risk of cartilage graft infection. This approach

however may lead to further scar contracture of skin and soft tissue during the time between the two stages. Therefore, we preferred simultaneous removal of the implant along with reconstruction, which was preceded by a pathogen sensitive intravenous antibiotic treatment.

After implant removal, we first needed to correct dorsum height and tip projection, which was initially achieved by the caudal part of the silicone implant. Secondly, we had to correct the overrotation by lengthening the entire nose. Finally, columellar and vestibular retraction by scarring required well-vascularized soft tissue replacement to cover the cartilaginous graft. All three problems were addressed with the L-shaped rib cartilage graft and the gingivobuccal flap. To maintain the soft tissue in the new position a strong stable support is required, therefore the anteriorly fixed L-shaped rib graft represents an ideal solution. However, the graft had to be fixed on the nasal spine with a wire. The second requirement for a stable reconstruction is the width of the columellar part of the L-shaped graft. It should be wide enough to present an adequate columella show. In addition, the L-shaped graft is maintained in position anteriorly and superiorly by close contact with the caudal septum. The shape of this graft is crucial for ideal and individual positioning and thus follows exact angles of the dorsum and the caudal septum.

With this technique, tip projection is augmented by a carved extension of the rib graft, similar to that of the initially created silicone implant (Fig. 7b).

Contemporary techniques used for nose lengthening include the extension spreader graft and the extended

Table 2 Anthropometric values of preoperative, early (8 months) and late (3 years) postoperative results as well as their differences (Δ) and percentage differences (Δ [%]) of case II

		NTP (cm)	NL (cm)	NTP ratio	NFA (°)	CFA (°)	NLA (°)
Pre-OP		1.6	2.68	0.59	134	147.3	121.6
Post-OP (8 months)		1.96	3.03	0.64	132.1	140	124.8
Post-OP (3 years)		1.77	3.32	0.53	135.7	136.2	116.3
8 months post-op	Δ	+0.36	+0.35	+0.05	- 1.9	- 7.3	+3.2
	Δ [%]	+22.5	+13.05	+8.47	- 1.42	- 4.95	+2.63
3 years post-op	Δ	+0.17	+0.64	- 0.06	+1.7	- 11.1	- 5.3
	Δ [%]	+10.6	+23.88	- 10.17	+1.26	- 7.54	- 4.36

caudal septal graft, often combined with various tip and dorsal onlay grafts. Theses techniques require a strong septal support to maintain the grafts in the proper position. The severe short nose often presents a week septum due to an infection and extremely retracted skin, which can twist the grafts. We believe that the L-shaped graft provides a better stability of the reconstruction. Moreover, the tip extension in our L-shaped graft allows a higher fixation of the upper lateral cartilages and the creation of a new dome higher than the level of the previous domes. This assures a good projection with a uniform repartition of the pressure under the skin. In case of any resorption, the large amount of cartilage of the L-shaped graft can still preserve the stability of the reconstruction.

Cases

Case I was successfully managed with optimal aesthetic and functional results. The gingivobuccal flap successfully covered the anterior septal cartilage and corrected the synechia of the upper part of the vestibule. Initially, the patient complained about nasal obstruction secondary to the thickness of the base of the flap. The problem resolved with a spontaneous atrophy of the flap after 6 months. Discomfort secondary to the scar in the gingivobuccal groove disappeared after 2 months of physiotherapy. No infection occurred despite the fact she was immunosuppressed in the context of kidney transplantation. A follow-up of 9 years showed a stable result with no long-term complications.

Anthropometric measurements confirmed the subjective aesthetical improvements. NL and NTP increased by 21.1 % and 34.7 %, respectively. The main reason for this improvement is rooted in the stability of the reconstructed cartilaginous framework with wires and the presence of individual skin elasticity, which allowed lengthening.

The unilateral gingivobuccal flap proved to be safe and very useful to replace the vestibular inner lining both on the medial side and the upper lateral wall of the nostril.

The length of nose in case II still maintained after a follow-up of 3 years. Comparison of the first with the last (3 years post-op) measurements revealed, that NL and NTP even increased by 23.8 % and 10.6 %, respectively. Despite wide subperiostal skin elevation, mobilization of the severely scarred skin envelope was limited. Additional lengthening would have required a regional flap, e.g. paramedian forehead flap to reconstruct the entire columella-dorso-tip or at least the dorsum unit. Unfortunately, the patient refused the paramedian forehead flap. Ultimately, the patient developed a limited distal necrosis of the left gingivobuccal flap without rib graft resorption that healed by secondary intention. This probably caused a minor tip deviation

to the left. Debulking of the contralateral flap was performed after 5 months to improve nasal breathing. Major improvements were observed only on the tip, infra-tip and columella, which showed better volume, contour and definition in the frontal view (Fig. 3).

In such cases of severe short noses, we usually observe a deficiency of inner lining of the membranous septum as well as between the ULC and LLC. In addition, scarring of the vestibule reduces the height of the nostril. An elevation of a large septo-muco-perichondrial flap would lengthen the nose to maximally 4 mm anteriorly. An anteriorly based septal flap would add an anterior lengthening with the disadvantage of crusting of a denuded posterior septum. Composite conchal grafts represent a reasonable additional method to add tissue between ULC and LLC. These grafts should only be placed in a well-vascularized surrounding tissue. In case II, we successfully integrated one composite graft between the right ULC and LLC.

In our opinion, the gingivobuccal flap is useful for the reconstruction of the membranous septum. This flap was previously described for septal perforations and was used in three stages [7]. The question arises whether a bilateral gingivobuccal flap is advised. This approach bears the risk to lose one of both. The median sublabial region must be respected on a distance of 2 cm in order to protect the branches of the superior labial artery (Fig. 5a), which will vascularize both the flaps.

In cases of bilateral gingivobuccal flaps use, an autonomization of both flaps ten days before - as described in Meyer's method to close septal perforations [8] - would probably decrease the risk of distal necrosis. However, this autonomization is not necessary in cases of unilateral usage of the gingivobuccal flap.

The major limitation of our technique is the confined mobilization of nasal skin envelope due to scar contractures.

The limitation of our study is the small number of patients.

Conclusions

Pronounced columellar retraction in severe short noses can be successfully managed with a combination of gingivobuccal flaps and a L-shaped costal cartilage grafting. Stabilization and exact design of the L-shaped rib graft is the key to successful lengthening of severe short noses, because the contracted skin leads to high pressure on the graft with the risk of displacement. The use of autologous materials decreases the risk of long-term extrusion through the tip. The gingivobuccal flap provides vascularization to the exposed rib cartilage on the columella and prevents its resorption.

It is important to assess the status of the skin elasticity preoperatively. In these particular cases the mobilization of the nasal skin envelope will not be sufficient to lengthen the nose to satisfactory extent and a paramedian frontal flap should be taken into consideration.

Consent

Written informed consent was obtained from the patient for the publication of this report and any accompanying images.

Competing interests
The authors declare that they have no competing interests.

Authors' contributions
Original idea by PP. PP, SS and IV operated the cases. SS gathered the data with IV. SS performed and revised figures. SS and PP wrote the paper. All authors read and approved the final manuscript.

Acknowledgment
The authors thank Marion Brun, photographer in the Department of Otorhinolaryngology, Head and Neck Surgery of CHUV, for her excellent media work. The authors thank also Dr. Mercy George and Dr. Volker Haxsen for editing the manuscript.

Interest of conflict
All authors declare no potential conflict of interest. No grant or funds have been received for this study.

References
1. Kim HS, Park SS, Kim MH, Kim MS, Kim SK, Lee KC. Problems associated with alloplastic materials in rhinoplasty. Yonsei Med J. 2014;55(6):1617–23. doi:10.3349/ymj.2014.55.6.1617.
2. Park JH, Mangoba DC, Mun SJ, Kim DW, Jin HR. Lengthening the short nose in Asians: key maneuvers and surgical results. JAMA Facial Plast Surg. 2013;15(6):439–47. doi:10.1001/jamafacial.2013.95.
3. Jung DH, Lin RY, Jang HJ, Claravall HJ, Lam SM. Correction of pollybeak and dimpling deformities of the nasal tip in the contracted, short nose by the use of a supratip transposition flap. Arch Facial Plast Surg. 2009;11(5):311–9. doi:10.1001/archfacial.2009.60.
4. Chalaye JC, Levignac J. Repair of cocaine-induced perforations of the nasal septum (or the glider-wing mucosal flap). Ann Chir Plast Esthet. 1985;30(3):229–35.
5. Ey W. Potentials of reconstructive plastic surgery in the area of the nose. Laryngol Rhinol Otol (Stuttg). 1983;62(1):1–5.
6. Meyer R, Kesselring UK. Surgical correction of the unusually short nose. Aesthetic Plast Surg. 1976;1(1):271–7. doi:10.1007/BF01570261.
7. Meyer R, editor. Secondary Rhinoplasty - Including Reconstruction of the Nose. 2nd ed.: Springer-Verlag Berlin Heidelberg 2002;2002. http://www.springer.com/gb/book/9783540658849.
8. Meyer R. Closure of septal perforations of every size and reconstruction of the septum. Aesthetic Plast Surg. 2002;26 Suppl 1:S15. doi:10.1007/s00266-002-4319-1.
9. Paulsen F, Waschke J. Sobotta, Atlas of Anatomy. Vol. 3, 15th ed. Elsevier GmbH: Urban & Fischer Verlag, Munich; 2011. http://store.elsevier.com/product.jsp?locale=en_EU&isbn=9780723437338.
10. Turner F, Zanaret M, Giovanni A. Evaluation of nasal tip projection. Fr ORL. 2007;92:282–7.
11. Goode RL. Proportions of the aesthetic face. In: Powell N, Humphreys B, editors. Personal Communication. New York: Thieme-Stratton Inc; 1983. p. 23–7.
12. Graham BS, Thiringer JK, Barrett TL. Nasal tip ulceration from infection and extrusion of a nasal alloplastic implant. J Am Acad Dermatol. 2001;44(2 Suppl):362–4.
13. Zeng Y, Wu W, Yu H, Yang J, Chen G. Silicone implant in augmentation rhinoplasty. Ann Plast Surg. 2002;49(5):495–9. doi:10.1097/01.SAP.0000020095.97899.EC.

29

Knowledge and risk perception of oral cavity and oropharyngeal cancer among non-medical university students

Nosayaba Osazuwa-Peters[1,2,3,4]* and Nhial T. Tutlam[4]

Abstract

Background: To assess non-medical university students' knowledge and perceived risk of developing oral cavity and oropharyngeal cancer.

Methods: A cross-sectional survey was conducted among non-medical students of a private Midwestern university in the United States in May 2012. Questionnaire assessed demographic information and contained 21 previously validated questions regarding knowledge and perceived risk of developing oral cavity and oropharyngeal cancer. Knowledge scale was categorized into low and high. Risk level was estimated based on smoking, drinking, and sexual habits. Bivariate associations between continuous and categorical variables were assessed using Pearson correlation and Chi-square tests, respectively.

Results: The response rate was 87% (100 out of 115 students approached). Eighty-one percent (81%) had low oral cavity and oropharyngeal cancer knowledge; and only 2% perceived that their oral cavity and oropharyngeal cancer risk was high. Risk perception was negatively correlated with age at sexual debut, r (64) = −0.26, $p = 0.037$; one-way ANOVA showed a marginally significant association between risk perception and number of sexual partners, $F(4, 60) = 2.48$, $p = 0.05$. There was no significant association between knowledge and perception of risk; however, oral cavity and oropharyngeal cancer knowledge was significantly associated with frequency of prevention of STDs ($p < 0.05$). Although 86% had heard about oral cavity and oropharyngeal cancer, only 18% had heard of oral mouth examination, and 7% of these reported ever having an oral cavity and oropharyngeal cancer exam.

Conclusions: Oral cavity and oropharyngeal cancer knowledge and risk perception is low among this student population. Since oral cavity and oropharyngeal cancer incidence is increasingly shifting towards younger adults, interventions must be tailored to this group in order to improve prevention and control.

Keywords: Oral cavity and oropharyngeal cancer, non-medical university students, knowledge, risk perception, sexual habits

Background

Oral cavity and oropharyngeal cancer is found around the oral cavity and oropharynx, and is the 6th most common cancer in the world, with estimated annual incidence of more than 405, 000 cases [1]. In 2012 in the United States, it was estimated that about 40,250 new cases of oral cancers will be diagnosed [2], thus meeting

qualification criteria to be regarded as a common cancer in the United States [3]. They account for almost 3% of all cancers, and are the 13th most common cancer in the United States [4, 5]. The causative factors linked to oral cancer include chronic use of tobacco and alcohol, which act independently and synergistically in the etio-pathogenesis of the disease [1, 6]. An increasing number of cases of non-smoking, non-drinking individuals have helped to establish another major causal factor - human papillomavirus (HPV), which was thought to account for up to 23% of cases of oropharyngeal cancer [7]. A newer study however indicates that at least 70% of the

* Correspondence: nosazuwa@slu.edu
[1]Brown School, Washington University in St. Louis, 1 Brookings Drive, Saint Louis, MO 63130, USA
[2]Saint Louis University Cancer Center, 3655 Vista Avenue, Saint Louis, Missouri 63110, USA
Full list of author information is available at the end of the article

oropharyngeal cancer incidence in the United States, in the last decade, may be causally linked to HPV [8].

Young adults of university age are known to engage in tobacco smoking and alcohol use, and may be frequently exposed to HPV infection, all of which are causal factors for oral cavity and oropharyngeal cancer [1, 6, 9]. Previous studies indicate that university students may have some knowledge of risks associated with tobacco smoking and alcohol [10–12]. However, while HPV remains the most prevalent sexually transmitted infection in the United States, knowledge of HPV among students remains quite low [13]. It has been reported that some college students even misinterpret HPV as HIV [13], and the latter remains a dominant topic of discussion in many sex education curricula across the United States [13, 14]. Over a decade ago in a Kaiser family survey, only 2% of the surveyed American population of young people not older than 18 years old, could identify that HPV was a sexually transmitted disease [14]. Knowledge of the link between oral cavity and oropharyngeal cancer and HPV seems even lower. Globally, the few studies that have examined students' knowledge of oral cavity and oropharyngeal cancer only looked at medical and dental students [15–20], who may presumably present with better knowledge scores due to their health-directed training. The only known study that compared undergraduates to medical students and to the general population focused exclusively on HPV as a causal factor for head and neck cancer [21]. No other study, to the best of the author's knowledge, has examined knowledge levels of oral cavity and oropharyngeal cancer exclusively among non-medical students, who may receive greater overall benefit from a customized health education program.

With the recent downward shift in the age of onset of oral cavity and oropharyngeal cancer, especially oropharyngeal cancer, from the typical sixth to seventh decade of life forty years ago [4, 8] to the third or fourth decade of life in the last twenty years [9, 22], there is a need for increased population based education about oral cavity and oropharyngeal cancer among university students, who represents a sizable population in the United States [23]. This study aims to examine non-medical university students' level of knowledge of oral cavity and oropharyngeal cancer and its risk factors, and to determine university students' perception of their risk of developing oral cavity and oropharyngeal cancer.

Methods

Study design

A cross-sectional study was conducted between May and June 2012 in a private, research university in the Midwest. Approval for this study was sought and obtained as protocol ID: 201205057 from the Institutional Review Board of the university prior to commencement of study.

Study participants

Participants for the study included conveniently sampled male and female students in the university, both undergraduate and graduate students. Students were recruited to voluntarily participate in the study from the university main library and cafeteria. There was no compensation for participating in the study.

Eligibility criteria

University students 18 years or older were eligible to take part in the study. In addition, participants needed to be able to consent to study in order to participate.

Exclusion criteria

In order to assess the level of oral cavity cancer knowledge among non-medical university students, all medical, nursing, and public health students were excluded from the study. Additionally, all students who were previously enrolled in a head and neck cancer study, or for those students less than 18 years old, were excluded from the study. In addition, those who had been previously diagnosed with oral head and neck cancer were ineligible to participate.

Data collection

Questionnaire

The study employed a previously validated 58-item, paper-based questionnaire adapted from previous studies [12, 15, 16, 19].

Demographic variables

The survey included demographic questions such as age, sex, relationship status, race, and educational level.

Risk factor-related variables

Students were asked *"Do you smoke?" "If yes, how many cigarettes do you smoke daily?"* and *"If you are a current smoker, how long have you been smoking?"* Additionally, students who were smokers were asked to gauge their relative risk of developing oral cavity and oropharyngeal cancer compared to other smokers of same age and sex. Students were also asked *"Do you drink alcohol?" "How often do you drink?" "If you still drink, how long have you been drinking?"* and *"If you have stopped drinking, when did you stop?"* Finally, students who drank alcohol were asked to gauge perceived oral cavity and oropharyngeal cancer risk.

To elicit risk factors for oral HPV, students were asked the following: *"Have you ever had sexual intercourse?", "At what age did you first have sexual intercourse",* and *"How many sexual partners have you had in your lifetime".* Finally, students were asked how frequently they used STD prevention during sexual intercourse, on a scale from "never" to "always".

Knowledge of oral cavity and oropharyngeal cancer

Students were asked 14 questions to gauge their knowledge of oral cavity and oropharyngeal cancer. General questions that elicited awareness included *"In your opinion, oral cavity and oropharyngeal cancer is more common in which age group?" "In your opinion, in which gender is oral cavity and oropharyngeal cancer more common?* and *"Does early diagnosis improve recovery from oral cavity and oropharyngeal cancer?"* Additionally, some questions focused on the pathophysiology of oral cavity and oropharyngeal cancer, such as: *"In your opinion, where are the most likely locations of oral cavity and oropharyngeal cancer?" "In your opinion, which of these could cause oral cavity and oropharyngeal cancer?" "How do you imagine oral cavity and oropharyngeal cancer looks like in the mouth?" "Can oral cavity and oropharyngeal cancer manifest without initial complaint, pain, or symptom?" and "Is oral cavity and oropharyngeal cancer a contagious disease?".* There were also Likert scale-styled questions that asked whether students thought HPV infection, tobacco and alcohol use, eating spicy foods, and exposure to sunlight increased an individual's chance of developing oral cavity and oropharyngeal cancer. Answers in the knowledge portion of the questionnaire were then scored as 1 for 'correct' and 0 for 'incorrect'. Each student's answers were summed to create a scale, "knowledge score."

Risk assessment

There were 4 risk perception questions on a 5-point Likert scale, and participants were asked to compare themselves to other smokers or drinkers of the same age and sex to describe what they thought their chances of developing oral cavity and oropharyngeal cancer in the future were, from most likely to least likely. There was also a question that assessed perceived severity of a potential cancer lesion: *"What would you do if you had a painless, abnormal swelling in your mouth for more than 2 weeks?"*

Data analysis

Our final sample size represents a convenience sample of 100 students out of 115 students approached to take the survey, yielding a response rate of 86.96%. Outcome of interest was oral cavity and oropharyngeal cancer knowledge level, a continuous variable which was derived from the knowledge score formed. Pearson's correlation, Chi-Square, and one-way ANOVA assessed bivariate associations between co-variables and outcome of interest. For the purpose of binary logistic regression analyses, knowledge score was categorized as low vs. high; low being knowledge score of 0 – 7, and high being 8 – 14. Crude measures of

association was performed for all covariates in the data. Data was analyzed using SPSS version 20 (Chicago, IL, USA). A two-tailed alpha of .05 was applied as a standard of significance in all analyses.

Results

There were 100 participants in the study out of 115 students approached, yielding a response rate of 87%. There were 58% male students in the survey, and 46% of the students were undergraduates (See Table 1 for demographic characteristics of the population). Demographic data yielded 37% Caucasians, 37% Asians, and 19% African-

Table 1 Sociodemographic characteristics of study population (N = 100)

Characteristics	N	%
Race		
African American	19	19
Asian	37	37
Caucasian	37	37
Hispanic/Latino	3	3
Mixed	4	4
Age Groups		
16 - 20	23	23
21 -25	44	44
26 - 30	23	23
31& over	10	10
Gender		
Male	58	58
Female	41	41
Unknown	1	1
Smoking Status		
Smoker	3	3
Never smoked	93	93
Quit smoking	3	3
Trying to quit	1	1
Drinking status		
Drinker	65	65
Non-drinker	34	34
Stopped drinking	1	1
Marital Status		
Married	13	13
Single	87	87
Level of study		
Undergraduate	46	46
Masters	34	34
Doctoral	18	18
Other	2	2

Americans in the study. A majority of students (93 %) reported that they were non-smokers, while 35% were non-drinkers. Sixty-eight percent had initiated sexual intercourse, and the youngest age of sexual debut was 14 years old. For oral cavity and oropharyngeal cancer knowledge, 81% had a low score (between 0–7), while only 19% had a high score (8–14). Yet, only 2% perceived that their oral cavity and oropharyngeal cancer risk was high. Risk perception was negatively correlated with age at sexual debut ($r(64) = -0.26$, p = 0.037; see Fig. 1).

There was no significant association between oral cavity and oropharyngeal cancer knowledge and perception of risk; however, knowledge was significantly associated with frequency of prevention of STDs $F(1, 65) = 4.90$, p = 0.03, A one-way ANOVA showed a significant positive association between risk perception and number of sexual partners, $F(4, 60) = 2.48$, $p = 0.05$; see Fig. 2).

Although 86% claimed to have heard about oral cavity and oropharyngeal cancer, only 7% of these reported ever having an oral cavity and oropharyngeal cancer examination (See Table 2).

Discussion

In the population we surveyed, only 3% of students who participated in this study reported they were current smokers. Previous studies have revealed that between 14% and 62% of university students may be considered smokers in the United States [23–27]. We note that this was self-reported data, and social desirability may lead to underreporting. However, another explanation could be that the university where the survey was conducted had implemented a comprehensive smoking ban on campus, and although we do not have information on smoking rates prior to the ban, it has been reported that such bans are associated with decreased smoking rates [28].

We found in our study that oral cavity and oropharyngeal cancer knowledge was not significantly associated with smoking or drinking rates, but was associated with a sexual risk factor for developing oral cavity and oropharyngeal cancer, and with frequency of prevention of STDs. It was also demonstrated that there were significant associations between risk perception and number of sexual partners, as well as the age of sexual debut. This is interesting finding, as literature shows that a significant proportion of young people who are experimenting with oral sex in fact consider oral sex less risky, and/or are more likely to have multiple oral sexual partners than vaginal sexual partners [29]. These sexual habits put them at a higher risk for developing oral cavity and oropharyngeal cancer, especially HPV-associated oropharyngeal cancer. It will remain crucial then to devise strategies to increase the awareness of cancer risks associated with sexual behavior. In this study, a majority of students self-reported that they have never heard of HPV. As HPV is a major driver of overall oral cavity and oropharyngeal cancer incidence, it will be important that information regarding HPV

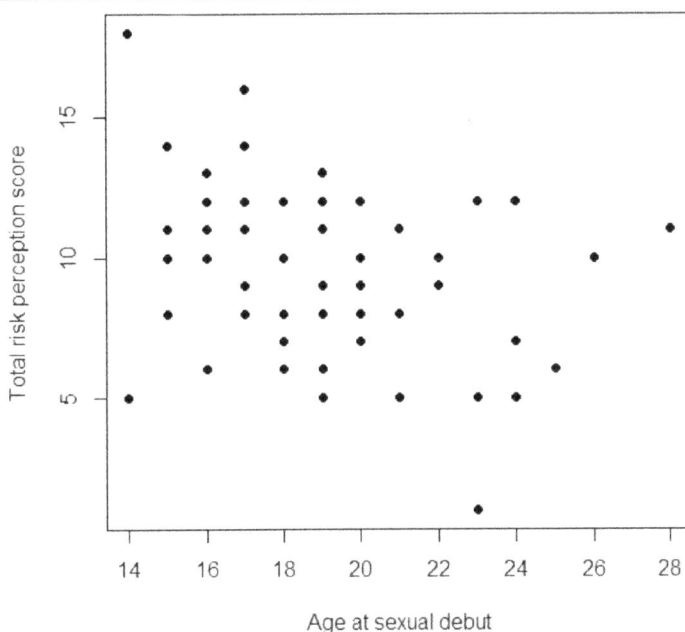

Fig. 1 Correlation between students" perception of risk and age at sexual debut. This figure shows a significant, negative correlation between age at sexual debut and risk perception of students

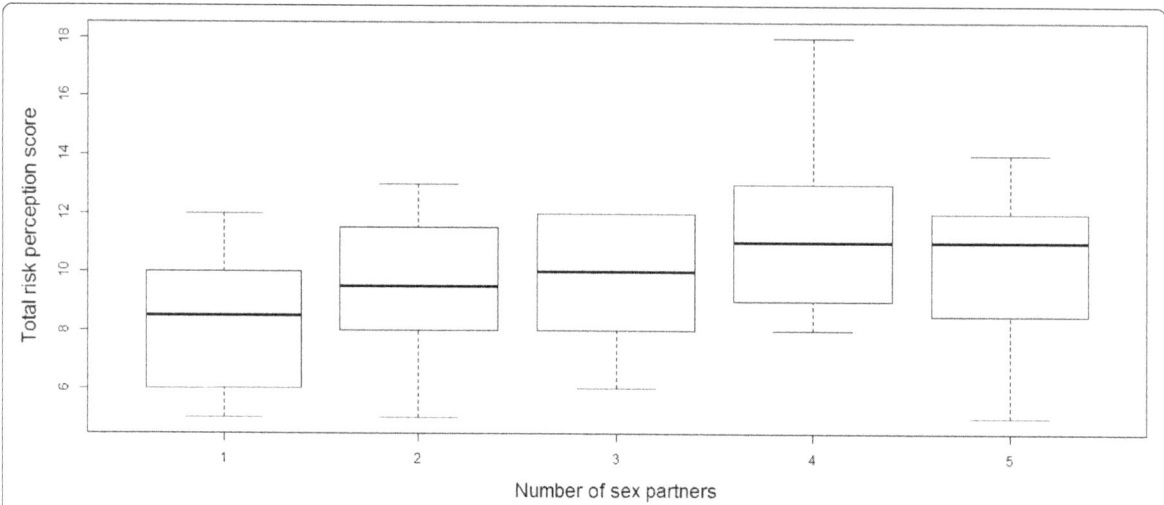

Fig. 2 Association between number of sexual partners and perception of oral cavity and oropharyngeal cancer risk. This figure shows that students with 3 or more sexual partners were more likely to have a high risk perception

and sexual risk taking become an essential component of all oral cavity and oropharyngeal cancer prevention efforts. At least two-thirds of this study population may benefit from interventions stressing the need for HPV vaccines as part of the HPV vaccine catch up age range, which may hold some promise in not only preventing HPV strains that cause cervical cancer, but also oropharyngeal cancers [30, 31].

Table 2 Oral cavity and oropharyngeal cancer and HPV knowledge questions

	Yes	No	Don't know
Characteristics	N (%)	N (%)	N (%)
Have you heard of oral cavity and oropharyngeal cancer?	86 (86)	12(12)	2 (2)
Have you ever heard of oral cavity and oropharyngeal cancer mouth exam?	18 (18)	66 (66)	16 (16)
Have you ever had an oral cavity and oropharyngeal cancer exam?	7 (7)	83 (83)	10 (10)
Certain types of HPV lead to oral cavity and oropharyngeal cancer	63 (63)	12 (12)	25 (25)
HPV is the same as HIV	1 (1)	76 (76)	23 (23)
Most types of HPV cannot clear up on their own	61 (61)	16 (16)	23 (23)
A person usually has symptoms when infected with HPV	14 (14)	62 (62)	24 (24)
Chance of getting HPV increase with number of sex partners	75 (75)	2 (2)	23 (23)
There is an HPV vaccine for both men and women	53 (53)	24 (24)	23 (23)

Only 7% reported to have had an oral cavity and oropharyngeal cancer examination. The American Cancer Society recommends that oral cavity and oropharyngeal cancer screening should be part of the periodic check for adults when they visit a dentist or other clinicians [32]. And while there remains insufficient evidence to accept or reject routine mouth screenings by primary care physicians in asymptomatic individuals, both the US Preventive Health Services Task Force (USPSTF) and the American Dental Association concede that dentists, otolaryngologists, primary care physicians and other clinicians may decide to screen high-risks groups, based on lifestyle factors or age, and those who may have reasons to suspect a lesion in their mouth [33–35]. This highlights the need for frontline healthcare providers, especially primary care physicians and dentists, to better understand the oral cavity and oropharyngeal cancer risk profiles of their patients, in order to reduce missed opportunities in the clinic for prevention of oral cavity and oropharyngeal cancer via regular oral cancer screenings and education.

There were some limitations in this study. Primarily, the study was non-experimental, and although Caucasians, African-Americans, and Asians were almost equally surveyed, there were few Latinos present in the study. Additionally, study participants stemmed from a single university, yielding a relatively small sample size. Thus, we may not be able to generalize results in the context of university students' population in the United States. Data analysis may have revealed more robust associations between variables if the study had compared medical vs. non-medical students to test whether the assumption that medical students are likely to have better oral cavity and oropharyngeal cancer knowledge is true. Notwithstanding these limitations, this project has helped to generate baseline information on the amount of knowledge non-medical students possess regarding oral cavity and oropharyngeal cancer, as well as perception of their risk of developing oral cavity and oropharyngeal cancer. It may be the first study in the United States to exclusively assess oral cavity and oropharyngeal cancer knowledge and knowledge of risk factors (smoking, drinking, and HPV) among a university student population that does not include medical and dental students. Furthermore, in an age where HPV-associated head and neck cancers are increasing in epidemic proportions, our finding that sex-related oral cavity and oropharyngeal cancer risk factors may be more salient among university students than traditional risk factors, such as tobacco and alcohol, is hugely important for future educational interventions, and is worth exploring further.

Conclusions

Oral cavity and oropharyngeal cancer knowledge and risk perception is low among this student population, and among the risk factors assessed in this population, it is to be concluded that sexual risks are more salient than the traditional oral cavity and oropharyngeal cancer risk factors of tobacco and alcohol use. Therefore, while tobacco cessation efforts and campus-wide smoking bans remain in place to continue addressing smoking rates, these efforts alone may not impact the prevalence of oral cavity and oropharyngeal cancer risk factors among university students. Increasing the awareness about other non-smoking related risk factors, especially those related to sexual behavior, may prove to be more effective in preventing oral cavity and oropharyngeal cancer among university-aged students. Inasmuch as health behavior is associated with risk perception, and oral cavity and oropharyngeal cancer incidence is increasingly shifting towards younger adults, interventions must be tailored to this group in order to improve prevention and control. Prevention of oral cavity and oropharyngeal cancers may pose a difficult challenge without first improving the knowledge of oral cavity and oropharyngeal cancers among high risk groups, particularly university-aged youth in the United States. In addition, since oral cavity and oropharyngeal cancer risk factors are largely prevalent among young adults, it may be of value to increase awareness of cancer risk factors and primary prevention strategies among elementary, middle and high school students, as many of the risk behaviors are likely to be initiated even before college age [36].

Competing interests

No competing financial or non-financial interests to declare.

Authors' contributions

Original idea by NOP. NOP designed and conducted the survey and gathered the data. NOP and NTT performed statistical analysis, and interpretation. NOP and NTT produced tables and figures. NOP and NTT wrote the manuscript, and both authors read and approved the final manuscript.

Acknowledgements

Part of this study was presented at the American College of Epidemiology's Annual Meeting in Louisville, Kentucky on September 21–24, 2013.
We would like to acknowledge the support of Kimberly J Johnson, PhD, Mark A Varvares, MD, FACS, and Mario Schootman, PhD, as well as Rebecca Rohde and Beth B. Tobo, MPH, for helping to proof-read this manuscript.

Author details

[1]Brown School, Washington University in St. Louis, 1 Brookings Drive, Saint Louis, MO 63130, USA. [2]Saint Louis University Cancer Center, 3655 Vista Avenue, Saint Louis, Missouri 63110, USA. [3]Department of Otolaryngology-Head and Neck Surgery, Saint Louis University, School of Medicine, 6th Floor Desloge Building, 3635 Vista Avenue, Saint Louis, MO 63110, USA. [4]Department of Epidemiology, Saint Louis University, College for Public Health and Social Justice, 3545 Lafayette Avenue, Saint Louis, Missouri 63108, USA.

References

1. Warnakulasuriya S. Global epidemiology of oral and oropharyngeal cancer Oral Oncol. 2009;45(4–5):309–16.
2. American Cancer Society. Cancer Facts & Figures 2012. Atlanta: American Cancer Society; 2012.
3. National Cancer Institute. Common cancer types. http://www.cancer.gov/cancertopics/types/commoncancers.
4. Silverman S. Demographics and occurrence of oral and pharyngeal cancers: the outcomes, the trends, the challenge. J Am Dent Assoc. 2001;132 suppl 1:7S–11S.
5. National Cancer Institute, SEER cancer statistics review 1975–2008. http://seer.cancer.gov/archive/csr/1975_2008/
6. Moreno-Lopez LA, Esparza-Gomez GC, Gonzalez-Navarro A, Cerero-Lapiedra R, Gonzalez-Hernandez MJ, Dominguez-Rojas V. Risk of oral cancer associated with tobacco smoking, alcohol consumption and oral hygiene: a case–control study in Madrid. Spain Oral Oncol. 2000;36(2):170–4.
7. Gillison ML, Koch WM, Capone RB, Spafford M, Westra WH, Wu L, et al. Evidence for a causal association between human papillomavirus and a subset of head and neck cancers. J Natl Cancer Inst. 2000;92(9):709–20.
8. Chaturvedi AK, Engels EA, Pfeiffer RM, Hernandez BY, Xiao W, Kim E, et al. Human papillomavirus and rising oropharyngeal cancer incidence in the United States. J Clin Oncol. 2011;29(32):4294–301.
9. Patel SC, Carpenter WR, Tyree S, Couch ME, Weissler M, Hackman T, et al. Increasing incidence of oral tongue squamous cell carcinoma in young white women, age 18 to 44 years. J Clin Oncol. 2011;29(11):1488–94.
10. Torabi MR, Yang J, Li J. Comparison of tobacco use knowledge, attitude and practice among college students in China and the United States. Health Promot Int. 2002;17(3):247–53.
11. Raychowdhury S, Lohrmann DK. Oral cancer risk behaviors among Indiana college students: a formative research study. J Am Coll Health. 2008;57(3):373–7.
12. Mallett KA, Bachrach RL, Turrisi R. Are all negative consequences truly negative? Assessing variations among college students' perceptions of alcohol related consequences. Addict Behav. 2008;33(10):1375–81.
13. Lambert EC. College students' knowledge of human papillomavirus and effectiveness of a brief educational intervention. J Am Board Fam Pract. 2001;14(3):178–83.
14. Klug SJ, Hukelmann M, Blettner M. Knowledge about infection with human papillomavirus: a systematic review. Prev Med. 2008;46(2):87–98.
15. Chowdhury MT, Pau A, Croucher R. Bangladeshi dental students' knowledge, attitudes and behaviour regarding tobacco control and oral cancer. J Cancer Educ. 2010;25(3):391–5.

16. Cannick GF, Horowitz AM, Drury TF, Reed SG, Day TA. Assessing oral cancer knowledge among dental students in South Carolina. J Am Dent Assoc. 2005;136(3):373–8.
17. Reed SG, Duffy NG, Walters KC, Day TA. Oral cancer knowledge and experience: a survey of South Carolina medical students in 2002. J Cancer Educ. 2005;20(3):136–42.
18. Boroumand S, Garcia AI, Selwitz RH, Goodman HS. Knowledge and opinions regarding oral cancer among Maryland dental students. J Cancer Educ. 2008;23(2):85–91.
19. Ogden GR, Mahboobi N. Oral cancer awareness among undergraduate dental students in Iran. J Cancer Educ. 2011;26(2):380–5.
20. Carter LM, Ogden GR. Oral cancer awareness of undergraduate medical and dental students. BMC Med Educ. 2007;7:44.
21. White LJ, Creighton Jr FX, Wise JC, Hapner ER. Association between HPV and head and neck cancer: differences in understanding among three distinct populations. Am J Cancer Prevent. 2014;2(1):14–9.
22. Schantz SP, Yu GP. Head and neck cancer incidence trends in young Americans, 1973–1997, with a special analysis for tongue cancer. Arch Otolaryngol Head Neck Surg. 2002;128(3):268–74.
23. Cronk NJ, Harris KJ, Harrar SW, Conway K, Catley D, Good GE. Analysis of smoking patterns and contexts among college student smokers. Subst Use Misuse. 2011;46(8):1015–22.
24. Everett SA, Husten CG, Kann L, Warren CW, Sharp D, Crossett L. Smoking initiation and smoking patterns among US college students. J Am Coll Health. 1999;48(2):55–60.
25. Rigotti NA, Moran SE, Wechsler H. US college students' exposure to tobacco promotions: prevalence and association with tobacco use. Am J Public Health. 2005;95(1):138–44.
26. Rigotti NA, Regan S, Majchrzak NE, Knight JR, Wechsler H. Tobacco use by Massachusetts public college students: long term effect of the Massachusetts Tobacco Control Program. Tob Control. 2002;11 suppl 2:ii20–4.
27. Rigotti NA, Lee JE, Wechsler H. US college students' use of tobacco products: results of a national survey. JAMA. 2000;284(6):699–705.
28. Seo DC, Macy JT, Torabi MR, Middlestadt SE. The effect of a smoke-free campus policy on college students' smoking behaviors and attitudes. Prev Med. 2011;53(4–5):347–52.
29. Gillison ML. Human papillomavirus-related diseases: oropharynx cancers and potential implications for adolescent HPV vaccination. J Adolesc Health. 2008;43(4):S52–60.
30. Osazuwa-Peters N. Human papillomavirus (HPV), HPV-associated oropharyngeal cancer, and HPV vaccine in the United States-Do we need a broader vaccine policy? Vaccine. 2013;31(47):5500–5.
31. Herrero R, Quint W, Hildesheim A, Gonzalez P, Struijk L, Katki HA, et al. Reduced prevalence of oral human papillomavirus (HPV) 4 years after bivalent HPV vaccination in a randomized clinical trial in Costa Rica. PloS One. 2013;8(7), e68329.
32. American Cancer Society. Cancer Facts & Figures 2015. Atlanta: American Cancer Society; 2015.
33. Neville BW, Day TA. Oral cancer and precancerous lesions. CA Cancer J Clin. 2002;52(4):195–215.
34. Moyer VA. Screening for oral cancer: U.S. Preventive Services Task Force recommendation statement. Ann Intern Med. 2014;160(1):55–60.
35. American Cancer Society. American Cancer Society Guidelines for the Early Detection of Cancer. http://www.cancer.org/healthy/findcancerearly/cancerscreeningguidelines/american-cancer-society-guidelines-for-the-early-detection-of-cancer.
36. Eaton DK, Kann L, Kinchen S, Shanklin S, Flint KH, Hawkins J, et al. Youth risk behavior surveillance-United States, 2011. MMWR Surveill Summ. 2012;61(4): 1–162.

30

Acoustic rhinometry and video endoscopic scoring to evaluate postoperative outcomes in endonasal spreader graft surgery with septoplasty and turbinoplasty for nasal valve collapse

Bree Erickson[1], Robert Hurowitz[2], Caroline Jeffery[1], Khalid Ansari[1], Hamdy El Hakim[1], Erin D. Wright[1], Hadi Seikaly[1], Sam R. Greig[1] and David W. J. Côté[1*]

Abstract

Background: Nasal obstruction is a common complaint seen by otolaryngologists. The internal nasal valve (INV) is typically the narrowest portion of the nasal cavity, and if this area collapses on inspiration the patient experiences significant symptoms of nasal obstruction. The nasal obstruction is further compounded if the INV is narrower than normal. Previous studies have evaluated the effectiveness of techniques to alleviate structural nasal obstruction, but none have looked specifically at spreader grafts measured by acoustic rhinometry or validated grading assessment of dynamic INV collapse. Our objective was to evaluate the application of acoustic rhinometry coupled with visual endoscopic grading of the INV, and validated subjective measurements, in patients undergoing endonasal spreader graft surgery with septoplasty and turbinoplasty.

Methods: This is a prospective clinical study conducted within a tertiary care rhinoplasty practice. Patients undergoing septoplasty and bilateral inferior turbinoplasty with bilateral endonasal spreader graft placement for observed internal nasal valve collapse were recruited. Baseline, early and intermediate postoperative measures were obtained. The primary outcome was grading of the INV collapse on video endoscopy. Secondary outcomes included cross-sectional area at the INV measured by acoustic rhinometry, subjective Nasal Obstruction Symptom Evaluation (NOSE) and Sino-Nasal Outcome Tool (SNOT-22) scores.

Results: A total of 17 patients, average age of 34.5 ± 12.2 years, undergoing septoplasty, bilateral endonasal spreader grafts, and bilateral turbinoplasty were included in the study. Postoperative measurements were performed at an average of 8.1 ± 1.6 weeks and 17.7 ± 4.2 weeks. Patients had significant improvement for INV collapse grading, cross-sectional area, NOSE and SNOT-22 scores in both the early and intermediate follow up. Endoscopic grading had moderate inter-rater agreement ($\kappa = 0.579$) and average intra-rater agreement ($\kappa = 0.545$).

(Continued on next page)

* Correspondence: drdavidcote@me.com
This study was presented at the Canadian Society of Otolaryngology – Head and Neck Surgery Annual Meeting (June 2015, Winnipeg MB).
[1]Department of Surgery, Division of Otolaryngology – Head and Neck Surgery, University of Alberta, 1E4 Walter C Mackenzie Centre, 8440-112 Street NW, Edmonton, AB T6G 2B7, Canada
Full list of author information is available at the end of the article

(Continued from previous page)

Conclusions: This study is the first to demonstrate a statistically significant improvement of objective measurement of internal nasal valve function, both static and dynamic, and subjective improvements. This supports endonasal cartilagenous spreader grafts with septoplasty and inferior turbinoplasty for patients with nasal obstruction with internal nasal valve collapse.

Keywords: Internal nasal valve collapse, Spreader graft, Septoplasty, Turbinoplasty, Acoustic rhinometry

Background

Nasal obstruction is a common complaint of patients seeking consultation with otolaryngologists [1]. The internal nasal valve (INV) is typically the narrowest portion of the nasal cavity and is bounded by the septum, the upper lateral cartilage (ULC), the inferior turbinate, and the nasal floor. A normal INV angle is between 10 and 15°, and a smaller angle can result in a predisposition to symptoms of nasal obstruction [2]. Collapse of the INV on inspiration can cause significant nasal obstruction. In fact, based on the Bernoulli principle, the degree of narrowing of the INV directly correlates to the tendency to collapse and obstruct.

The static area of the INV can be enlarged through various techniques depending on the cause of narrowing. Septoplasty removes and straightens obstruction caused by the nasal septum. Inferior turbinoplasty reduces the bulk of the inferior turbinates, especially at the turbinate head, where it is a contributing boundary of the INV. Endonasal spreader graft placement is a procedure used to address INV collapse [3]. The technique involves harvesting cartilage and creating grafts approximately 2–3 mm in width and 2 mm in height and 7–10 mm in length. The graft is placed into a submucosal pocket inferior to the superior edge of the ULC, running dorsally up the length of the ULC. The intent is to stent open the INV angle in order to prevent collapse during inspiration [3].

Studies evaluating the effectiveness of nasal surgery techniques to alleviate structural nasal obstruction often lack objective evidence. In particular, no study has looked specifically at endonasal spreader graft placement [4–9]. Our objective was to evaluate the utility of acoustic rhinometry and visual endoscopic grading of the INV, as well as subjective measurements, in patients undergoing spreader graft surgery with septoplasty and turbinoplasty.

Methods

Prior to commencement of this study, ethics approval was obtained from the University of Alberta Health Research Ethics Board (Pro00041956). Informed consent to participate in this study was obtained from each of the participants. Inclusion criteria included patients over the age of 17 seen in a single tertiary care otolaryngology practice. Patients' primary complaint was nasal obstruction and all were diagnosed with structural causes of nasal obstruction, including septal deviation and internal nasal valve collapse. Patients were excluded if they required revision septoplasty or formal septorhinoplasty. Other exclusion criteria included concomitant diagnosis of other causes of nasal obstruction requiring additional adjunct procedures (e.g. external nasal valve collapse, nasal polyposis, etc.). Surgical method involved a standard submucosal resection of the septum with placement of endonasal spreader grafts as previously described [3]. Intraturbinal turbinoplasty was performed in all patients using a Medtronic microdebrider with turbinoplasty blade as described by Lee in 2013 [10].

The primary outcome was grading of the INV collapse on video endoscopy. Secondary outcomes included cross-sectional area at the INV measured by acoustic rhinometry protocol, subjective Sino-Nasal Outcome Tool (SNOT-22) and Nasal Obstruction Symptom Evaluation (NOSE) scores. Patients underwent preoperative measurements as well as early and intermediate postoperative measurements at 6 to 12 weeks and at 12 to 16 weeks, respectively.

Acoustic rhinometry was performed with the A1 Acoustic Rhinometer (GM Instruments Ltd., Kilwinning, Scotland) utilizing recommendations as set out by the consensus report on acoustic rhinometry developed by Clement et al. in 2005 [11]. Acoustic rhinometry is a technique used to measure the cross-sectional area of the nasal cavity as a function of the distance into the nasal cavity from the nasal sill. This measurement is performed by analyzing the amplitude of the reflection of sound waves projected into the nose. The minimum cross-sectional area identified within the first 3 cm of the nose typically corresponds with the INV. A single experienced technician performed the measurements. Topical spray consisting of 0.1 % xylometazoline and 4 % lidocaine was administered 5 min prior to measurement. Nosepiece sizing was chosen to provide an appropriate acoustic seal for each patient without altering nasal anatomy. Measurements were performed during a breathing pause by the patient. Three repeated measurements were performed on each side and the minimum cross-sectional area value was averaged from the readings.

Rigid endoscopy was next performed, using 0° 4 mm Olympus rigid endoscope and video recorded. The patient was asked to inhale repetitively as the video was recorded examining bilateral INV.

Finally, patients were asked to complete the NOSE scale and SNOT-22 at the time of their measurements pre- and postoperatively. The Nasal Obstruction Symptom Evaluation (NOSE) Scale was developed and validated by Stewart et al. in 2004 [12]. This survey was initially developed for assessment of septoplasties but can be used for any corrective technique for nasal obstruction of varying cause. The Sino-Nasal Outcome Tool (SNOT-22), however, was developed for patients with chronic sinusitis and therefore not limited to nasal obstruction alone, although it has been shown to be an effective measurement in patients undergoing septoplasty [13, 14].

Collapse of the INV occurs when the lateral nasal wall moves inwards during inspiration. This dynamic change in INV dimensions has been described as a percentage of full collapse with a grading scheme developed by Most et al. in 2008 and validated in 2013 by Tsao et al. [15, 16]. The grading scheme consists of grades 1 through 3, as <33 %, 33–66 % collapse, and >66 % collapse towards the septum respectively. Four independent otolaryngologists performed analysis of the video endoscopy. The videos were divided into preoperative, postoperative, right and left, and then randomized. The reviewers were blinded to the patients and operative status and asked to grade the degree of INV collapse based on Tsao et al. validated grading method published in 2013 [16]. The final grading of each video was calculated by averaging the grades from the four reviewers.

Statistical methods
Statistical analysis of measurements was performed using SPSS version 22.0 (SPSS Inc., Chicago IL, USA). Descriptive statistics were performed to assess the data. Test for normality on difference of data sets was calculated using Kolmogorov-Smirnov and Shapiro-Wilk tests. Paired t-test was performed to compare the preoperative and postoperative data for video grading scores, acoustic measurements of INV cross-sectional area, and patient-completed surveys NOSE and SNOT-22 scores. Statistical significance was defined as $p < 0.05$. Fleiss kappa calculation for inter- and intra-rater

agreement was performed using the online calculator developed by Geertzen in 2012 for inter-rater agreement with multiple raters [17].

Results
A total of 17 patients undergoing septoplasty, bilateral endonasal spreader grafts, and bilateral turbinoplasty were included in the study. Demographics included a male to female ratio of 16:1 and an average age of 34.5 ± 12.2 years. Average early follow up time was 8.1 ± 1.6 weeks and 17.7 ± 4.2 weeks for intermediate follow up. No postoperative complications occurred in any of the patients. Measurements for early and intermediate follow up time were obtained for 14 and 12 patients respectively. Preoperative and postoperative measurement means are presented in Table 1. All sets of data, were normally distributed, and therefore preoperative and postoperative comparisons were performed with paired t-test. Calculations comparing preoperative and postoperative data sets for all variables were shown to have a significant improvement (Tables 2 and 3). Inter-rater agreement was found to be moderate between the four graders, with a kappa value of 0.579. Intra-rater agreement was also moderate with an average kappa value of 0.545 ($\kappa_1 = 0.610$, $\kappa_2 = 0.534$, $\kappa_3 = 0.574$, $\kappa_4 = 0.461$).

Discussion
This is the first study that provides objective evidence of the utility of endonasal spreader grafts, when performed in conjunction with nasal septoplasty and inferior turbinoplasty, in addressing the internal nasal valve. Both static and dynamic measurements were obtained along with subjective symptomatic improvement. Several studies have previously investigated objective measures of improvement with spreader graft surgery using cadaver models [4, 5]. Huang et al., in 2006, studied an endoscopic approach to spreader grafts on cadaveric heads using 8 specimens. They found significantly improved nasal valve area (mean change 0.28 cm^2) using acoustic rhinometry measurements. Craig et al., in 2014, also performed spreader graft placement on 6 cadaveric heads and also found a significant improvement in INV area (mean change 0.10 cm^2). Rigid nasal endoscopy was used in this study, but only to classify the INV as normal

Table 1 Preoperative and postoperative mean values for measured variables

Variable	Preoperative (N = 17)			Early postoperative (N = 14)			Intermediate postoperative (N = 12)		
	Mean	Range	SD	Mean	Range	SD	Mean	Range	SD
INV collapse grading	2.23	1–3	0.67	1.37	1–2.5	0.46	1.54	1–3	0.70
INV cross-sectional area (cm^2)	0.519	0.02–1.10	0.278	0.614	0.19–1.32	0.277	0.552	0.17–1.01	0.230
NOSE	14.0	10–20	3.3	5.9	2–10	2.9	7.7	0–15	4.5
SNOT-22	34.1	13–71	16.5	16.9	1–55	15.4	22.7	1–57	19.8

SD standard deviation, *INV* internal nasal valve, *NOSE* nasal obstruction symptom evaluation scale, *SNOT* sino-nasal outcome tool

Table 2 Comparison of preoperative and early postoperative values (paired t-test)

Variable	Mean of difference	95 % CI	Significance
INV collapse grading	0.857	0.542–1.172	<0.001
INV cross-sectional area (cm²)	0.095	0.001–0.189	0.047
NOSE	8.1	6.1–10.2	<0.001
SNOT-22	17.3	10.2–24.4	<0.001

CI confidence interval, *INV* internal nasal valve, *NOSE* nasal obstruction symptom evaluation scale, *SNOT* sino-nasal outcome tool

or narrow, not as a means to measure improvement. Of note, this study did find that there was greater improvement in the INV with narrow classification (cross-sectional area less than 0.50 cm²) than in those with normal based on a normal classification. A statistically significant 51 % improvement was found for narrow INV, whereas only a 1 % improvement for normal preoperative INV was found. Neither of these above mentioned studies were able to assess dynamic changes or subjective assessments as these were performed in cadaveric models. Of note, there has been no establishment of a clinically significant improvement in INV area in the current literature.

Few studies have examined both the objective and subjective outcomes of surgery for nasal obstruction. Haavisto et al., in their 2012 paper, examined the use of acoustic rhinometry and rhinomanometry as well as a visual analogue scale to evaluate improvement in unilateral nasal obstruction in 30 patients undergoing septoplasty [6]. Objective measure of patients improved significantly and a trend toward improvement in patient satisfaction was also found, though not statistically significant. Mengi et al., in 2011, however did show a significant improvement in NOSE scores, minimal cross-sectional area measured by acoustic rhinometry, and nasal resistance values measured by rhinomanometry after septoplasty in 44 patients [7].

Edizer et al. evaluated 26 patients undergoing septorhinoplasty for objective improvement in nasal airway using acoustic rhinometry and subjective improvements using a 10-point visual analog scale [8]. Although the patients all underwent septorhinoplasty, not all had preoperative complaints of nasal obstruction. The study

found significant improvement in symptom scoring but not in cross-sectional area. Zoumalan et al., in 2012, also evaluated objective and subjective measurements of 31 septorhinoplasty patients [9]. This study also used acoustic rhinometry and a 10-point rating scale for the measurements. Thirteen patients underwent spreader grafts, but it is unclear as to what other techniques were used in their septorhinoplasty procedures. Our study is the first to provide data on a procedure specifically aimed at correcting the INV static area and dynamic collapse.

Our study highlights not only the utility of endonasal spreader grafts with septoplasty and turbinoplasty, but also the significant quality of life issues that accompany nasal obstruction due to INV collapse. In 2009, Gillett et al. showed that normal subjects who are free of sinonasal disease have an average SNOT-22 score of 7 [18]. The patients in the study had preoperative average NOSE and SNOT-22 scores of 14.1 and 34.8 respectively, both of which are significant for symptomatic disease.

A potential limitation of this study is the reliability of acoustic rhinometry. Various studies have shown varying degrees of reliability of acoustic rhinometry as compared to computed tomography scans and magnetic resonance imaging, assessing both cross-sectional area and volume of the nasal cavity [19–22]. These studies have shown significant correlation between acoustic rhinometry and imaging for the anterior portion of the nose but not the posterior. This finding was confirmed in a more recent study using high-resolution computed tomography scanning by Numminen et al. [23]. A statistically significant correlation was found between the minimum cross-sectional areas in the first 10 mm and 11–40 mm of the nasal cavity. There was a weaker correlation in the posterior portion of the nose. A well-defined measurement protocol, similar to the one used in our study, was employed for acoustic measurement. Using a single experienced technician, appropriately sized nasal coupling pieces, and consistent technique strengthened our measurement reliability. In addition, the study specifically examines the most anterior portion of the nasal cavity, which is the most accurately measured area.

The inter-rater agreement for this study was calculated as fair to good, with a kappa value of 0.579. This is less robust than the kappa of 0.77 found by the validating paper for this grading scheme. It will be interesting in the future to observe what other groups are able to attain for inter-rater agreement for this grading scheme to better determine its clinical utility.

Finally, due to the combined techniques of septoplasty and turbinoplasty with the endonasal spreader graft placement, it is not possible to determine how much of the objective and subjective success is attributable to the spreader grafts alone. Potentially, the increase in cross-sectional area may be more attributable to the correction

Table 3 Comparison of preoperative and intermediate postoperative values (paired t-test)

Variable	Mean of difference	95 % CI	Significance
INV collapse grading	0.859	0.528–1.190	<0.001
INV cross-sectional area (cm²)	0.075	0.005–0.145	0.036
NOSE	6.9	4.9–8.9	<0.001
SNOT-22	19.1	12.5–25.7	<0.001

CI confidence interval, *INV* internal nasal valve, *NOSE* nasal obstruction symptom evaluation scale, *SNOT* sino-nasal outcome tool

Acoustic rhinometry and video endoscopic scoring to evaluate postoperative outcomes...

205

of septal deviation and reduction of the turbinates whereas the decrease in INV collapse seen on video endoscopy should be attributable to the spreader graft placement. However, the increased INV area may improve the degree of INV collapse due decreased Bernoulli effect.

This study included a specific group of patients who demonstrated nasal obstruction from both static and dynamic causes. Although previously Mengi et al. found significant increase in INV area from septoplasty alone, this is not applicable to our patient population that had demonstrated INV collapse [7]. As described by Rhee et al. in their 2010 consensus statement on diagnosis and management of nasal valve compromise there are thought to be some cases where septoplasty and/or turbinate surgery can be used to treat nasal valve collapse without surgery to support the lateral wall [24]. Ideally a randomized controlled trial of septoplasty and turbinoplasty with and without spreader graft placement could better show the effectiveness of spreader graft placement. This future research would be justified to determine which cases of INV collapse truly require endonasal spreader grafts for surgical correction.

Observation of the demographics of the patients in this study reveals a significant preponderance of male patients. This preponderance is seen in the study by Haavisto et al. addressing surgical correction of nasal obstruction but has not been noted elsewhere [6]. Further review of patient populations may reveal that male patients either exhibit more nasal obstruction or seek surgical correction of this obstruction more often than their female counterparts.

Conclusion

This study provides an agreement of objective measurement of internal nasal valve function, both static and dynamic, with subjective patient improvement supporting endonasal cartilagenous spreader grafts in combination with septoplasty and inferior turbinoplasty as a safe and effective approach for patients complaining of nasal obstruction with internal nasal valve collapse.

Ethics approval

Prior to commencement of this study ethics approval was obtained from the University of Alberta Health Research Ethics Board.

Competing interests

Division of Otolaryngology – Head and Neck Surgery, University of Alberta, the authors declare that they have no competing interests.

Authors' contributions

BE, RH, CJ, HS, HE, EW, SG, KA, and DC contributed through design, acquisition of data, and manuscript. CJ, RH, and DC contributed through conception. BE, RH, and DC contributed through analysis and interpretation of data. KA and DC contributed through administrative support and supervision. All authors read and approved the final manuscript.

Authors' information

Presentation: this study was presented at the Canadian Society of Otolaryngology-Head and Neck Surgery Annual Meeting (June 6, 2015, Winnipeg MB)

Acknowledgements

There are no acknowledgements.

Author details

[1]Department of Surgery, Division of Otolaryngology – Head and Neck Surgery, University of Alberta, 1E4 Walter C Mackenzie Centre, 8440-112 Street NW, Edmonton, AB T6G 2B7, Canada. [2]Faculty of Medicine and Dentistry, University of Alberta, Edmonton, AB, Canada.

References

1. Jessen M, Malm L. Definition, prevalence and development of nasal obstruction. Allergy. 1997;52(40 Suppl):3–6.
2. Mink P. Le nez comme voie respiratoire. Presse Otolaryngol Belg. 1903;21:481–96.
3. Pontius AT, Williams 3rd EF. Endonasal placement of spreader grafts in rhinoplasty. Ear Nose Throat J. 2005;84(3):135–6.
4. Huang C, Manarey CR, Anand VK. Endoscopic placement of spreader grafts in the nasal valve. Otolaryngol Head Neck Surg. 2006;134(6):1001–5.
5. Craig J, Goyal P, Suryadevara A. Upper lateral strut graft: a technique to improve the internal nasal valve. Am J Rhinol Allergy. 2014;28(1):65–9.
6. Haavisto LE, Sipila JI. Acoustic rhinometry, rhinomanometry and visual analogue scale before and after septal surgery: a prospective 10-year follow-up. Clin Otolaryngol. 2013;38(1):23–9.
7. Mengi E, Cukurova I, Yalcin Y, Yigitbasi OG, Karaman Y. Evaluation of operation success in patients with nasal septal deviation with quality of life scale and objective methods. Kulak Burun Bogaz Ihtis Derg. 2011;21(4):184–91.
8. Edizer DT, Erisir F, Alimoglu Y, Gokce S. Nasal obstruction following septorhinoplasty: How well does acoustic rhinometry work? Eur Arch Otorhinolaryngol. 2013;270(2):609–13.
9. Zoumalan RA, Constantinides M. Subjective and objective improvement in breathing after rhinoplasty. Arch Facial Plast Surg. 2012;14(6):423–8.
10. Lee JY. Efficacy of intra- and extraturbinal microdebrider turbinoplasty in perennial allergic rhinitis. Laryngoscope. 2013;123(12):2945–9.
11. Clement PA, Gordts F. Standardisation Committee on Objective Assessment of the Nasal Airway, IRS, and ERS. Consensus report on acoustic rhinometry and rhinomanometry. Rhinology. 2005;43(3):169–79.
12. Stewart MG, Witsell DL, Smith TL, Weaver EM, Yueh B, Hannley MT. Development and validation of the nasal obstruction symptom evaluation (NOSE) scale. Otolaryngol Head Neck Surg. 2004;130(2):157–63.
13. Buckland JR, Thomas S, Harries PG. Can the sino-nasal outcome test (SNOT-22) be used as a reliable outcome measure for successful septal surgery? Clin Otolaryngol Allied Sci. 2003;28(1):43–7.
14. Piccirillo JF, Merritt Jr MG, Richards ML. Psychometric and clinimetric validity of the 20-item sino-nasal outcome test (SNOT-20). Otolaryngol Head Neck Surg. 2002;126(1):41–7.
15. Most SP. Trends in functional rhinoplasty. Arch Facial Plast Surg. 2008;10(6):410–3.
16. Tsao GJ, Fijalkowski N, Most SP. Validation of a grading system for lateral nasal wall insufficiency. Allergy Rhinol. 2013;4(2):e66–8.
17. Geertzen J. Inter-rater agreement with multiple raters and variables. https://nlp-ml.io/jg/software/ira/. Updated 2012. Accessed March 25, 2015.
18. Gillett S, Hopkins C, Slack R, Browne JP. A pilot study of the SNOT 22 score in adults with no sinonasal disease. Clin Otolaryngol. 2009;34(5):467–9.
19. Hilberg O, Jensen FT, Pedersen OF. Nasal airway geometry: comparison between acoustic reflections and magnetic resonance scanning. J Appl Physiol. 1993;75(6):2811–9.
20. Min YG, Jang YJ. Measurements of cross-sectional area of the nasal cavity by acoustic rhinometry and CT scanning. Laryngoscope. 1995;105(7 Pt 1):757–9.
21. Gilain L, Coste A, Ricolfi F, Dahan E, Marliac D, Peynegre R, et al. Nasal cavity geometry measured by acoustic rhinometry and computed tomography. Arch Otolaryngol Head Neck Surg. 1997;123(4):401–5.

22. Dastidar P, Numminen J, Heinonen T, Ryymin P, Rautiainen M, Laasonen E. Nasal airway volumetric measurement using segmented HRCT images and acoustic rhinometry. Am J Rhinol. 1999;13(2):97–103.
23. Numminen J, Dastidar P, Heinonen T, Karhuketo T, Rautiainen M. Reliability of acoustic rhinometry. Respir Med. 2003;97(4):421–7.
24. Rhee J, Weaver E, Park S, Baker S, Helger J, Kriet D, et al. Clinical consensus statement: diagnosis and management of nasal valve compromise. Otolaryngol Head Neck Surg. 2010;143:48–59.

31

Balloon dilation of the eustachian tube: a tympanometric outcomes analysis

Blair Williams[1], Benjamin A. Taylor[1], Neil Clifton[2] and Manohar Bance[1*]

Abstract

Background: Eustachian tube dysfunction (ETD) is a common medical issue, occurring in at least 1 % of the adult population. Patients suffering from ET dysfunction typically present with complaints of hearing loss or sensation of pressure or plugged ear, which can lead to impaired quality of life. Over time ETD can result in conductive hearing loss or choleastatoma formation. Effective theraputic options for ET dysfunction are few. Eustachian tube balloon dilation is a novel surgical technique being used to treat ETD.
The aim of our study is to objectively measure the success of Eustachian tube balloon dilation by comparing pre and post-operative middle ear pressures using tympanometric testing.

Methods: RA retrospective chart review was preformed on all patients who underwent balloon dilation of the Eustachian tube by authors NC or MB from 2010 to 2014. Pre and post-operative tympanograms were analyzed and categorized based on type (Type A, Type B, Type C). Success was defined by an improvement in tympanogram type: Type B or C to Type A, or Type B to type C. Pre and post-operative tympanograms were further analyzed using middle ear pressure values. Follow-up ranged from 3 to 15 months.

Results: Twenty-five ears (18 patients) were included in the study. Overall 36 % of ears had improvement in tympanogram type, and 32 % had normalization of tympanogram post-operatively. The Jerger tympanogram type improved significantly following the procedure ($p = 0.04$). Patients also had statistically significant improvement in measured middle ear pressure post-operatively ($P = 0.003$).

Conclusion: The natural history of Eustachian tube dysfunction is poorly understood, and evidence for current treatments are limited. Eustachian tube balloon dilation is a safe procedure, and produces significant improvement in tympanogram values up to 15 months post-operatively. Further refinement of patient selection and standardization of technique is required to optimize the effect of this therapy. Longterm follow-up data will clarify the persistence of the effect.

Keywords: Eustachian tube, Eustachian tube balloon dilation, Balloon dilation, Eustachian tube dysfunction, Tuboplasty

Background

The Eustachian tube (ET) is a conduit between the middle ear space and the nasopharynx, which opens in a physiologically complex and poorly understood manner to provide ventilation to the middle ear, and so equalize middle ear and ambient pressures. In this report, we refer by "Eustachian tube dysfunction" only to dilatory Eustachian tube dysfunction, i.e. failure to open and ventilate the middle ear, as opposed to patulous Eustachian tube, in which there is failure of closure of the Eustachian tube. Eustachian tube dysfunction is a common medical issue, occurring in at least 1 % of the adult population [1]. ET dysfunction can lead to impaired quality of life due to persistent sensation of ear fullness, ear pain, and inability to tolerate air travel or scuba diving. With time, ET dysfunction can lead to conductive hearing loss and cholesteatoma formation.

Patients suffering from ET dysfunction typically present with complaints of hearing loss or sensation of pressure

* Correspondence: m.bance@dal.ca
[1]Division of Otolaryngology – Head & Neck Surgery, Department of Surgery, Dalhousie University, Room 3184, 1276 South Park Street, Halifax, NS B3H 2Y9, Canada
Full list of author information is available at the end of the article

or plugged ear, which can be chronic or recurrent. Findings of ET dysfunction can include serous effusion, conductive hearing loss (on tuning fork or audiometric testing), or negative middle ear pressure (on pneumatic otoscopy or tympanometry). Later, there may be findings of sequelae of this dysfunction, such as retraction pockets, perforations, chronic drainage or cholesteatoma. The underlying etiology and natural history of ET dysfunction is poorly understood. There is a lack of clear diagnostic criteria, which further impairs our ability to study the disease and potential therapies. Anti-reflux therapy or nasal steroid sprays are often used first line treatments, without much evidence to support their efficacy. A randomized, placebo controlled study examining the effect of nasal steroid spray on ET dysfunction found no significant difference between treatment and placebo [2]. Similarly, a recent systematic review found no significant effect of any intervention including observation, nasal steroids, and various surgical techniques [3].

The standard surgical treatment of ET dysfunction is myringotomy and tympanostomy tube placement in the tympanic membrane (TM). This technique allows equalization of middle ear pressure and drainage of fluid via the TM, effectively bypassing the ET. This approach effectively relieves symptoms but does not treat the ET dysfunction. Tympanostomy tubes often need to be replaced multiple times if ET dysfunction persists. This places a burden on the health care system and adds to patient discomfort and inconvenience. Tympanostomy tubes also have some risk of perforations of the tympanic membrane, with associated conductive hearing loss. Other novel surgical therapies have emerged, which focus on the ET itself.

In select patients there is redundant mucosa in the area of the opening of the ET, impairing its dilation. Ablation of this tissue with laser [4] or microdebrider [5] has shown promise in small studies but these interventions are not appropriate for all patients. Other novel therapies have focused on the cartilaginous portion of the ET [6]. Of particular note, a recent, promising innovation is balloon dilation of this portion of the ET.

Eustachian tuboplasty by balloon dilation involves the cannulation of the cartilaginous portion of the ET via the nasopharynx with a balloon catheter. This catheter is inflated to multiple atmospheres of pressure (typically 10–12 bar) for a short amount of time and then removed. The surgical technique is also variable in the literature. Balloons used range between 3–7 mm in diameter, and are of variable lengths. They are typically inflated for 1–2 min. Currently, no evidence exists regarding the optimal balloon diameter, pressure, or duration of inflation.

Numerous studies have demonstrated the safety of this procedure. A systematic review preformed in 2014 showed no adverse outcomes in 103 patients who had undergone balloon dilation of the Eustachian tube [3]. While some short term success has been reported, there is little data regarding long-term outcomes [7–12]. The criteria for measuring surgical success are inconsistent across studies, with outcomes often consisting of subjective symptomatic impressions or non-validated subjective scoring systems. The primary outcome for the present study was middle ear pressure improvement following ET dilation in patients with chronic ET dysfunction. This was accomplished by comparing pre- and post-operative tympanogram values.

Methods

Approval for this study was obtained from our Nova Scotia Health Authority Research Ethics Board. Data were collected via retrospective chart review. All patients who underwent balloon ET dilation by authors NC or MB, from 2010 to 2014, were reviewed. The procedures were preformed at two different centers but the surgical technique was consistent. The Belfiel® Eustachian tube dilatation system (Spiggle and Theis, Overath, Germany) was used. Under general anesthesia the Eustachian tube orifice was identified endoscopically, and cannulated with a 20 mm long, 3 mm diameter balloon. The balloon was inflated for 2 min at 10 bar and then removed. Surgeon MB also placed tympanostomy tubes in a subset of patients. These patients were not selected, but rather requested concurrent placement of tympanostomy tubes, as this was the standard therapy they were accustomed to. There was no other selection criterion for patients who received a ventilation tube and those who did not.

Patients were selected for ET balloon dilation if they had long-standing Eustachian tube dysfunction (ETD) treated with multiple sets of tympanostomy tubes, and were interested in pursuing a longer-term solution. Patients were excluded from analyses if they had a normal pre-operative tympanogram or an 'open' post-operative tympanogram (i.e., a perforation or patent tympanostomy tube). These patients could not be included as a main outcome measure was improvement on the tympanogram, which couldn't be measured for improvement in these cases. If the tympanostomy tube extruded or the perforation healed during the study period, the results were included in analysis. Patients were also excluded if no post-operative tympanograms were performed.

Tympanogram results were collected retrospectively from pre-operative visits and all visits up to 15 months post-operatively. Follow up time points were 2–3 months, 6–9 months, and 12–15 months post operatively. In-hospital audiologists preformed Tympanometric testing. Values were generated using a tympanometer, which produced waveforms and peak pressure values. Tympanograms were then assessed by audiologists (blinded) and

Table 1 Summary of pre and post-operative improved tympanograms based on type (A, B, or C)

Pre-op tymp	Post-op tymp	Proportion	Percentage
B	A	2/5	40 %
C	A	6/20	30 %
B	C	1/5	20 %
Improvement in Type		9/25	36 %
Normalization of Tympanogram		8/25	32 %

again by the attending surgeon (not blinded). Although standard definitions of Type A, B and C tympanograms were used, there is the possibility of interpretation bias. The pre-operative and most recent post-operative tympanograms were categorized based on type (Type A, Type B, Type C) and compared using the Wilcoxon Signed Rank Test. Success was defined by an improvement in tympanogram type: Type B or C to Type A, or Type B to type C.

Data analysis

Each patient was analyzed by comparing their pre-operative tympanogram and their most recent post-operative tympanogram value. The data was broken down for two different analyses. First, the change in tympanogram Jerger type was analyzed, as this is the most clinically familiar parameter. For this, we counted how many tympanograms evolved from one type (A, B, or C) to another type post-treatment. Data for a second analysis were regrouped to better assess the Type C tympanograms, by analyzing by the actual measured middle ear pressure before and after balloon dilatation. Type C tympanograms were defined as those with the maximum compliance peak at less than -150 dPa. The negative tympanogram values were grouped by 100 daPa intervals. This was assessed first for all patients, (i.e those who did, and did not, receive ventilation tubes in aggregate). Then we repeated

the analysis for just the subset that had received ventilation tubes concurrently. This was performed, despite the low numbers, so that we could see if this group had different outcomes compared to the group without concurrent ventilation tubes. Tympanograms for this subset were preformed after the tubes had extruded and the tympanic membrane had healed, not while the tubes were in place. The data were non-parametric, repeated measures so a Wilcoxon Signed rank test was selected to determine statistical significance. Type B tympanograms do not generate a numerical value so our data set could not be analyzed using parametric tests.

Results

A total of 25 ears were included. Patients ranged in age from 18–68 years, with a mean age of 40.6 years. Follow-up time ranged from 3 to 15 months with a mean follow-up of 7.1 months. All patients had recurrent serous otitis media or negative pressure and retraction, requiring ventilation tube insertions. Nine patients underwent bilateral operations (18 ears), and 6 patients had had previous tympanostomy tube insertion. Previous mastoid surgery or tympanoplasty had been preformed on 4 patients.

Tympanograms were preformed at each follow up visit, and the most recent post-operative tympanograms were used for analysis. A summary of the results experienced by individual patients is summarized in Table 1. Overall, 36 % of patients improved their tympanogram type and 32 % had their tympanogram normalize to Type A. Figure 1 shows pre-operative and post-operative results by tympanogram type. The type improved significantly following the procedure ($p = 0.04$). Figure 2 illustrates the results with negative tympanograms (type C) categorized by 100 daPa intervals. Figure 2 appears to show a clearer difference between pre and post operative status. Again, the improvement was significant ($p = 0.003$).

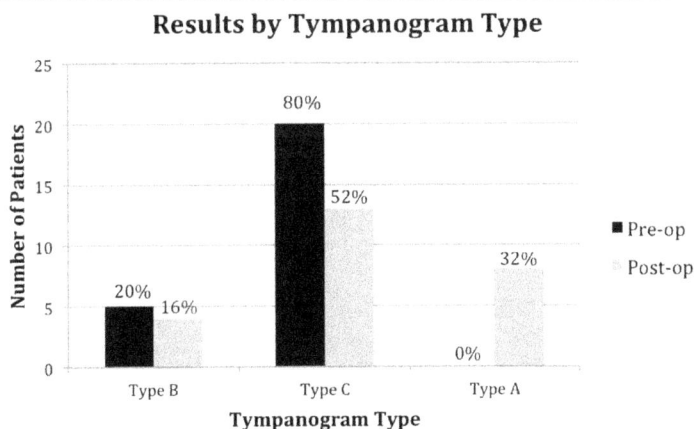

Fig. 1 Pre and post-operative assessment of tympanogram type

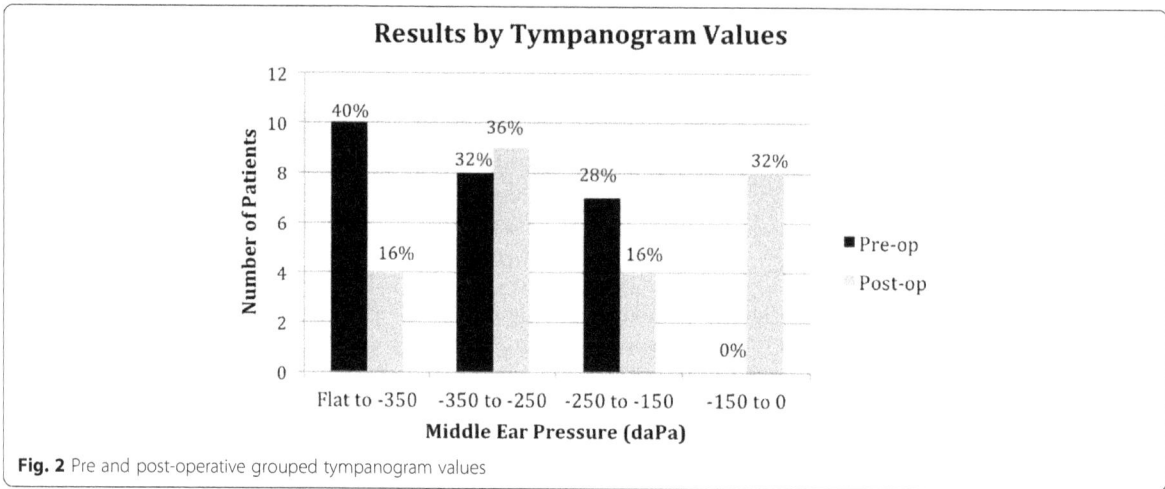

Fig. 2 Pre and post-operative grouped tympanogram values

At one centre, 5 of 11 ears had concurrent tympanostomy tube placement with ET dilation. In this group, 60 % had normalization of middle ear pressure. In the remaining 6 of 11 ears, 67 % improved in tympanogram type and 50 % normalized. Data on the timing of tympanostomy tube extrusion was not available. Figure 3 illustrates the proportion of abnormal tympanograms pre operatively and at multiple post operative follow up points. The proportion of abnormal tympanograms was highest pre-operatively and decreased most between pre operative and 2–3 month follow up points. All follow up points had a lower proportion of abnormal tympanograms compared to pre-operative measures. This was generated through tympanometric analysis at all follow up points. The most negative middle ear pressure pre operatively ($n = 18$, mean = −295 DaPa, SD = 77.38) with the most improvement seen at the 2-3 month follow up point ($n = 15$, mean = −164 DaPa, SD = 105.09). Middle ear pressure at 6–9 months ($n = 9$, mean = −255, SD = 90.08) and at 12-15 months ($n = 8$, mean = −213, SD 124.64) also remained less negative compared to pre-operative state.

No adverse events occurred as a result of ET balloon dilation.

Discussion

Eustachian tube balloon dilation has emerged as a surgical option, which targets the cartilaginous portion of the ET. Histopathological analysis preformed after balloon dilation shows decreased inflammation in the surface epithelium and submucosal tissues. The net reduction of inflammation is the hypothesized mechanism for improvement in clinical Eustachian tube function post-operatively [5]. Recent studies have shown promise in both short term and long-term outcomes, but variability in operative approach, sample size, patient follow-up, and outcome measurements make it difficult to interpret with certainty [3, 6–12]. Many studies focus not on tympanometric outcomes, but on ability to valsalva, opening pressures, or subjective outcomes. We feel the most important end-point is whether or not there is return of middle ear ventilation, and have used middle ear pressure as a surrogate measure for this. Our study relied on objective measurements using

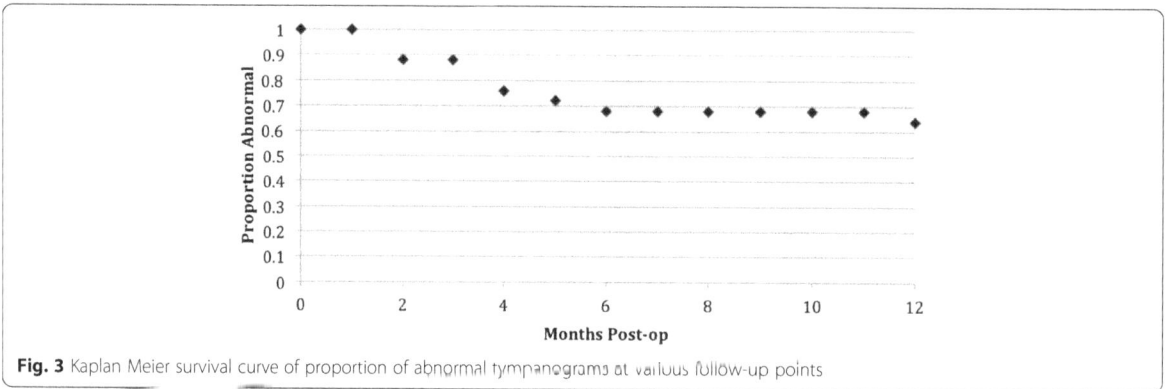

Fig. 3 Kaplan Meier survival curve of proportion of abnormal tympanograms at various follow-up points

tympanogram values, and had follow-up to 15 months post operatively.

Overall, 36 % of patients showed an improvement in tympanogram type post-operatively (Table 1) and this improvement was significant ($p = 0.04$, Fig. 1). Similarly, tympanogram measurement categorized by 100 daPa intervals also showed statistically significant improvement post-operatively ($p = 0.003$, Fig. 2). Follow-up time ranged from 3 to 15 months with a mean follow-up of 7.1 months, and the most recent post-operative tympanograms were used for analysis. A recent systematic review of Eustachian tube balloon dilation showed a conversion to type A tympanograms in 36 to 96 % of patients [3]. Silvola et. al reported type A tympanograms in 23 (56 %) patients post operatively, compared to 1 (2 %) pre-operatively, with a similar follow-up time [7]. The lesser benefit in found our study might be due to variability in patient selection, or surgical approach. Silvola et. al reported use of a 7 mm diameter balloon, whereas we used a 3 mm balloon.

Other studies of interest reported outcomes in a summative Eustachian Tube Score (ETS). This score relies on subjective symptoms and tubomanometry to measure successful opening of the Eustachian tube post-operatively with pressurization of the nasopharynx. A higher score indicates improvement in subjective symptoms and lower opening pressures on tubomanometry. For 1076 balloon dilation procedures, Schroder et. al found significant improvement in 71 % of patients at 2 months post-operatively, 73 % at 1 year, and 82 % at 2 years procedures [8]. In a study of 380 cases, Dalchow et. al also showed a mean increase in ETS at 12 months post-operatively [9].

We present the first Canadian data on balloon dilatation of the ET. In our study, the concurrent placement of tympanostomy tubes at the time of ET dilation does not appear to improve outcomes, though sample size of those who received a ventilation tube was small. No literature has shown outcomes of ET balloon dilation with concurrent myringotomy.

Limitations of our study include relatively small sample size, limited longitudinal follow up, and lack of a control group. Due to these limitations, and the lack of a control arm in our study, we cannot say, definitively, if our intervention improved ET function over time, compared to simple observation.

The use of objective outcome measurements is strength of the study, however, we did not collect associated subjective outcomes. Thus, while some middle ear pressures improved, we cannot say if this was related to relief of symptoms or improved quality of life. This consideration would be important for future studies.

Other future directions of this study include the effect of adjunctive interventions (i.e., tympanostomy tube insertion) preformed at the time of Eustachian tube balloon dilation and determining if there are patient factors that correlate with success. Further analysis of surgical protocol and equipment will aid in comparison of results among studies and improve the predictability of patient outcomes. It is important for clinicians to document their results with different diameter balloons, balloon pressures, and dilatation times, so that these parameters can be compared and the surgical approach optimized for success.

Conclusion

Eustachian tube dysfunction is a common entity that is difficult to treat. Eustachian tube balloon dilation produces modest improvement in tympanogram scores up to 14 months post-operatively. Further refinement of patient selection and standardization of technique is required to optimize the effect of this therapy.

Abbreviations
CSOM: Chronic serous otitis media; ET: Eustachian tube; ETD: Eustachian tube dysfunction; TM: Tympanic membrane.

Competing interests
The authors declare that they have no competing interests.

Authors' contributions
BW preformed retrospective review, analysis, refined and edited manuscript. BT preformed writing of manuscript and formatting. NC provided guidance for the study. MB provided guidance for the study, assisted with manuscript. All authors read and approved the final manuscript.

Authors' information
BW is a Senior Resident in the Division of Otolaryngology – Head and Neck Surgery at Dalhousie University, Halifax, Nova Scotia. BT is a Junior Resident in the Division of Otolaryngology – Head and Neck Surgery at Dalhousie University, Halifax, Nova Scotia. NC is an Otolaryngologist, Assistant Professor, and Head of Surgery at St Martha's Regional Hospital, Antigonish, Nova Scotia. MB is an Otologist/Neurotologist, Professor and Division Head of Otolaryngology – Head and Neck Surgery at Dalhousie University, Halifax, Nova Scotia.

Acknowledgements
None.

Author details
[1]Division of Otolaryngology – Head & Neck Surgery, Department of Surgery, Dalhousie University, Room 3184, 1276 South Park Street, Halifax, NS B3H 2Y9, Canada. [2]Division of Otolaryngology – Head and Neck Surgery, Department of Surgery, St Martha's Regional Hospital, Halifax, Canada.

References
1. Browning GG, Gatehouse S. The prevalence of middle ear disease in the adult British population. Clin Otolaryngol Allied Sci. 1992;17:317–21.
2. Gluth MB, McDonald DR, Weaver AL, Bauch CD, Beatty CW, Orvidas LJ. Management of eustachian tube dysfunction with nasal steroid spray: a prospective, randomized, placebo-controlled trial. Arch Otolaryngol Head Neck Surg. 2011;137:449–55.
3. Llewellyn A, Norman G, Harden M, et al. Interventions for adult Eustachian tube dysfunction: a systematic review. Health Technol Assess. 2014;18(46):1–180.
4. Caffier PP, Sedlmaier B, Haupt H, Göktas O, Scherer H, Mazurek B. Impact of laser eustachian tuboplasty on middle ear ventilation, hearing, and tinnitus in chronic tube dysfunction. Ear Hear. 2011;32:132–9.
5. Metson R, Pletcher SD, Poe DS. Microdebrider eustachian tuboplasty: A preliminary report. Otolaryngol–Head Neck Surg Off J Am Acad Otolaryngol-Head Neck Surg. 2007;136:422–7.

6.   Kivekäs I, Chao WC, Faquin W, et al. Histopathology of balloon-dilation
     Eustachian tuboplasty. Laryngoscope. 2015;125(2):436–41.
7.   Silvola J, Kivekäs I, Poe DS. Balloon Dilation of the Cartilaginous Portion of
     the Eustachian Tube. Otolaryngol–Head Neck Surg Off J Am Acad
     Otolaryngol-Head Neck Surg. 2014;151:125–30.
8.   Schröder S, Lehmann M, Ebmeyer J, Upile T, Sudhoff H. Balloon
     Eustachian Tuboplasty (BET): our experience of 622 cases. Clin
     Otolaryngol. 2015. doi:10.1111/coa.12429. [Epub ahead of print] PubMed
     PMID: 25867023.
9.   Dalchow CV, Loewenthal M, Kappo N, Jenckel F, Loerincz BB, Knecht R. First
     results of Endonasal dilatation of the Eustachian tube (EET) in patients with
     chronic obstructive tube dysfunction. Eur Arch Otorhinolaryngol. 2015.
     [Epub ahead of print] PubMed.
10. Catalano PJ, Jonnalagadda S, Yu VM. Balloon catheter dilatation of
     Eustachian tube: a preliminary study. Otol Neurotol Off Publ Am Otol Soc
     Am Neurotol Soc Eur Acad Otol Neurotol. 2012;33:1549–52.
11. Jurkiewicz D, Bień D, Szczygielski K, Kantor I. Clinical evaluation of balloon
     dilation Eustachian tuboplasty in the Eustachian tube dysfunction. Eur Arch
     Oto-Rhino-Laryngol Off J Eur Fed Oto-Rhino-Laryngol Soc EUFOS Affil Ger
     Soc Oto-Rhino-Laryngol - Head Neck Surg. 2013;270:1157–60.
12. Ockermann T, Reineke U, Upile T, Ebmeyer J, Sudhoff HH. Balloon dilatation
     Eustachian tuboplasty: a clinical study. Laryngoscope. 2010;120:1411–6.

32

Endoscopic ear surgery in Canada: a cross-sectional study

Michael Yong[1], Tamara Mijovic[2] and Jane Lea[3]*

Abstract

Background: Endoscopic ear surgery is an emerging technique with recent literature highlighting advantages over the traditional microscopic approach. This study aims to characterize the current status of endoscopic ear surgery in Canada and better understand the beliefs and concerns of the otolaryngology – head & neck surgery community regarding this technique.

Methods: A cross-sectional survey study of Canadian otolaryngologists was performed. Members of the Canadian Society of Otolaryngology were contacted though an online survey carried out in 2015.

Results: The majority of participants in this study (70 %) used an endoscope in their practice, with a large proportion utilizing the endoscope for cholesteatoma or tympanoplasty surgery. To date, 38 Canadian otolaryngologists (70 % of respondents) have used an endoscope for at least 1 surgical case, but only 6 (11 %) have performed more than 50 endoscopic cases. Of the otolaryngologists who use endoscopes regularly, the majority still use the microscope as their primary instrument and use the endoscope only as an adjunct during surgery. However, the general attitude surrounding endoscopes is positive; 81 % believe that endoscopes have a role to play in the future of ear surgery and 53 % indicated they were likely to use endoscopes in their future practice. Participants who were earlier in their practice or who had more exposure to endoscopic techniques in their career were more likely to have a positive stance towards endoscopic ear surgery ($p < 0.05$, $p < 0.01$, respectively). The main concern regarding endoscopic ear surgery was the technical challenge of one-handed surgery, while the primary perceived advantage was the reduced rates of residual or recurrent disease.

Conclusions: Endoscopic ear surgery is a new technique that is gaining momentum in Canada and there is enthusiasm for its incorporation into future practice. Further investment in training courses and guidance for those looking to start or advance the use of endoscopes in their practice will be vital in the years to come.

Keywords: Endoscopic ear surgery, Middle ear surgery, Otology, Survey, Canada

Background

The use of endoscopes in ear surgery began approximately forty years ago; however, it is only recently that enthusiasm for this technique has grown. Acceptance of endoscopic ear surgery techniques has likewise grown [1], albeit slowly and with initial great resistance. Over the past decade, numerous studies have been published on the overall efficacy of endoscopic ear surgery as compared to the traditional microscopic approach, thus promoting wider usage of the endoscope [2–6]. The endoscope has been supported as a tool for improving the visual exposure of hidden structures and deep recesses, obtaining a wider angle of view, and achieving a minimally-invasive operation with greater healthy tissue preservation [4–6]. The ability to view blind spots during surgeries for diseases such as cholesteatoma has also been shown to decrease residual disease and recurrence rates when compared to surgeries which used the microscope alone [6, 7].

While some authors are optimistic that endoscopes will become increasingly utilized and important in otologic surgery due to the cumulative advances in technique and quality of equipment [4–6], there are still some concerns over safety and efficiency that contribute to the reluctance of some ear surgeons to adopt usage of

* Correspondence: jlea@providencehealth.bc.ca
[3]University of British Columbia, Division of Otolaryngology – Head and Neck Surgery, ENT Clinic, 1081 Burrard Street, St. Paul's Hospital, Vancouver, BC V6Z 1Y6, Canada
Full list of author information is available at the end of the article

this technique. Careful control of hemorrhage, anti-fogging methods, reducing potential endoscope-associated thermal injury, and compensation for the loss of depth perception are challenges that need addressing when maximizing the safety of the procedure [5, 8, 9]. In addition, the cost of endoscopic equipment and the need for specialized training and experience is a hurdle that can further deter surgeons who already practice exclusively with the microscope from embracing this new technique [5, 8].

At the present time, there are no studies that characterize the usage patterns of endoscopes among those who perform ear surgery in Canada. Given the improvements in technology and changes made to the endoscopic technique over the past four decades, an assessment of the current attitudes towards endoscopic ear surgery will provide some valuable insight on the role this approach currently plays and may play in the future. The objective of this study was to provide an analysis of the current usage of endoscopic ear surgery techniques among Canadian otolaryngologists, as well as obtain a better understanding of the attitudes and learning experiences surrounding endoscopic ear surgery in Canada.

Methods

Following approval by the UBC Behavioural Research Ethics Board (ID H14-03499), members of the Canadian Society of Otolaryngology were contacted by email and invited to participate in an on-line survey. Subject invitation and recruitment were facilitated using the Canadian Society of Otolaryngology's e-mail listserv and took place during a 6-week period from March 2015 to April 2015. Consent was obtained from each study participant to use the anonymous study data collected for the purposes of publication.

This cross-sectional study involved an online survey questionnaire administered through FluidSurveys (Ottawa, ON, Canada). It was composed of eleven main questions (Additional file 1) aimed at characterizing the subjects' surgical experience, use of endoscopes in ear surgery, and perceived advantages and concerns with endoscopic ear surgery techniques. This survey was not pre-validated because no similar characterizations of endoscope usage have been previously conducted.

Statistical analysis

Descriptive statistics were used to characterize the current use of endoscopes and identify the concerns and attitudes held by otolaryngologists regarding the use of endoscopes in ear surgery.

Study participants were divided into categories based on the number of years in practice and the number of endoscopic ear cases performed. These two categorical sub-groups were then used as factors against which the

responses to various continuous and categorical variable survey questions were analyzed. In particular, three main questions regarding the likelihood to use endoscopes in the future, overall learning experience with endoscopes, and belief in a role for endoscopes in ear surgery in the future were chosen for statistical analysis. Furthermore, three additional questions regarding concerns, advantages, and ease of use were analyzed for descriptive purposes.

Odds ratio calculations comparing various pre-determined sub-groups were conducted for three key questions which were felt to best represent the overall attitude towards using endoscopes in ear surgery (Questions 7, 10, and 11). In addition, cross-tabulations (Pearson's chi-square test and Fishers exact test for small sample sizes) were conducted for the categorical data in Questions 7 and 10 and one-way ANOVA analysis was conducted for the continuous variable data in Question 11. Rigorous statistical analysis excluded data from resident physicians due to lack of adequate sample size. These data were still included in the reported percentages in the descriptive statistics. All data was analyzed using Excel 2013 (Version 15.0, Microsoft®).

Results

Study participants

The survey was sent to 703 individuals; 484 active, 50 emeritus, and 169 resident members of the Canadian Society of Otolaryngology. At the conclusion of the 6-week study period, 80 surveys were completed. Of these 80 responses, 16 were incomplete with no usable data and discarded. Of the remaining 64 responses, 10 were from otolaryngologists who did not perform ear surgery and were therefore excluded, leaving 54 responses for analysis. Of the 54 study participants, 16 (30 %) were otologists, 21 (39 %) were general otolaryngologists, 12 (22 %) were paediatric otolaryngologists, and 5 (8 %) were trainees (residents and fellows). Figure 1 describes the distribution of the number of years subjects have been in practice.

Use of endoscopes in ear surgery practice

Among the respondents who perform ear surgery, 70 % indicated that they use endoscopes in their practice. Figure 2 describes the number of endoscopic cases that respondents have performed. Based on our survey, there are currently 38 surgeons in Canada who have performed at least one endoscopic ear case, but only 6 surgeons have completed more than 50 cases. Of the surgeons who indicated that they use an endoscope, 68 % used the endoscope in the clinic and in the operating room, while smaller numbers of surgeons used the endoscope only in clinic (8 %) or only in the operating room (24 %) (Fig. 3).

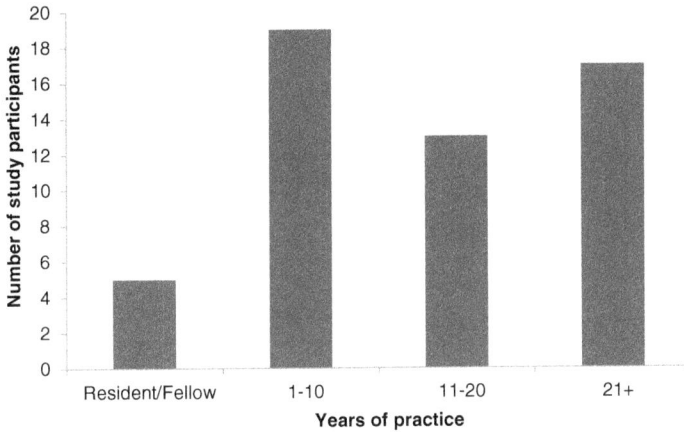

Fig. 1 Distribution of study participants by number of years in practice

Cholesteatoma (97 %) and tympanoplasty (71 %) were the two most common applications for the endoscope among respondents (Fig. 4). Ossicular reconstruction was a more infrequent application, while skull base and stapedotomy were very uncommon uses. Specifically for cholesteatoma surgery, 42 % of surgeons still primarily use the microscope with the endoscope as an adjunct, 36 % mainly use the endoscope, and 21 % only use the endoscope to check for residual disease at the end of the case (Fig. 5).

Attitude towards endoscopes in ear surgery

The majority of participants (81 %) recognize a role for the endoscope in ear surgery. The recognition of a role for endoscopes was seen across sub-groups including those who do not perform endoscopic surgery (57 %) and those who were well into their practice (65 %).

There was no statistically significant difference among the sub-groups.

Overall, participants had a positive stance on endoscopic ear surgery with over 50 % indicating that they were likely to use endoscopes for ear surgery in their future practice (Table 1). There was a significant difference in the likelihood of using endoscopes in the future based on number of years in practice ($p < 0.05$), as well as based on number of endoscopic cases performed to date ($p < 0.01$). Study participants indicated that they were more inclined to use endoscopes for ear surgery in their future practice if they were earlier in their practice with 11 to 20 years of experience (OR 2.33, 95 % CI 0.05–11.81) and significantly more inclined with only 1 to 10 years of experience (OR 18.67, 95 % CI 1.88–185.41, $p < 0.01$) when compared to those with 21 years or more of experience. Participants also responded that they would be more likely to use endoscopes in the future as their endoscopic ear surgery

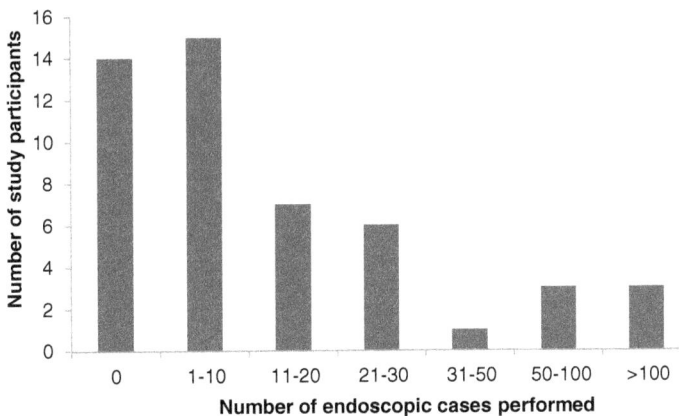

Fig. 2 Distribution of study participants by number of endoscopic ear cases performed

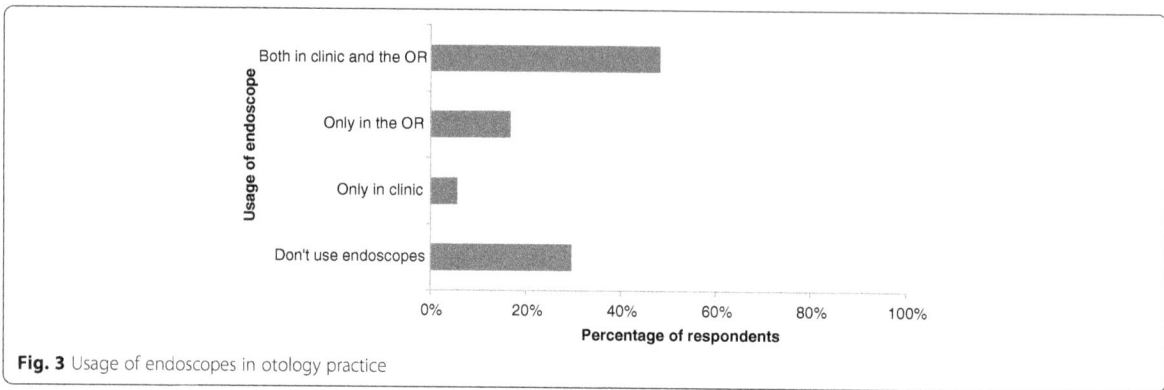

Fig. 3 Usage of endoscopes in otology practice

experience increased; when compared to those who had not performed any endoscopic surgery, participants were more likely to use an endoscope in the future if they had done between 1 and 20 endoscopic cases (OR 2.92, 95 % CI 0.55–15.56) and significantly more likely to use endoscopes in the future if they had done more than 20 endoscopic cases (OR 31.29, 95 % CI 1.72–897.14, $p < 0.05$).

Participants also appeared to be more likely to find endoscopic ear surgery easier than microscopic surgery if they were earlier in their practice and if they had done more endoscopic ear cases to date, but no significant difference was found between these sub-groups (Fig. 6).

Concerns and challenges surrounding endoscopic ear surgery

Single-handed surgery was the main prevailing concern regarding endoscopic ear surgery (44 %), followed by efficiency/operative time (32 %), technical difficulty (25 %), cost (24 %), and managing bleeding (24 %). No concerns over endoscopic surgery were expressed by 36 % of participants.

Advantages of endoscopic ear surgery

Reduced recurrence and residual disease rate was the most frequent perceived advantage (59 %), followed by ease of teaching trainees (36 %), faster patient recovery (31 %), ease of use (25 %), and less post-operative pain (25 %). No advantage to endoscopic ear surgery over microscopic ear surgery was expressed by 17 % of participants.

Discussion

The field of ear surgery has seen rapid technological advancement that has greatly impacted the field of otology, first with the invention of the operating microscope, and more recently with the emergence of minimally-invasive endoscopic techniques. Numerous advantages of the endoscope as compared to the microscope have been described and it has become clear that despite some of the disadvantages of the endoscopic approach, such as technical skill necessary and increased training requirements, many ear surgeons recommend a move towards minimally-invasive endoscopic ear surgery techniques.

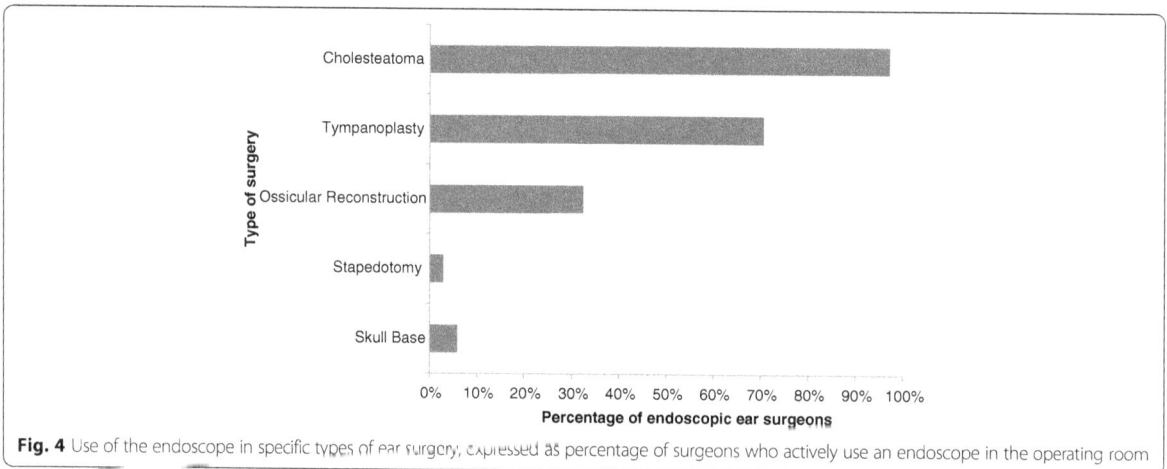

Fig. 4 Use of the endoscope in specific types of ear surgery, expressed as percentage of surgeons who actively use an endoscope in the operating room

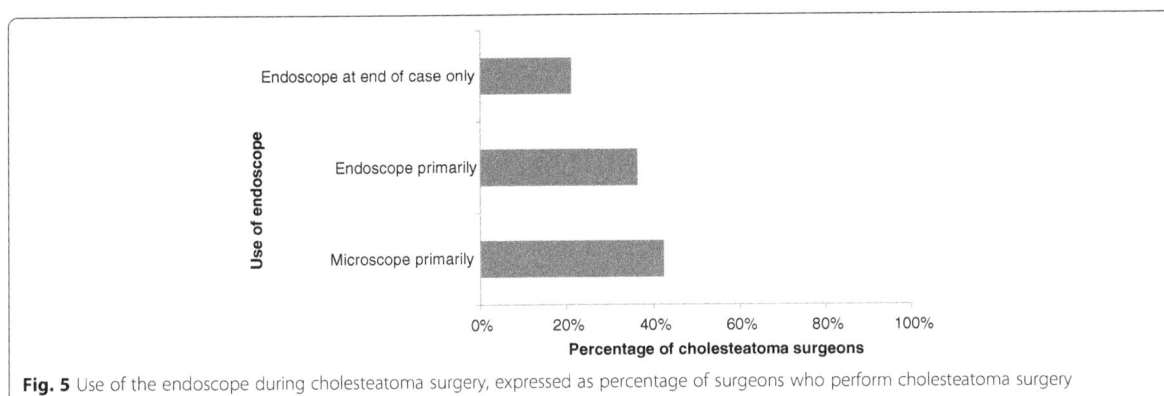

Fig. 5 Use of the endoscope during cholesteatoma surgery, expressed as percentage of surgeons who perform cholesteatoma surgery

Although the response rate of our study limits our ability to accurately characterize the use of endoscopic ear surgery in Canada, this survey shows an interest among otolaryngologists in Canada regarding endoscopic ear surgery techniques with several surgeons already adopting and implementing the technique in the operative setting. In addition, there appears to be prevailing optimism regarding the future role of the endoscope in otologic surgery, even among those not currently using endoscopes. Based on our survey, the most common application for the endoscope in the operating room is among cholesteatoma and tympanoplasty procedures. This finding is consistent with previous literature which describes reduced cholesteatoma recurrence rates when using an endoscope and the advantages of minimally-invasive surgery in surgeries such as tympanoplasty [4, 6, 10 11]. However, among our respondents it seems that the microscope is still the instrument of choice in Canada for these procedures due to the amount of study participants indicating that they use the endoscope only as a adjunct or to check for residual disease at the end of a case. While the endoscope is being used for other purposes such as ossicular reconstruction, skull base surgery, and stapedotomy, it appears that the endoscopic approach in these procedures is not common practice among the subgroup of Canadian otolaryngologists who responded to the survey.

Challenges surrounding the technical skill required continue to deter some surgeons from using endoscopes [8]. The main concerns regarding the use of endoscopes in ear surgery based on this study were single-handed surgery, efficiency, cost, and technical difficulty; similar concerns have been raised in previously published literature, especially the challenge of one-handed surgery and the initial technical difficulty of implementing and using endoscopic equipment for the surgeon and operative team [6, 8, 11]. Nonetheless, most surgeons indicated that they were likely to use endoscopes for ear surgery in their future practice. In particular, those surgeons who were earlier in their practice and had performed more endoscopic ear cases to date were the most enthusiastic. This supports the concept that surgeons who have a younger practice and a baseline skill level with endoscopes appear to be more likely to invest resources in acquiring endoscopic equipment that may put them

Table 1

	Mean Rating (0 – Strongly Disagree, 5 – Strongly Agree)	Odds Ratio	95 % Confidence Interval	One-Way ANOVA
Overall ($n = 50$)	3.9	-	-	-
Years in Practice				$p = 0.014$
21+ ($n = 13$)	3.2	1	-	
11-20 ($n = 12$)	4.1	2.33	0.05–11.81	
1–10 ($n = 17$)	4.6	18.67	1.88–185.41*	
Trainee ($n = 5$)	3.8	N/A	-	
Number of Endoscopic Ear Cases				$p = 0.0030$
0 ($n = 8$)	3	1		
1–20 ($n = 22$)	3.9	2.92	0.55–15.56	
21+ ($n = 12$)	4.8	31.29	1.72–897.14*	

Likelihood of using endoscopes in the future, with responses separated by years of practice and by number of endoscopic ear cases performed
*$p < 0.05$

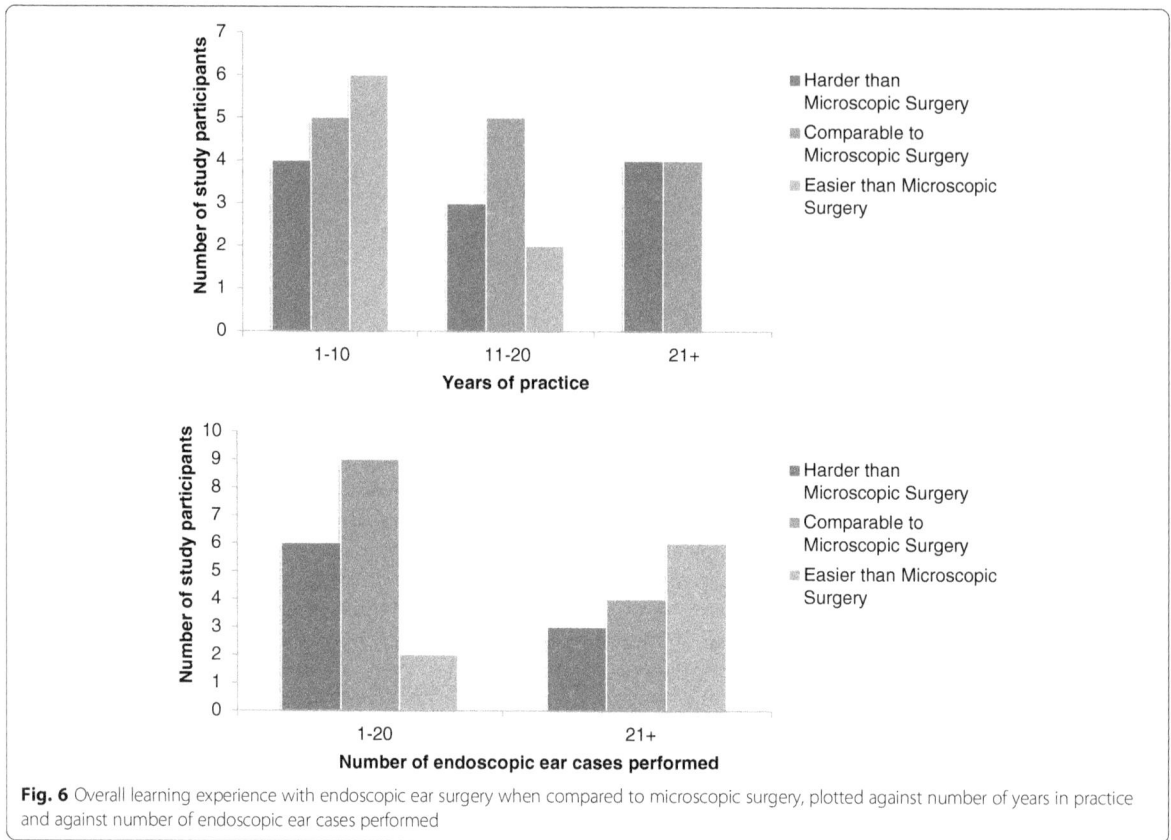

Fig. 6 Overall learning experience with endoscopic ear surgery when compared to microscopic surgery, plotted against number of years in practice and against number of endoscopic ear cases performed

in a better position to overcome some of the concerns that deter usage of the endoscope in ear surgery. In the authors' experience, the cost of implementing endoscopic ear surgery is often quite minimal as most centres are often already well-equipped with endoscopic sinus surgery equipment and already have standard otologic operative instruments which, when combined, are more than adequate to get started with the technique.

There is a challenging learning curve when transitioning from the microscope to the endoscope in ear surgery. As expected, this study shows a trend, albeit not statistically significant, that implies that junior staff and those with more endoscopic ear experiences find endoscopic techniques easier than microscopic approaches. This concept has been supported by authors who have described their own endoscopic learning experience and who have also provided guidance to surgeons who are seeking to implement endoscopic techniques into their practice for the first time [8, 11, 12]. Further investment in endoscopic training programs may allow more surgeons to overcome the hurdles that currently preclude them from incorporating endoscopes into their ear surgery practice.

Once some of the initial technical and learning difficulties of endoscopic ear surgery can be overcome, many authors advocate that the benefits of using the endoscope are multifaceted [2, 6, 8, 11]. The proposed benefits of endoscopic surgery based on current literature align well with the views of Canadian otolaryngologists, particularly with respect to the reduced rate of residual or recurrent cholesteatoma and the ease of obtaining better surgical visualization [6, 7]. Other advantages such as reduced post-operative pain and faster patient recovery are also in agreement with literature articles studying these outcomes in ear surgery patients [10, 12, 13].

There was considerable agreement among respondents that endoscopes have a role to play in the future of ear surgery. The fact that there was no significant difference in these results based on either number of years in practice or experience with the endoscope suggests that there is a general acceptance and support for the use of endoscopes in ear surgery among the subgroup of Canadian otolaryngologists participating in the survey. This finding supports previous literature which promotes the use of endoscopes in the field of ear surgery [6–8, 10–11, 14], and, at the very least, indicates that investing further resources into teaching and promoting the use of endoscopes will likely be met with enthusiasm.

This study has a number of limitations. Survey data was collected in a non-randomized manner and was entirely dependent on the voluntary response rate among otolaryngologists who were subscribed to the Canadian Society of Otolaryngology listserv. The survey was sent to 703 Canadian Society of Otolaryngology members and while 64 responded, only 54 actually performed ear surgery in their current practice. Although the response rate was low at 9 %, one must take into account the current subspecialized nature of otolaryngology in Canada within both community and academic environments. Many Canadian otolaryngologists with interests in subspecialty fields such as rhinology/sinus, head and neck, and facial plastics likely ignored the email given that ear surgery is not within their scope of current practice. The response rate, although quite low, is therefore still difficult to fully interpret. Among the active members of the Canadian Society of Otolaryngology, 36 are fellowship trained in otology and 18 have an interest in otology without formal fellowship training. It may not be coincidence that this sum equals 54, which is the exact number of survey responses analyzed for this study. This survey may therefore be biased towards surgeons with a subspecialty interest in otology and likely a practice with higher volumes of more complex otologic surgery. Accordingly, the results need to be interpreted within that context and not extrapolated to the wider otolaryngology community within Canada. The small response rate also meant that in cases where subgroup analysis was necessary, some sample sizes were too small to conduct rigorous statistical analyses. Finally, the amount of trainees completing the survey was too small to be included in rigorous statistical analysis calculations and, thus, was only included in the graphical statistics.

Conclusion

This is the first study aimed toward comprehensively characterizing the current state of endoscopic ear surgery in Canada. Patterns of endoscope use, attitudes, learning experiences and perceived advantages and challenges regarding endoscopic ear surgery were documented and quantified among Canadian otolaryngologists. Although care should be taken when generalizing these findings to all Canadian otolaryngologists considering the aforementioned study limitations, a number of valuable overall assessments can be offered. Findings show that a considerable number of ear surgeons currently use endoscopes to some capacity in their practice and that, despite some reservations, there is an overall enthusiasm for the endoscopic approach to otologic surgery. Furthermore, there is a general feeling among survey respondents that endoscopes will likely have a role to play in the future of otologic surgery. Given the

continuous improvement in endoscopic technology and increasing acceptance of endoscopic ear surgery, investment in training courses and guidance for those looking to start or advance their use of the endoscope in their practice will be vital in the years to come.

Ethics approval

Ethics approval was obtained from the UBC Behavioural Research Ethics Board (ID H14-03499) and consent was obtained from survey participants by email using the CSO listserv.

Additional file

Additional file 1: Endoscopic ear surgery in Canada survey.
(DOC 25 kb)

Abbreviations
CSO: Canadian Society of Otolaryngology; OR: Odds ratio; ANOVA: Analysis of variance.

Competing interests
The authors declare that they have no competing interests.

Authors' contributions
JL conceived of the study, facilitated survey administration and data gathering, and oversaw editing of the manuscript. TM assisted with data analysis and contributed to drafting the manuscript. MY facilitated study design and survey administration, conducted raw data processing and statistical analysis, and contributed to drafting the manuscript. All authors read and approved the final manuscript.

Acknowledgements
We would like to thank Ms. Donna Humphrey from the administrative staff at the Canadian Society of Otolaryngology for her assistance in administering the survey.

Author details
[1]University of British Columbia, Division of Otolaryngology – Head and Neck Surgery, 4th Floor, 2775 Laurel Street, Vancouver General Hospital, Vancouver, BC V5Z 1 M9, Canada. [2]McGill University, Department of Otolaryngology – Head and Neck Surgery, Royal Victoria Hospital - D05.5712, 1001 Décarie Boul, Montreal H4A 3 J1, Canada. [3]University of British Columbia, Division of Otolaryngology – Head and Neck Surgery, ENT Clinic, 1081 Burrard Street, St. Paul's Hospital, Vancouver, BC V6Z 1Y6, Canada.

References
1. Yung MM. The use of rigid endoscopes in cholesteatoma surgery. J Laryngol Otol. 1994;108(4):307–9.
2. El-Meselaty K, Badr-El-Dine M, Mourad M, Darweesh R. Endoscope affects decision making in cholesteatoma surgery. Otolaryngol Head Neck Surg. 2003;129(5):490–6.
3. Lade H, Choudhary SR, Vashishth A. Endoscopic vs microscopic myringoplasty: a different perspective. Eur Arch Otorhinolaryngol. 2014;271(7):1897–902.
4. Marchioni D, Villari D, Mattioli F, Alicandri-Ciufelli M, Piccinini A, Presutti L. Endoscopic management of attic cholesteatoma: a single-institution experience. Otolaryngol Clin N Am. 2013;46(2):201–9.
5. Badr-el-Dine M, James EL, Panetti G, Marchioni D, Presutti L, Nogueira JF. Instrumentation and technologies in endoscopic ear surgery. Otolaryngol Clin N Am. 2013;46(2):211–25.
6. Badr-el-Dine M. Value of ear endoscopy in cholesteatoma surgery. Otol Neurotol. 2002;23:631–5.

7.　Ayache S, Tramier B, Strunski V. Otoendoscopy in cholesteatoma surgery of the middle ear: what benefits can be expected? Otol Neurotol. 2008;29(8):1085–90.

8.　Pothier DD. Introducing endoscopic ear surgery into practice. Otolaryngol Clin N Am. 2013;46(2):245–55.

9.　Kozin ED, Lehmann A, Carter M, Hight E, Cohen M, Nakajima HH, et al. Thermal effects of endoscopy in a human temporal bone model: implications for endoscopic ear surgery. Laryngoscope. 2014;124(8):E322–9.

10.　Tarabichi M. Endoscopic management of cholesteatoma: long-term results. Otolaryngol Head Neck Surg. 2000;122:874–81.

11.　Youssef TF, Poe DS. Endoscope-assisted second-stage tympanomastoidectomy. Laryngoscope. 1997;107:1341–4.

12.　James AL. Endoscopic middle ear surgery in children. Otolaryngol Clin N Am. 2013;46:233–44.

13.　Shaia WT, Diaz RC. Evaluation in surgical management of superior canal dehiscence syndrome. Curr Opin Otolaryngol Head Neck Surg. 2013;21(5):497–502.

14.　Presutti L, Nogueira JF, Alicandri-Ciufelli M, Marchioni D. Beyond the middle ear: endoscopic surgical anatomy and approaches to inner ear and lateral skull base. Otolaryngol Clin N Am. 2013;46:189–200.

33

Rinne test: does the tuning fork position affect the sound amplitude at the ear?

Oleksandr Butskiy[1,3,5]*, Denny Ng[2], Murray Hodgson[2,4] and Desmond A. Nunez[1,3,5]

Abstract

Background: Guidelines and text-book descriptions of the Rinne test advise orienting the tuning fork tines in parallel with the longitudinal axis of the external auditory canal (EAC), presumably to maximise the amplitude of the air conducted sound signal at the ear. Whether the orientation of the tuning fork tines affects the amplitude of the sound signal at the ear in clinical practice has not been previously reported. The present study had two goals: determine if (1) there is clinician variability in tuning fork placement when presenting the air-conduction stimulus during the Rinne test; (2) the orientation of the tuning fork tines, parallel versus perpendicular to the EAC, affects the sound amplitude at the ear.

Methods: To assess the variability in performing the Rinne test, the Canadian Society of Otolaryngology – Head and Neck Surgery members were surveyed. The amplitudes of the sound delivered to the tympanic membrane with the activated tuning fork tines held in parallel, and perpendicular to, the longitudinal axis of the EAC were measured using a Knowles Electronics Mannequin for Acoustic Research (KEMAR) with the microphone of a sound level meter inserted in the pinna insert.

Results: 47.4 and 44.8 % of 116 survey responders reported placing the fork parallel and perpendicular to the EAC respectively. The sound intensity (sound-pressure level) recorded at the tympanic membrane with the 512 Hz tuning fork tines in parallel with as opposed to perpendicular to the EAC was louder by 2.5 dB (95 % CI: 1.35, 3.65 dB; $p < 0.0001$) for the fundamental frequency (512 Hz), and by 4.94 dB (95 % CI: 3.10, 6.78 dB; $p < 0.0001$) and 3.70 dB (95 % CI: 1.62, 5.78 dB; $p = .001$) for the two harmonic (non-fundamental) frequencies (1 and 3.15 kHz), respectively. The 256 Hz tuning fork in parallel with the EAC as opposed to perpendicular to was louder by 0.83 dB (95 % CI: −0.26, 1.93 dB; $p = 0.14$) for the fundamental frequency (256 Hz), and by 4.28 dB (95 % CI: 2.65, 5.90 dB; $p < 0.001$) and 1.93 dB (95 % CI: 0.26, 3.61 dB; $p = .02$) for the two harmonic frequencies (500 and 4 kHz) respectively.

Conclusions: Clinicians vary in their orientation of the tuning fork tines in relation to the EAC when performing the Rinne test. Placement of the tuning fork tines in parallel as opposed to perpendicular to the EAC results in a higher sound amplitude at the level of the tympanic membrane.

Keywords: Tuning fork, Physical examination, Rinne test

Background

Historically, up to 20 tuning fork tests were used in the diagnosis of hearing loss [1]. Anecdotally only two tests, Webber and Rinne, continue to be routinely taught in medical schools and used clinically by otologists and primary care physicians. The Rinne test is recommended as part of an otological physical exam to detect conductive hearing loss [2]. In patients with otosclerosis, the Rinne test is used to determine stapes surgery candidacy [3]. Olotaryngologists have advocated for further study of the sources of variation in performing the Rinne test given its widespread clinical use [4].

Audiology society recommendations [5] instructions aimed at medical student and non-specialist on performing the Rinne test in general and otolaryngology textbooks [6], instructions intended for otolaryngology residents in speciality textbooks [7], and peer reviewed

* Correspondence: butskiy.alex@gmail.com
[1]Division of Otolaryngology – Head and Neck Surgery, Vancouver General Hospital, Vancouver, BC, Canada
[3]Department of Surgery, University of British Columbia, Vancouver, BC, Canada
Full list of author information is available at the end of the article

publications [4, 8] all describe placing the vibrating tuning fork tines in parallel with the longitudinal axis of external auditory canal (or parallel to the frontal plane of the skull). In comparison to perpendicular placement of the tines, placement of the tines parallel to the ear canal is thought to result in higher sound intensities (i.e., sound pressure levels) at the patient's eardrum [5].

Mathematical calculations and sound field recordings conclude that a higher amplitude sound is delivered to the ear when the fork is placed parallel to as opposed to perpendicular to the EAC [9, 10]. These lines of evidence show a 5 dB difference in the sound intensity produced by the two different positions of the tuning fork [10]. However, there are several known tuning fork vibration modes, and these mathematical models and experimental studies have only tested the individual vibration modes. A tuning fork activated by a physician likely produces a sound that is a product of at least seven known vibration modes [11]. The sound intensities of a tuning fork placed parallel to and perpendicular to the EAC during the Rinne test have not been compared before.

The present study had two goals: To determine if (1) Canadian otolaryngologists demonstrate variability in performance of the Rinne test, specifically focusing on the tuning fork placement during air conduction testing; (2) orientation of the tuning fork tines, parallel to as compared to perpendicular to the EAC, affects the amplitude of sound (at fundamental and harmonic frequencies) at the level of the tympanic membrane.

Methods

To assess the variability in performance of the Rinne test amongst Canadian otolaryngologists, we conducted an e-mail survey through the Canadian Society of Otolaryngology – Head and Neck Surgery member e-mail list. Prior to conducting the survey, ethics approval from our institution was sought, but was deemed unnecessary by the research ethics board. The survey was e-mailed out once to the member list on April 22nd, 2015 and the results were collected until June 2nd, 2015. The survey consisted of four multiple-choice questions and a comment section.

An experimental simulation of the air conduction component of the Rinne test was used to measure the sound intensity at the level of the tympanic membrane for both parallel and perpendicular positions of the tuning fork. Two aluminum tuning forks (512 Hz and 256 Hz) of the same design were used in the experiment (Fig. 1).

The experimental design is summarized in Fig. 2. The protocol for tuning fork activation and placement was based on the most common responses from the email survey. One of the testers was blinded to the study

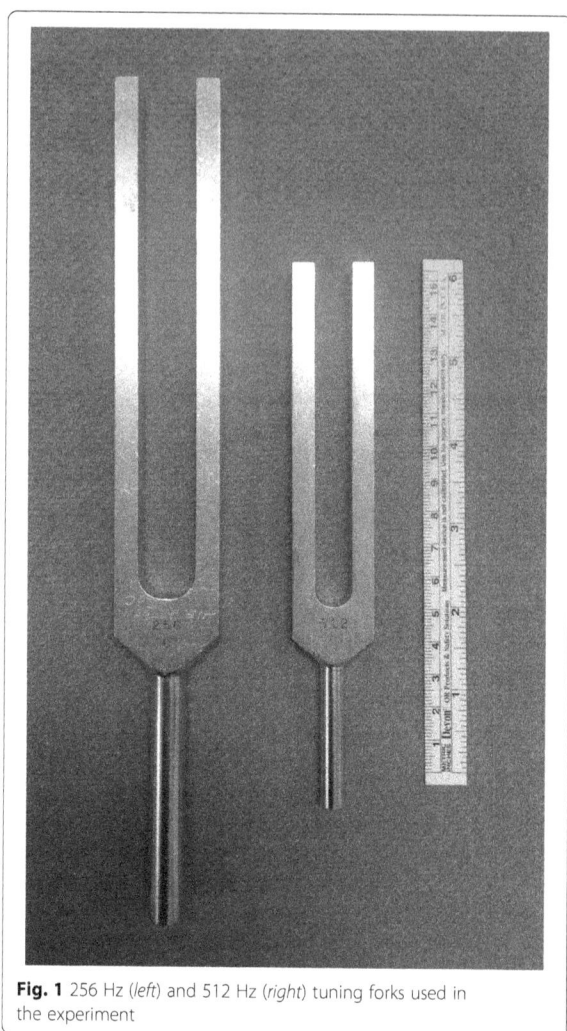

Fig. 1 256 Hz (*left*) and 512 Hz (*right*) tuning forks used in the experiment

question. A visual reference was used to train the testers to consistently place the edge of the vibrating tuning fork 30–49 mm lateral to the ear canal (Fig. 3a, c). In addition, the testers were trained to align the middle of tuning fork with the EAC viewed in the coronal plane (Fig. 3b, d). To ensure consistent tuning fork placement throughout the experiment, the placement of the tuning fork was re-checked using a visual reference after each of 50 consecutive activations.

The sound intensities produced by the tuning fork during individual activations were recorded with a RION NA-28 Sound Level Meter (RION Co., Ltd., Tokyo, Japan) with its microphone inserted into the EAC hole in the pinna insert of a KEMAR Manikin Type 45BA (G.R.A.S. Sound & Vibration, Holte, Denmark). The sound spectra of the tuning forks were measured in 1/3 octave bands. Each measurement was triggered when the 1/3 octave band of interest (256 or 512 Hz) exceeded

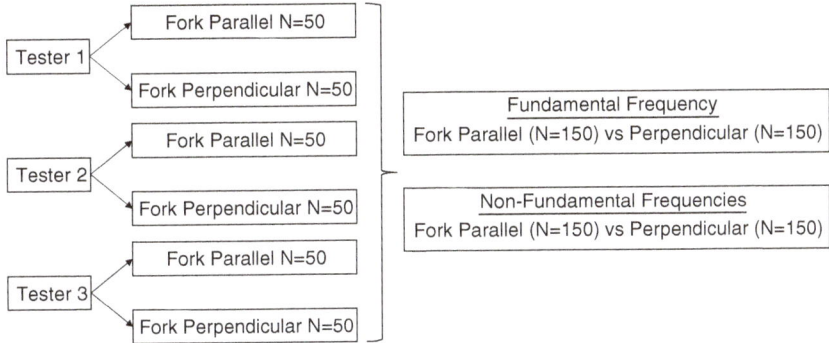

Protocol
1. Activate the fork by a strike on the knee
2. Place the fork 30-49mm away from the mannequin ear
3. Record the amplitudes of the fundamental and non-fundamental frequencies

Tester 1
Fork Parallel N=50
Fork Perpendicular N=50

Tester 2
Fork Parallel N=50
Fork Perpendicular N=50

Tester 3
Fork Parallel N=50
Fork Perpendicular N=50

Fundamental Frequency
Fork Parallel (N=150) vs Perpendicular (N=150)

Non-Fundamental Frequencies
Fork Parallel (N=150) vs Perpendicular (N=150)

Fig. 2 The experimental design

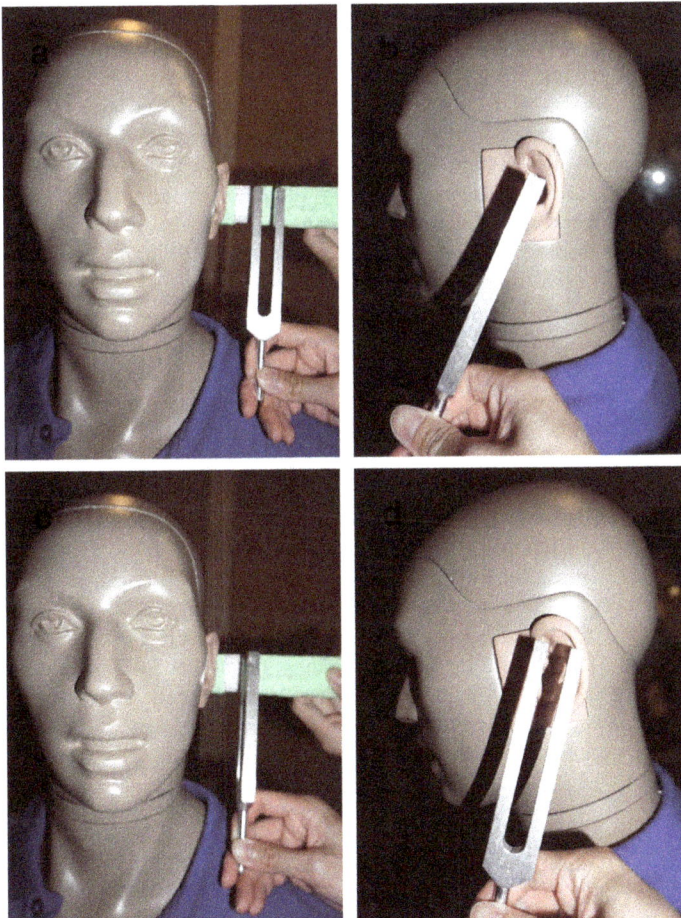

Fig. 3 Simulation of the Rinne Test: placement of the 512 Hz tuning fork parallel (**a**, **b**) and perpendicular (**c**, **d**) to the ear canal

70 dB. This helped reduce variability associated with different excitations, and positionings, of the tuning fork. Once triggered, the measurements were taken over 3 s and averaged.

An independent-samples t-test was used to compare the parallel and perpendicular placements of the tuning fork with respect to the measured amplitudes of the fundamental frequencies (512 and 256 Hz) and dominant harmonic frequencies. The dominant harmonic frequencies were identified by visual inspection of the averaged sound spectrum of each tuning fork activation.

Results
(1) Email survey
Out of 512 active members of the CSO-HNS, 116 physicians responded to the survey for a response rate of 23 % (Tables 1, 2, 3, and 4). 113 responders reported practicing in Canada. The highest proportion of the responders reported using a 512 Hz tuning fork (73 %; 85 responders), activating the fork by a strike on the knee (45.7 %; 55 responders), and holding the fork 3 to 4 cm away from the ear (44.8 %; 52 responders). 55 (47.4 %) of the surveyed physicians reported placing the fork parallel, and 52 (44.8 %) reported placing the fork perpendicular to the ear canal.

(2) Simulation of the Rinne air conduction testing
The average amplitudes of the sound spectra produced by 512 and 256 Hz tuning forks placed parallel and perpendicular to the ear canal are presented in Fig. 4. Visual inspection of the sound spectra of each tuning fork identified two dominant harmonic frequencies for the 512 Hz tuning fork (1 and 3.15 kHz) and three dominant harmonic frequencies for the 256 Hz tuning fork (500 Hz, 1.6, and 4 kHz).

The statistical comparison of parallel and perpendicular placements of the 512 and 256 Hz tuning forks with respect to the amplitude of the fundamental frequencies and dominant harmonic frequencies are summarized in Tables 5 and 6. The sound intensity recorded at the tympanic membrane with the 512 Hz tuning fork tines in parallel with as opposed to perpendicular to the EAC was louder by 2.5 dB (95 % CI: 1.35, 3.65 dB; $p < 0.0001$) for the fundamental frequency (512 Hz), and by 4.94 dB (95 % CI: 3.10, 6.78 dB; $p < 0.0001$) and 3.70 dB (95 % CI: 1.62, 5.78 dB; $p = .001$) for the two harmonic frequencies (1 and 3.15 kHz) respectively (Table 5). The

Table 1 Canadian Society of Otolaryngology - Head and Neck Surgery e-mail survey results (116 Responders)

What Frequency of tuning fork do you use to administer the Rinne test?		
256 Hz	512 Hz	Other
16	83	17

Table 2 Canadian Society of Otolaryngology - Head and Neck Surgery e-mail survey results (116 Responders)

How do you mostly activate the tuning fork for the Rinne test?				
Elbow Strike	Knee Strike	Striking a soft coated surface	Finger Pinch	Other
38	53	10	3	12

256 Hz tuning fork in parallel with the EAC as opposed to perpendicular to was louder by 0.83 dB (95 % CI: -0.26, 1.93 dB; $p = 0.14$) for the fundamental frequency (256 Hz), and by 4.28 dB (95 % CI: 2.65, 5.90 dB; $p < 0.001$) and 1.93 dB (95 % CI: 0.26, 3.61 dB; $p = .02$) for the two harmonic frequencies (500 and 4 kHz) respectively (Table 6). For the 1.6 kHz harmonic frequency of the 256 Hz tuning fork, the perpendicular placement of the tuning fork was louder than parallel placement of the tuning fork by 0.11 dB (95 % CI: -1.58, 1.8 dB; $p = 0.89$).

Discussion
The results of the e-mail survey show that despite the use of the Rinne test by the majority of the responding otolaryngologists, the air conduction testing techniques in use are not uniform. The survey suggests that the majority of Canadian otolaryngologists prefer the 512 Hz tuning fork, activate the fork by the strike of the knee, and place the fork approximately 3 to 4 cm away from the ear canal when testing air conduction. Despite the traditional teaching on the placement of the tuning fork tines during air conduction testing, the results of the survey show a roughly equal use of parallel and perpendicular tuning fork placement amongst the responders. Whilst some of the responders did not understand what was meant by parallel and perpendicular placement of the fork, these findings suggest that Canadian Otolaryngologists vary in their orientation of the tuning fork tines.

The results of the survey should be interpreted with caution. Only a limited number of physicians responded to the survey (23 % response rate). Furthermore, the question design only allowed for a limited number of responses. Therefore, the complete variability in air conduction testing by Canadian otolaryngologists has likely not been captured by the survey. Despite these limitations, the survey provided useful information for designing the experimental part of the study.

To our knowledge, the sound spectra for the 512 and 256 Hz tuning forks activated in clinical practice for the

Table 3 Canadian Society of Otolaryngology - Head and Neck Surgery e-mail survey results (116 Responders)

How far from the ear do you hold the tuning fork?					
12 cm	3–4 cm	5–6 cm	7 0 cm	9–10+ cm	other
45	52	11	4	0	4

Table 4 Canadian Society of Otolaryngology - Head and Neck Surgery e-mail survey results (116 Responders)

During the Rinne test, are the tines of the fork parallel or perpendicular to the auditory canal?

Parallel	Perpendicular	Other
55	52	9

purposes of the Rinne test have not been documented previously. The sound spectra (Fig. 4) and the knowledge of the dominant harmonic frequencies are valuable for interpreting Rinne test results for patients with different levels of hearing loss across the frequency spectrum.

The experimental findings support the traditional teaching that parallel placement of tuning fork tines with respect to the EAC produces higher sound amplitude at

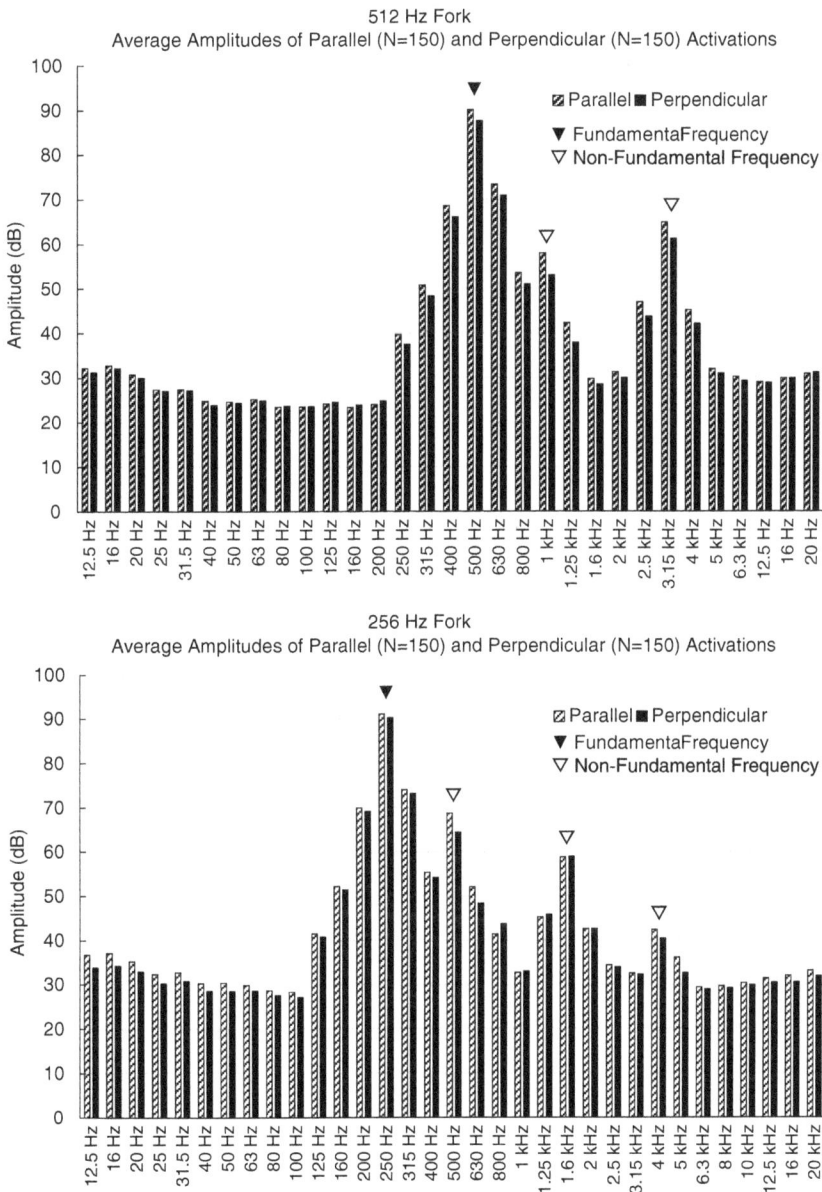

Fig. 4 Average amplitudes obtained by activating 512 and 256 Hz tuning forks in parallel (*shaded bars*) and perpendicular (*solid bars*). The fundamental frequencies are marked with solid arrow heads; the main non-fundamental frequencies are marked with empty arrow heads

Table 5 Sound amplitudes produced by parallel and perpendicular placement of 512Hz fork at the selected frequencies

Frequency Measured	Mean Amplitude (±SD)		Mean Difference (95 % CI)	p-value
	Parallel (N = 150)	Perpendicular (N =150)		
500 Hz	90.04 dB (±4.46 dB)	87.53 dB (±5.63 dB)	2.50 dB (±1.15 dB)	<0.0001
1 kHz	57.86 dB (±7.64 dB)	52.92 dB (±8.50 dB)	4.94 dB (±1.84 dB)	<0.0001
3.15 kHz	64.76 dB (±7.32 dB)	61.05 dB (±10.69 dB)	3.70 dB (±2.08 dB)	.001

SD Standard Deviation, *CI* Confidence Interval

the level of the tympanic membrane than perpendicular placement of the tines. For the 512 Hz tuning fork, the difference between the two positions of the tuning fork was measured to be 2.5 dB for the fundamental frequency. This is less than the 5 dB difference predicted by the mathematical models [10]. The smaller than expected difference could be due to the complex interactions of the tuning fork vibration modes not accounted for by the mathematical models. Alternatively, this smaller difference could be explained by the inherent variability in activations of the tuning fork by a strike on the knee.

The measured 0.83 dB fundamental frequency amplitude difference between the parallel and perpendicular placement of the 256 Hz tuning fork was smaller than the 2.5 dB difference measured for the 512 Hz tuning fork. Even though the amplitude for the parallel placement of the 256 Hz tuning fork was again greater than for the perpendicular placement, this difference did not reach statistical significance. The explanation for the lack of statistical significance likely lies in the difference of geometry between the 512 and 256 Hz fork. Due to the need to keep the design of the 512 and 256 Hz tuning forks consistent, the 256 Hz tuning fork was larger than the 512 Hz tuning fork (Fig. 1). Given, its larger dimensions, the difference in the amplitude between the parallel and perpendicular placement of the 256 Hz tuning fork was likely negated by the wider vibration field of the larger tines: when testing the parallel position of the tuning fork, placing the edge of the 256Hz fork 30 to 49 cm away from the EAC positions the centre of the tuning fork further away from the EAC as compared to the same placement of the smaller 512Hz tuning fork (Fig. 5). We tested this explanation by performing a separate experiment with a different design of the 256 Hz

tuning fork, where the dimensions of the 256 Hz fork were similar to the 512 Hz fork. In this separate experiment, not presented in this report, a statistically significant difference of 3.7 dB in favour of the parallel placement of the tuning fork was found.

Loudness perception is a complicated psychoacoustic phenomenon influenced not only by the amplitude but also by the frequency of the sound, its spectral distribution, its duration and time structure, and by its overall acoustic environment [12]. Assuming that all other variables influencing the perception of loudness are kept constant, a normal hearing individual should be able to discriminate a difference in amplitude as small as 1.5 dB [13, 14]. The amplitude resolution of 1.5 dB is preserved in hearing-impaired patients with most types of conductive and sensorineural hearing loss. The only apparent exception is the lower amplitude resolution seen in patients with acoustic neuroma (4.5 dB) [13, 14]. These facts suggest that the amplitude difference between in parallel and perpendicular to the EEC tuning fork placement observed in this study can be perceived by most patients undergoing the Rinne test. Thus, the position of the tuning fork with respect to the EAC during the Rinne test represents a significant variable that can potentially influence the sensitivity and specificity of the test. Further investigation is needed to test whether the position of the tuning fork during the Rinne test affects the its results in patients with hearing loss.

Conclusions

Despite widespread use of the Rinne test by Canadian otolaryngologists, the Rinne test techniques practiced are non-uniform. Orientation of the tuning fork tines with respect to the EAC during air conduction testing is an important source of variation in performing the

Table 6 Sound amplitudes produces by parallel and perpendicular placement of 256Hz fork at the selected frequencies

Frequency Measured	Mean Amplitude (±SD)		Mean Difference (95 % CI)	p-value
	Parallel (N = 150)	Perpendicular (N =150)		
250 Hz	91.14 dB (±4.06 dB)	90.30 dB (±5.47 dB)	0.83 dB (±1.09 dB)	.14
500 kHz	68.67 dB (±7.30 dB)	64.39 dB (±6.99 dB)	4.28 dB (±1.62 dB)	<0.001
1.6 kHz	58.80 dB (±7.13 dB)	58.92 dB (±7.73 dB)	−0.11 dB (±1.69 dB)	.89
4 kHz	42.35 dB (±8.52 dB)	40.42 dB (±6.05 dB)	1.93 dB (±1.67 dB)	.02

SD Standard Deviation, *CI* Confidence Interval

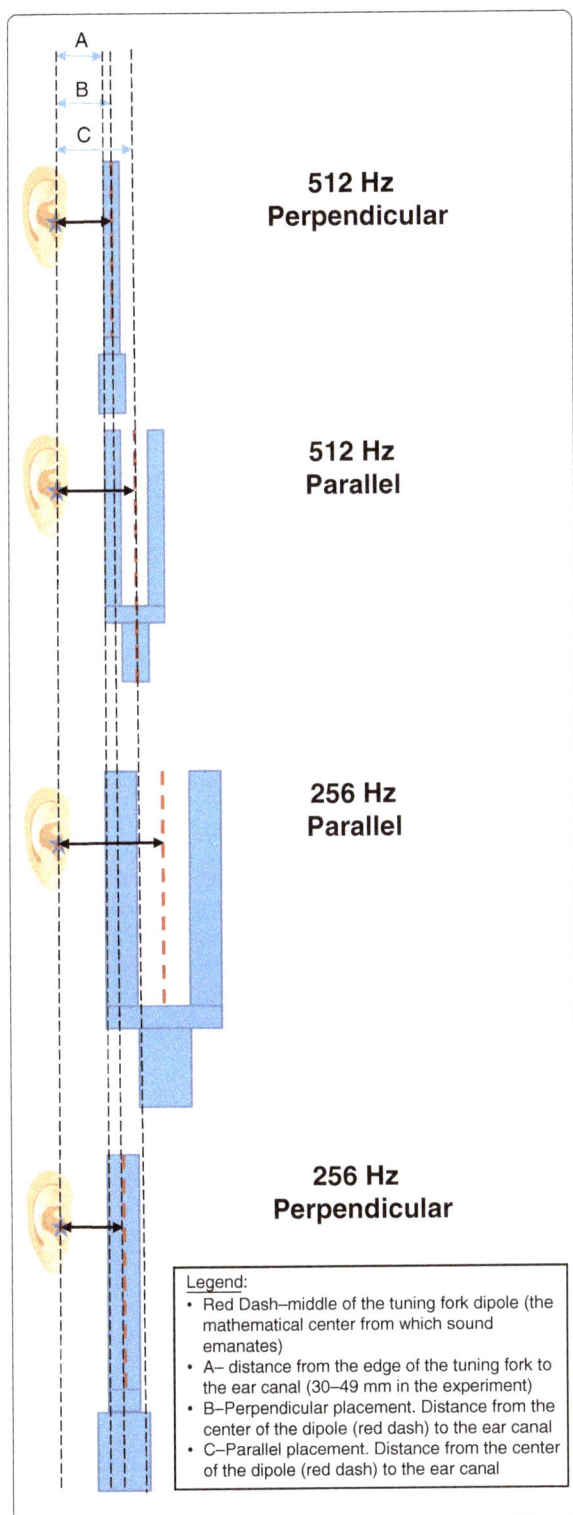

A

B

C

**512 Hz
Perpendicular**

**512 Hz
Parallel**

**256 Hz
Parallel**

**256 Hz
Perpendicular**

Legend:
- Red Dash—middle of the tuning fork dipole (the mathematical center from which sound emanates)
- A– distance from the edge of the tuning fork to the ear canal (30–49 mm in the experiment)
- B–Perpendicular placement. Distance from the center of the dipole (red dash) to the ear canal
- C–Parallel placement. Distance from the center of the dipole (red dash) to the ear canal

Fig. 5 The influence of tuning fork size on the distance from the centre of the tuning fork dipole to the ear canal. Parallel orientation produces a louder sound and when this is coupled with placement of the vibrating dipole closer to the ear canal in the smaller 512 Hz tuning fork the effect is most marked

Rinne test. Placement of the tuning fork tines in parallel as opposed to perpendicular to the ear canal produces a sound of higher amplitude at the level of the tympanic membrane. Physicians are encouraged to pay attention to the orientation of tuning fork's tines with respect to the long axis of the EAC when testing air conduction during the Rinne test.

Abbreviations
EAC: external ear canal.

Competing interests
The authors declare that they have no competing interests.

Authors' contributions
OB: study conception, literature search, study design, data collection, data analysis, manuscript drafting and revision. DN: study design, acoustic experiment set up, and data collection. MH: study design, acoustic experiment set up. DN: study design, literature search, financial support, manuscript revision. All authors read and approved the final manuscript.

Acknowledgements
We thank Dr. Lorienne M. Jenstad for the use of her laboratory space and equipment.

Author details
[1]Division of Otolaryngology – Head and Neck Surgery, Vancouver General Hospital, Vancouver, BC, Canada. [2]Department of Mechanical Engineering, University of British Columbia, Vancouver, BC, Canada. [3]Department of Surgery, University of British Columbia, Vancouver, BC, Canada. [4]School of Population and Public Health, University of British Columbia, Vancouver, BC, Canada. [5]Gordon & Leslie Diamond Health Care Centre, 4th. Fl. 4299B-2775 Laurel Street, Vancouver, BC V5Z 1M9, Canada.

References
1. Ng M, Jackler RK. Early history of tuning-fork tests. Am J Otol. 1993;14:100–5.
2. Burkey JM, Lippy WH, Schuring AG, Rizer FM. Clinical utility of the 512-Hz Rinne tuning fork test. Am J Otol. 1998;19:59–62.
3. Shea PF, Ge X, Shea JJ. Stapedectomy for far-advanced otosclerosis. Am J Otol. 1999;20:425–9.
4. MacKechnie CA, Greenberg JJ, Gerkin RC, McCall AA, Hirsch BE, Durrant JD, Raz Y. Rinne revisited: steel versus aluminum tuning forks. Otolaryngol–Head Neck Surg Off J Am Acad Otolaryngol-Head Neck Surg. 2013;149:907–13.
5. British Society of Audiology. Recommended procedure for Rinne and Weber tuning-fork tests. British Society of Audiology. Br J Audiol. 1987;21: 229–230. http://www.tandfonline.com/doi/abs/10.3109/03005368709076410.
6. Bickley L. Bates' Guide to Physical Examination and History-Taking. 11th ed. Philadelphia: Lippincott Williams & Wilkins; 2012.
7. Bunni J, Nunez D, Shikowitz M. The Essential Clinical Handbook for ENT Surgery: The Ultimate Companion for Ear, Nose and Throat Surgery Including a Chapter on Facial Plastic Surgery …. London: BPP Learning Media; 2013.
8. Sheehy JL, Gardner G, Hambley WM. Tuning fork tests in modern otology. Arch Otolaryngol Chic Ill 1960. 1971;94:132–8.
9. Rossing TD, Russell DA, Brown DE. On the acoustics of tuning forks. Am J Phys. 1992;60:620–6.
10. Russell DA. On the sound field radiated by a tuning fork. Am J Phys. 2000; 68:1139–45.

11. Vibrational Modes of a Tuning Fork. [http://www.acs.psu.edu/drussell/Demos/TuningFork/fork-modes.html]
12. Florentine M. Loudness. In: Florentine M, Popper AN, Fay RR, editors. Loudness. New York: Springer; 2011. p. 1–15. Springer Handbook of Auditory Research, vol. 37.
13. Zwicker E, Fastl H. Psychoacoustics: Facts and Models, Springer Science & Business Media. 2013.
14. Fastl H, Schorn K. Discrimination of level differences by hearing-impaired patients. Audiol Off Organ Int Soc Audiol. 1981;20:488–502.

Permissions

List of Contributors

Brittany Greene and Linden Head
University of Ottawa Faculty of Medicine, 451 Smyth Road, Ottawa, Canada

Nada Gawad
University of Ottawa Faculty of Medicine, 451 Smyth Road, Ottawa, Canada
University of Toronto Department of Surgery, Faculty of Medicine, 1 King's
College Circle, Medical Sciences Building, Room 2109, Toronto, Canada.
Department of Surgery, The Ottawa Hospital, General Campus, 501 Smyth
Road, Ottawa, Canada

Stanley J Hamstra
Department of Surgery, The Ottawa Hospital, General Campus, 501 Smyth
Road, Ottawa, Canada
University of Ottawa Skills and Simulation Centre, The Ottawa Hospital, Civic Campus, Loeb Research Building, 1st floor, 725 Parkdale Avenue, Ottawa, Canada

Laurie McLean
Department of Otolaryngology Head and Neck Surgery, The Ottawa Hospital, General Campus, 501 Smyth Road, Ottawa, Canada

Sachio Takeno and Katsuhiro Hirakawa
Department of Otolaryngology, Head and Neck Surgery, Division of Clinical Medical Science, Programs for Applied Biomedicine, Graduate School of Biomedical Sciences, Hiroshima University, Hiroshima, Japan

Kazunori Kubota
Department of Otolaryngology, Head and Neck Surgery, Division of Clinical Medical Science, Programs for Applied Biomedicine, Graduate School of Biomedical Sciences, Hiroshima University, Hiroshima, Japan
Department of Otorhinolaryngology, Hiroshima University School of Medicine, 1-2-3 Kasumi, Minami-ku, Hiroshima 734-8551, Japan

Zeinab A Dastgheib
Department of Electrical & Computer Engineering, University of Manitoba, Room E3-512 Eng. Bldg., 75A Chancellor's Circle, Winnipeg, MB R3T 5V6, Canada

Brian Lithgow
EVestG Research Lab, Riverview Health Centre, Room PE446, 1 Morley Avenue, Winnipeg, MB R3L2P4, Canada

Brian Blakley
Department of Otolaryngology - Head and Neck Surgery, University of Manitoba, GB421 – 820 Sherbrook Street, Winnipeg, Manitoba R3A 1R9, Canada.

Zahra Moussavi
Department of Electrical & Computer Engineering, University of Manitoba, 75A Chancellor's Circle, Winnipeg, MB R3T 5V6, Canada

Kristine A Smith and Luke Rudmik
Division of Otolaryngology, Head and Neck Surgery, Department of Surgery;
University of Calgary, Calgary, Alberta, Canada

Doron D Sommer
Division of Otolaryngology, Head and Neck Surgery, Department of Surgery, McMaster University, Hamilton, Ontario, Canada

Sean Grondin
Division of Thoracic Surgery, Department of Surgery, University of Calgary, Calgary, Alberta, Canada

Brian Rotenberg
Department of Otolaryngology, Head and Neck Surgery, University of Western Ontario, London, Ontario, Canada

Marc A Tewfik
Department of Otolaryngology, Head and Neck Surgery; McGill University, Jewish General Hospital, Montreal, Quebec, Canada

Shaun Kilty
Department of Otolaryngology, Head and Neck Surgery, University of Ottawa, Ottawa, Ontario, Canada

Erin Wright
Division of Otolaryngology-Head & Neck Surgery, University of Alberta, Edmonton, Alberta, Canada

Arif Janjua and Chris Diamond
Division of Otolaryngology, Head and Neck Surgery, Department of Surgery, University of British Columbia, Vancouver, BC, Canada

John Lee
Department of Otolaryngology, Head and Neck Surgery, University of Toronto, Toronto, Ontario, Canada

Adrian I. Mendez, Hadi Seikaly, Vincent Biron, Lin-fu Zhu and David W. J. Côté
Division of Otolaryngology, Head and Neck Surgery, University of Alberta, 8440-112 Street, Room 1E4, WMC, Edmonton T6G 2B7, AB, Canada

Sarah C Hugh
Department of Otolaryngology – Head & Neck Surgery, University of Toronto, Toronto, ON, Canada

Jennifer Siu
School of Medicine, Queen's University, Kingston, ON, Canada

Thomas Hummel
Department of Otorhinolaryngology, Interdisciplinary Center Smell & Taste, Technische Universitat Dresden, Dresden, Germany

Vito Forte, Paolo Campisi, Blake C Papsin and Evan J Propst
Department of Otolaryngology – Head & Neck Surgery, University of Toronto, Toronto, ON, Canada

The Hospital for Sick Children, Toronto, ON, Canada

Katrina Anna Mason and Evgenia Theodorakopoulou
Barts and The London School of Medicine and Dentistry, The Blizard Institute of Cell and Molecular Science, 4 Newark Street, Whitechapel, E1 2AT London, UK

Perumal Gounder Chokkalingam and Annakan Navaratnam
Colchester Hospital University NHS Foundation Trust, Colchester, UK

Graeme B. Mulholland, Caroline C. Jeffery, Paras Satija and David W. J. Côté
Division of Otolaryngology-Head and Neck Surgery, 1E4 Walter MacKenzie Centre, University of Alberta, 8440 112 Street, Edmonton, AB T6G 2B7, Canada

Brian W. Blakley and Laura Chan
Department of Otolaryngology, University of Manitoba, GB420-820 Sherbrook Street, Winnipeg, MB R3A 1RJ, Canada

Masaya Akashi, Shungo Furudoi, Akiko Sakakibara, Takumi Hasegawa, Takashi Shigeta, Tsutomu Minamikawa and Takahide Komori
Department of Oral and Maxillofacial Surgery, Kobe University Graduate School of Medicine, Kusunoki-cho 7-5-1, Chuo-ku, Kobe 650-0017, Japan

Kazunobu Hashikawa
Department of Plastic Surgery, Kobe University Graduate School of Medicine, Kobe, Japan

Brandon Wickens and Murad Husein
Department of Otolaryngology – Head and Neck Surgery, Western University, London, Ontario, Canada

Jordan Lewis
Department of Medical Biophysics, Western University, London, Ontario, Canada

David P Morris
Division of Otolaryngology – Head and Neck Surgery, Department of Surgery, Dalhousie University, Halifax, Nova Scotia, Canada

Hanif M Ladak
Department of Otolaryngology – Head and Neck Surgery, Western University, London, Ontario, Canada
Department of Medical Biophysics, Western University, London, Ontario, Canada
Department of Electrical & Computer Engineering, Western University, London, Ontario, Canada

Sumit K Agrawal
Department of Otolaryngology – Head and Neck Surgery, Western University, London, Ontario, Canada
Department of Medical Biophysics, Western University, London, Ontario, Canada
Department of Electrical & Computer Engineering, Western University, London, Ontario, Canada
London Health Sciences Centre, Room B1-333, University Hospital, 339 Windermere Rd., London, Ontario N6A 5A5, Canada.

Eva Ekvall Hansson and Liselott Persson
Department of Health Sciences, Health Science Centre, Lund University, Baravägen 3, SE222 41 Lund, Sweden

Anders Beckman
Department of Clinical Sciences in Malmö, Clinical Research Centre, Lund University, Jan Waldenströmsgata 25, SE205 02 Malmö, Sweden

Paul Kerr
Department of Otolaryngology, Winnipeg, Manitoba, Canada

Candace L Myers, Mohamed Alessa and Pascal Lambert
Cancer Care Manitoba, Winnipeg, Manitoba, Canada

James Butler
Cancer Care Manitoba, Winnipeg, Manitoba, Canada
Department of Radiology, Winnipeg, Manitoba, Canada

Andrew L Cooke
Cancer Care Manitoba, Winnipeg, Manitoba, Canada
Department of Radiation Oncology, CancerCare Manitoba, 675 McDermot Avenue, Winnipeg, Manitoba R3E 0 V9, Canada

Timothy Cooper, Vincent L Biron and Hadi Seikaly
Division of Otolaryngology - Head and Neck Surgery, Department of Surgery, University of Alberta, 1E4 University of Alberta Hospital, 1E4 Walter Mackenzie Center, 8440 112 St., Edmonton, AB T6G 2B7, Canada

David Fast
Faculty of Science 1–001 CCIS, University of Alberta, Edmonton, AB T6G 2E9, Canada

Raymond Tam
Faculty of Medicine and Dentistry, University of Alberta, 2J2 WC Mackenzie Health Sciences Centre, Edmonton, AB T6G 2R7, Canada

Thomas Carey
Department of Head and Neck Surgery, University of Michigan, 5311B Med Sci I, Ann Arbor, MI 48109-5616, USA

Maya Shmulevitz
Department of Medical Microbiology and Immunology, University of Alberta, 6–142 J Katz Group Centre for Pharmacy & Health Research, Edmonton, AB T6G 2E1, Canada

Edward Park, Hosam Amoodi, Jafri Kuthubutheen, Joseph M. Chen, Julian M. Nedzelski and Vincent Y. W. Lin
Department of Otolaryngology – Head and Neck Surgery, Sunnybrook Health Sciences Centre, 2075 Bayview Avenue, Toronto, ON M4N 3M5, Canada

Andre R Le
Memorial University Faculty of Medicine, S-1758B 300 Prince Phillip Drive, St John's, NL A1B 3 V6, Canada

Gregory W Thompson and Benjamin John A Hoyt
Department of Otolaryngology – Head & Neck Surgery, Zone 3, Horizon Health Network, 700 Priestman St, Fredericton, NB E3B 5 N5, Canada

Maria K. Brake1
Department of Otolaryngology – Head and Neck Surgery, University of Toronto, Ontario, Canada

Jennifer Anderson
St. Michael's Hospital, Department of Otolaryngology – Head and Neck Surgery, University of Toronto, 30 Bond St. 8C-129, ON M5B 1 W8 Toronto, Canada

Hussain Alsaffar, Lindsay Wilson, Dev P. Kamdar, Faizullo Sultanov, Danny Enepekides and Kevin M. Higgins
Sunnybrook Health Sciences Centre, University of Toronto, Toronto, ON, Canada

Adrian Mendez, Hadi Seikaly and Vincent L. Biron
Department of Surgery, Division of Otolaryngology-Head and Neck Surgery, University of Alberta, Edmonton, AB, Canada

Lin Fu Zhu
Faculty of Medicine and Dentistry, University of Alberta, Edmonton, AB, Canada

David W. J. Côté
Department of Surgery, Division of Otolaryngology-Head and Neck Surgery, University of Alberta, Edmonton, AB, Canada 1E4 Walter C Mackenzie Centre, 8440-112 Street NW, Edmonton, AB T6G 2B7, Canada

Oleksandr Butskiy
Division of Otolaryngology Head and Neck Surgery, Department of Surgery, Vancouver General Hospital & University of British Columbia, Vancouver, BC, anada

Donald W. Anderson
Division of Otolaryngology Head and Neck Surgery, Department of Surgery, Vancouver General Hospital & University of British Columbia, Vancouver, BC, Canada
Gordon & Leslie Diamond Health Care Centre, 4th. Fl. 4299B-2775 Laurel Street, Vancouver, BC V5Z 1 M9, Canada

Hui Xu
Stomatology Department, Affiliated Yantai Yuhuangding Hospital of Qingdao University Medical College, Yantai City, Shandong Province, China

Fa-ya Liang
Otorhinolaryngology Head and Neck Surgery Department, Sun Yat-sen Memorial Hospital of Sun Yat-sen University, Guangzhou, China

Liang Chen
Otorhinolaryngology Head and Neck Surgery Department, Affiliated Yantai Yuhuangding Hospital of Qingdao University Medical College, Yantai City, Shandong Province, China
Otology Department, Affiliated Yantai Yuhuangding Hospital of Qingdao University Medical College, Yantai City, Shandong Province, China

Xi-cheng Song, Qing-quan Zhang and Yan Sun
Otorhinolaryngology Head and Neck Surgery Department, Affiliated Yantai Yuhuangding Hospital of Qingdao University Medical College, Yantai City, Shandong Province, China

Michael Chi Fai Tong
Otorhinolaryngology Head and Neck Surgery Department, The Chinese University of Hong Kong, New Territories, Hong Kong, China

Jiun Fong Thong
Otorhinolaryngology Head and Neck Surgery Department, Singapore General Hospital, Singapore, Singapore

Emily Kay-Rivest
Department of Otolaryngology – Head and Neck surgery, McGill University, Montreal, QC, Canada

Elliot Mitmaker
Department of General surgery, McGill University, Montreal, QC, Canada.

Richard J. Payne, Michael P. Hier, Alex M. Mlynarek, Jonathan Young and Véronique-Isabelle Forest
Division of Head and Neck Surgery, Department of Otolaryngology – Head and Neck surgery, Jewish General Hospital, Mc Gill University, Montreal, QC H3T 1E2, Canada

Saad Ansari and Brian W. Rotenberg
Department of Otolaryngology-Head & Neck Surgery, Western University, London, ON, Canada

Leigh J. Sowerby
Department of Otolaryngology-Head & Neck Surgery, Western University, London, ON, Canada
Department of Otolaryngology-Head & Neck Surgery, St. Joseph's Hospital,
Room B2-501, 268 Grosvenor Street, London, ON N6A 4V2, Canada

D. Forner, T. Phillips, M. Rigby, R. Hart, M. Taylor and J. Trites
Division of Otolaryngology – Head and Neck Surgery, Department of Surgery, Dalhousie University, Halifax, Canada

Benjamin A. Taylor, Robert D. Hart, Matthew H. Rigby, Jonathan Trites, S. Mark Taylor and Paul Hong
Division of Otolaryngology Head and Neck Surgery, Department of Surgery, IWK Health Centre, Dalhousie University, 5850 University Avenue, Halifax, NS B3K 6R8, Canada

J. Mierzwinski, AJ Fishman, T. Grochowski, S. Drewa and M. Drela
Department of Otolaryngology, Audiology and Phoniatrics, Children's Hospital of Bydgoszcz, Chodkiewicza 44, 85-667 Bydgoszcz, Poland.

P. Winiarski
Department of Otolaryngology, Head and Neck Surgery, University Hospital of Bydgoszcz, Ujejskiego 52, 85-168 Bydgoszcz, Poland

I. Bielecki
Department of Pediatric Otolaryngology, University Children's Hospital of Katowice, ul Medyków 16, 40-752 Katowice, Poland

Benjamin Mossman and Stuart Mossman
Department of Neurology, Wellington Hospital, Riddiford Street, Private Bag 7902, Wellington South, Wellington, New Zealand

Gordon Purdie
Dean's Department, University of Otago, Wellington, New Zealand

Erich Schneider
Institute of Medical Technology, Brandenburg University of Technology Cottbus, Senftenberg, Germany

Serkan Sertel
Department of Otorhinolaryngology, Head & Neck Surgery, University Hospital CHUV, Rue du Bugnon 46, 1011 Lausanne, Switzerland
Department of Otorhinolaryngology, Head & Neck Surgery, University of Heidelberg, Heidelberg, Germany

Ioana Irina Venara-Vulpe and Philippe Pasche
Department of Otorhinolaryngology, Head & Neck Surgery, University Hospital CHUV, Rue du Bugnon 46, 1011 Lausanne, Switzerland

Nosayaba Osazuwa-Peters
Brown School, Washington University in St. Louis, 1 Brookings Drive, Saint Louis, MO 63130, USA
Saint Louis University Cancer Center, 3655 Vista Avenue, Saint Louis, Missouri 63110, USA
Department of Otolaryngology-Head and Neck Surgery, Saint Louis University, School of Medicine, 6th Floor Desloge Building, 3635 Vista Avenue, Saint Louis, MO 63110, USA
Department of Epidemiology, Saint Louis University, College for Public Health and Social Justice, 3545 Lafayette Avenue, Saint Louis, Missouri 63108, USA

Nhial T. Tutlam
Department of Epidemiology, Saint Louis University, College for Public Health and Social Justice, 3545 Lafayette Avenue, Saint Louis, Missouri 63108, USA

Bree Erickson, Caroline Jeffery, Khalid Ansari, Hamdy El Hakim, Erin D. Wright, Hadi Seikaly, Sam R. Greig and David W. J. Côté
Department of Surgery, Division of Otolaryngology – Head and Neck Surgery, University of Alberta, 1E4 Walter C Mackenzie Centre, 8440-112 Street NW, Edmonton, AB T6G 2B7, Canada

Robert Hurowitz
Faculty of Medicine and Dentistry, University of Alberta, Edmonton, AB, Canada

Blair Williams, Benjamin A. Taylor and Manohar Bance
Division of Otolaryngology – Head & Neck Surgery, Department of Surgery, Dalhousie University, Room 3184, 1276 South Park Street, Halifax, NS B3H 2Y9, Canada

Neil Clifton
Division of Otolaryngology – Head and Neck Surgery, Department of Surgery, St Martha's Regional Hospital, Halifax, Canada

Michael Yong
University of British Columbia, Division of Otolaryngology – Head and Neck Surgery, 4th Floor, 2775 Laurel Street, Vancouver General Hospital, Vancouver, BC V5Z 1 M9, Canada

Tamara Mijovic
McGill University, Department of Otolaryngology – Head and Neck Surgery, Royal Victoria Hospital - D05.5712, 1001 Décarie Boul, Montreal H4A 3 J1, Canada

Jane Lea
University of British Columbia, Division of Otolaryngology – Head and Neck Surgery, ENT Clinic, 1081 Burrard Street, St. Paul's Hospital, Vancouver, BC V6Z 1Y6, Canada

Oleksandr Butskiy and Desmond A. Nunez
Division of Otolaryngology – Head and Neck Surgery, Vancouver General Hospital, Vancouver, BC, Canada
Department of Surgery, University of British Columbia, Vancouver, BC, Canada
Gordon & Leslie Diamond Health Care Centre, 4th. Fl. 4299B-2775 Laurel Street, Vancouver, BC V5Z 1M9, Canada

Denny Ng
Department of Mechanical Engineering, University of British Columbia, Vancouver, BC, Canada

Murray Hodgson
Department of Mechanical Engineering, University of British Columbia, Vancouver, BC, Canada
School of Population and Public Health, University of British Columbia, Vancouver, BC, Canada

Index

www.ingramcontent.com/pod-product-compliance
Lightning Source LLC
Chambersburg PA
CDIIW001939190326
41458CB00009B/2778